Chronic inflammation - The Greatest Threat to our Health

5 simple steps to protect you and your family

"Inflammation is an underlying contributor to virtually every chronic disease... rheumatoid arthritis, Crohn's disease, diabetes and depression, along with major killers such as heart disease and stroke."

Scientific American (2009)

"The connection between inflammation and cancer has moved to center stage in the research arena."

Massachusetts Institute of Technology's Whitehead Institute for Biomedical Research (2009)

Why this book?

Healthcare and the healthcare business is dominated by the pharmaceutical 'magic bullet' model. When the symptoms of a non-communicable, degenerative disease such as cancer or heart disease appear, doctors will generally reach for drugs.

But this strategy is too little and far too late. Most drugs treat symptoms rather than the root causes of disease, and by the time symptoms emerge the disease has already progressed a long way; the 'age-related' diseases develop silently for many years before they finally emerge, and start to cause pain or disability. The drug model has also signally failed to prevent the gathering tides of diabetes, dementia, allergy, cancer, osteoporosis …

Now, however, we have an alternative. The latest science shows that we can head trouble off at the pass, and stop disease from starting. We know now that all these diseases are driven by a silent killer called chronic inflammation, and we know also that this is due largely to nutritional and lifestyle choices that can be changed quite easily.

This book will not take long to read, because the message is simple. If you take action against chronic inflammation, you and your family take a major step towards living healthier, longer lives. The actions to take are equally simple – and the positive changes start to take effect within weeks.

Section 1 (the first 36 pages) spells out the causes of chronic inflammation, and shows you how to avoid them. Section 2 (the rest of the book) presents the science behind the recommendations for life scientists, health care professionals and the worried well.

CONTENT

SECTION 1. Putting Out the Flames of Disease - Fast Start

The ancient Greek, Roman and Islamic physicians believed that our bodies contained just four different humours, or liquids, and that all illnesses were due to an imbalance between these four. This simple theory lasted some 2000 years, until the advent of modern medicine in the 19th century. Then began a series of detailed investigations into how and what we are; which produced a hugely complex mass of information, numerous medical specialities and specialists, and the wide range of specific (and toxic) drugs still in use today.

The pharmaceutical approach, although often effective in suppressing the symptoms of disease, has failed to prevent the terrifying increases in degenerative diseases which are overwhelming our health care services today. Heart disease, diabetes, cancer, dementia, allergy, auto-immune disease, neuro-developmental disorders, mental illnesses – the so-called diseases of civilisation – all are running out of control, and affecting more and more of us, and at earlier and earlier ages.

But now – and just in time – a new unifying theory of disease has emerged, one which leaves harmful drugs behind and which focusses on the foods we eat. It is surprisingly simple, and could almost be compared to a modern and scientific version of the old humour theory. There are five basic elements in this new Grand Unifying Theory of disease.

1. It is widely recognised that the 'diseases of civilisation 'are hugely influenced by nutritional factors.
2. Recent research has shown that almost all of these diseases have a single common element; chronic inflammation, a process that damages and destroys healthy tissue in every organ that it touches.
3. The key anti-inflammatory compounds in our diet are the 1-3, 1-6 beta glucans found in yeasts and mushrooms; the omega 3 fatty acids which occur in oily fish; and the polyphenols, valuable nutrients found in fruits and vegetables.
4. The study of dietary shift (the way our diet changes over time) has revealed that levels of these anti-inflammatory nutrients are at an all-time low. In particular, the ratio of omega 3 to omega 6 fatty acids in the diet has fallen dramatically, and our intake of polyphenols has crashed. The decline in these anti-inflammatory nutrients matches the increasing rates of the inflammatory diseases referred to above.
5. When the key anti-inflammatory nutrients are put back into the diet, rates of these diseases (in both animals and humans) fall by up to 90%. We become almost immune to degenerative disease, and our chances of successful ageing increase very dramatically.

You will probably not hear much of this from your doctors, as they are not taught this new science at medical school. When I was at medical school I only learned about drugs, and nutrition was neglected. Four decades on, not much has changed. Perhaps this is because Big Pharma has not yet worked out how to profit from these new ideas. Perhaps it is because the regulators, who are busy preventing the development of these new nutritional programs, are excessively influenced by pharmaceutical thinking.

Best not to wait. The new science is surprisingly easy to understand, and even easier to put into practice. The ground rules are broadly in line with the familiar guidelines – eat more fruit, vegetables and oily fish, cut down on fried and grilled foods, reduce salt and alcohol, no smoking – but are made vastly more potent by the use of two anti-inflammatory supplements. One of these is a beta glucan formulation, the other is a fish oil / polyphenol combination.

The fish oil / polyphenol combination is particularly powerful, and is based on work done at the Universities of Trondheim (Norway) and Milan (Italy). Senior academics at these sites developed an accurate and sensitive lab test which reveals the balance of omega 3 to 6 fatty acids in the blood; and a perfectly balanced nutritional oil which combines purified fish oils with a polyphenol-rich olive oil. This balanced oil, which combines the health benefits of the Eskimo and the Mediterranean diets, has powerful anti-inflammatory effects – and as a result, dramatic and easily observed health benefits. These can be easily measured by using the validated Trondheim test.

There is a considerable body of science behind this story, and it is all developed in the following pages. Section 1 is a Fast Start, a quick guide to improving your health which will get you on the right track in a single day. It is based on courses of lectures which have been given to doctors, providing an easy guide to the new medical model. Section 2 is an in-depth analysis which is aimed at life scientists (and the educated lay-person), bringing them up to date with current research and showing how it all fits together into a surprisingly coherent body of evidence. It covers such topics as the epidemiology of inflammation; the role of the microbiota; the involvement of telomeres; the sudden death problem; the role of the innate immune system – and many others.

All of this is based on published science, and is starting to be taught at various academic venues all over the world. It is a detailed and comprehensive guide to vastly better health, and puts the control of your health back into your own hands.

Oxford, June 2013.

Chapter 1: Chronic inflammation - the main cause of premature ageing and death

"Low-grade inflammation is associated with everything from heart disease and diabetes to Alzheimer's and arthritis, and may even be the cause of most chronic diseases."

University of California Berkeley, School of Public Health (2010)

Don't confuse ageing with getting older. We can't change the passage of time (chronological ageing), but we can change the rate at which our bodies age (biological ageing.) If you choose to do this you won't just look and feel younger, you will also cut the risk of degenerative disease and increase your prospects of a healthy and extended middle and old age.

Ageing used to be seen as the steady accumulation of damage to body cells. This was a 'wear and tear' model that went hand in hand with the concept of 'age-related diseases'; crudely, the longer you lived the more your tissues and organs would wear out. This idea lead to a terrible medical fatalism; after all, if your symptoms are due to wear and tear, there is little that medics can do other than try to make the symptoms more bearable – and that is what most modern drugs do.

Fortunately the 'wear and tear' theory has been demolished, as there are plenty of individuals – and whole populations – who lived to ripe old ages in great good health. In fact, current research reveals that almost all the 'age-related' diseases - from declining mental powers to coronary artery disease, from cancer to hypertension, from arthritis to diabetes and stroke - do not have to occur as we age, and are not a necessary part of the ageing process. It shows that all these diseases have one driver in common: chronic sub-clinical inflammation, a condition which is not inevitable at all and which is surprisingly easy to prevent. (Chronic and sub-clinical means continuous and un-noticeable, until the chronic inflammation has caused so much tissue damage that the symptoms of disease finally emerge.)

"Inflammatory factors predict virtually all bad outcomes in humans. They predict heart attacks, heart failure, becoming diabetic; becoming fragile in old age; cognitive function decline, even cancer to a certain extent."

Russell Tracy, professor of pathology and biochemistry at the University of Vermont, College of Medicine

Chronic inflammation is clearly a condition to be avoided. Unfortunately, given the way we live today, it is a gradually accumulating condition that is now found in almost every adult over the age of about 30 – and increasingly, even in in teenagers.

Some people are at increased risk. If you are over 50: over-weight: a smoker, or exposed to polluted air: have been diagnosed with any long-term illness ending in '-itis' (which means 'inflammation'): a high performance athlete or a couch potato; or if confectionery, baked goods, and barbequed and deep-fired foods feature heavily in your diet, then you almost certainly have a level of chronic inflammation in your body that should be reduced now to protect your long term health.

Inflammation and ageing

Very few of us die of old age. The vast majority of us sicken and die prematurely, picked off by 'natural causes' long before our biological life span has run its course. Cell culture studies, and the small but growing numbers of individuals who live on healthily into their second century (1), indicate that our potential life span may be up to 30% longer than what we consider normal today. But why is such a long and healthy life such a rarity? Why do so few of us live out our biological potential?

We used to die, in the main, of infection, starvation or trauma. Twentieth century sanitation, medicine and social planning scored significant victories against these killers – although the infectious diseases show signs of making a comeback, due to the careless way we use antibiotics and the prospect of emergent viruses.

At the time of writing, however, the major causes of death are still the chronic degenerative diseases such as cardiovascular disease and cancer, conditions worsened by the parallel epidemic of overweight and obesity. What we need is a 21st century medicine which will slow or stabilise these conditions, prevent them from making our last years difficult, extend our healthy middle years and allow us to remain physically young into our 60's and beyond.

The new model of healthcare which has the potential to do this, known as pharmaco-nutritional medicine, is based on three simple and self-evident truths.

Firstly, all living tissue is dynamic – that is, it is constantly repairing and renewing itself. Skin cells are sloughed off and replaced every day; red blood cells last for around 4 months before they wear out and new ones take their place; you grow a new skeleton every ten years or so. This type of change is imperceptible and constant.

Cartilage in the joints is eroded and regenerated, atheroma is constantly deposited in the artery walls and is constantly being removed, calories are taken into the body in food every day, and every day transformed into heat, movement, and all the businesses of life.

Secondly, the body has incredible powers of regeneration and renewal, forged in the evolutionary fires of our Paleolithic past. If that were not the case, we would not have survived as a species. Our joints would wear thin by the age of 20, our arteries would solidify by 30, our brains would burn out by the age of 40. And for most of us, that is simply not the case.

But thirdly, it is equally true that as the years pass, these types of degenerative change eventually gather momentum, and emerge in increasing numbers of us as clinical disease. This trend is so commonplace as to almost beyond questioning – but we need to ask why this pattern is so prevalent. Just what is so different about old age?

During the first 20 or so years of life we are dominated by the processes of growth and renewal, a condition sometimes described as 'anabolic dominance'. As we age, however, growth and renewal slow, and the forces of breakdown and decay accelerate. By the time we have reached the roaring 40's they are beginning to outstrip growth and renewal, and we gradually shift from 'anabolic dominance' to 'catabolic dominance'.

Our ability to heal is compromised; wounds, for example, take longer to heal, and are more likely to become infected. The immune system becomes less effective. In general, the rate at which we can re-build and renew our tissues declines, and is overtaken by the processes of decay. Little by little, therefore, tissue damage begins to accumulate, rather like the slow erosion of a landscape; whether we are talking about the slow silting of an artery, the equally slow thinning of the cartilage in a hip or knee; or the silent dying of our brain cells. We become less active, are now typically consuming more calories than we utilise, and the majority of us begin to put on weight. We grow slow, ill and fat. By the time we emerge, blinking, into the 6th decade of life, 5 out of 6 of us have the symptoms of one or more of the degenerative diseases, and the majority of us are overweight.

These intertwined problems have two intertwined causes: malnutrition and inflammation.

The processes of growth and renewal depend on the presence in the body of a number of vital building blocks and co-factors derived from the diet. The building blocks include amino acids, amino sugars and the essential fatty acids, and the co-factors are, broadly, the classical vitamins and trace elements such as iron, selenium, magnesium and zinc. These micronutrients can be thought of as anabolic co-factors. Conversely, the processes of breakdown and decay are, in health, held in check by the Omega 3 fatty acids and phytonutrients such as the polyphenols, carotenoids, xanthophylls, the 1-3, 1-6 beta glucans and the fermentable starches. These compounds can reasonably be considered to be anti-catabolic agents, and are all essential to our long-term health. A really healthy diet would provide optimal amounts of all these compounds, and keep the processes of tissue wear and renewal in perfect balance.

Many people do try to eat a healthy diet, and believe that they are getting all the nutrients that they need. This is generally not the case. Indeed, there is a plenty of evidence that the majority of us are depleted in both the anabolic co-factors, and the anti-catabolic agents. This is not the near-absolute absence of a micronutrient that causes a deficiency disease (such as scurvy, an example of what is known as Type A Malnutrition), but a pattern of sub-optimal intakes of most of the micronutrients, often associated with calorie excess. This is termed Type B malnutrition;

and it is emerging as a common cause of the majority of the degenerative diseases, and much of the process of ageing as we know it.

The reasons for this prevalent pattern of multiple micronutrient depletion are structural and well established. Perhaps the single most important cause of Type B malnutrition is that we don't eat enough. This sounds paradoxical, given that we are getting fatter, but we actually eat far less than we used to. Read, for example, accounts written by the diarists James Boswell or Samuel Pepys of the vast lunches and dinners that were regularly consumed by our relatively recent ancestors. But then remember that those diners and lunchers walked or rode horse-back where we drive, climbed stairs where we take elevators, and burned calories to keep warm where we turn up the central heating.

Looked at through a longer lens, humans were 'designed' to live active lives and to consume 3500 thousand Kcalories or more per day. No longer hunter-gatherers, we live sedentary lives, working at a computer screen during the day and basking in the glow of the cathode ray tube at night. The result is that we burn, on average, 2000 to 25000 Kcalories a day. Our appetites have indeed shrunk but not quite to match, thanks in no small measure to the tricks of the food industry; leaving most of us in a slight but persistent state of calorie excess. This explains, over time, our weight gain.

But by cutting our food intakes in half, we have at a stroke halved our intakes of the essential micro-and phyto-nutrients. To make matters worse, our dietary habits are out of joint. We no longer eat much unprocessed food but increasingly rely on pre-processed, pre-cooked and ready to eat meals and snacks which in many cases are significantly less nutritious than the original ingredients would have been. Thanks again to the food industry and the regulators and legislators that they rent, our diet has become a nutritional wasteland. The average American, for example, currently obtains 13% of their calories from added sugars (93) and another 25% of their calories form soy oil (94). Fully a third of what we eat is nutritionally sterile[1]!

These and other factors have dramatically reduced our intakes of such valuable nutrients as the Omega 3 fatty acids and polyphenols; resulting in the widespread problem of Type B malnutrition we see today (2-4). These compounds have powerful anti-inflammatory actions in the body, so as we become more depleted we become more prone to inflammation.

A person who is depleted in anabolic co-factors and the anti-catabolic agents is heading for trouble. Tissue renewal is down, inflammation is raging, tissue decay and breakdown are up; he or she is now catabolically dominant, accumulating tissue damage, and heading towards clinical illness.

To make matters worse, Type B malnutrition generally worsens as we age, due to such factors

---

1. The amounts of vitamins K, E and choline in soy oil are very low

as dental problems, difficulties with swallowing, reduced calorific throughput (5), a deteriorating sense of taste and appetite, and often reduced finances. This neatly explains why we become progressively more catabolically dominant, and ever more likely to become diseased, as the years and decades pass.

Pharmaceutical models which developed from the concept of 'magic bullets' and the closely related idea of specificity are appropriate when dealing with infectious illness. They are not the right tools, however, for dealing with degenerative diseases caused by adverse life-style factors, and consequently many metabolic imbalances, going subtly wrong over many years. The huge increases in obesity, diabetes, asthma and allergy, auto-immune disease, autism, depression, osteoporosis, dementia and cancer, the recent declines in life expectancy reported in parts of the former Soviet Union, Italy, the UK and the USA, the relative fall in average height now occurring in the United States (6-7), and the persistent failure of the pharmaceutical model to find cures for any of these problems, are all telling us that we need a new way of looking at health; one which takes life-style and nutritional factors into account.

Seen from this perspective, the way to preventing disease and slowing ageing is simple and universal. It starts with using nutritional inputs to damp down the fires of inflammation, and avoiding known pro-inflammatory factors. This straightforward strategy allows the body's natural and amazing healing processes to come to the fore.

Not all inflammation, however, is bad.

Acute inflammation is usually a positive healing reaction

Chronic inflammation is harmful, but acute inflammation is usually positive. One example of acute inflammation is the reddening and warming of the skin following a cut, insect bite or sting.

Acute inflammation is a short term, protective immune response that is switched on to counteract harmful external threats. It's generally a very productive response – indeed without it we would not be alive - and the symptoms are usually short-lived and often visible externally. Once the inflammatory response has neutralized the threat, powerful *anti-inflammatory* compounds are released to begin the healing process.

But sometimes the acute inflammatory response is insufficient to clear the threat. If the threat that initially triggered the inflammation remains, or is constantly drip-fed into the body, as occurs with bad diets or a tobacco habit, this can result in continuous, low level of inflammation; aka **chronic** inflammation.

Chronic inflammation is harmful; it damages and destroys tissue

Chronic sub-clinical inflammation is a silent threat that simmers undetected in the body, progressively damaging tissues in the body wherever it occurs; in the heart, brain, joints, bowel, colon, prostate, lungs and skin - in potentially any organ.

Harvey Jay Cohen, of the Center for the Study of Ageing at Duke University in the U.S., likens inflammation to "little waves lapping on the shore. It's a relatively low level of activity that, sustained over time, wears away at the beach and stimulates other bad events."

This insidious and gradual process of tissue destruction is why chronic inflammation is now thought to be a main cause of almost all the age-related illnesses; and why chronic inflammation is associated with faster ageing, or 'inflammageing'.

Today's lifestyles create an excessive degree of chronic inflammation, and in this way condemn us to an increased risk of degenerative disease, accelerated ageing and premature death. This was confirmed by the recent (British) Whitehall II cohort study, in which researchers analysed the dietary habits of 3,775 men and 1,575 women and related this to chronic disease and mortality rates, over an average of 16 years (8).

People who ate a "Western-style" diet rich in fried and sugary foods and refined starches, aged more quickly and died younger than people who adhered to healthier diets. Ideal aging (being free of chronic illness, and having high performance in mental, physical, and mental agility tests), occurred almost exclusively in those few people (4% of the total!) who ate a healthier diet with plenty of fruits, vegetables, whole grains and fish.

The evidence is overwhelming. Reducing or preventing chronic inflammation is the key to cutting the risk of degenerative disease and maximise your chances of long term health. Fortunately you can reduce your levels of inflammation quickly and effectively.

Has chronic inflammation always been such a problem?

In a word, no. We know that most people today are very prone to inflammation, because so many people acquire and die of diseases caused by chronic inflammation. Heart disease and cancer, for example, are major causes of disease and death in our society; but it was not always so. The mid-Victorians, for example, had a life expectancy similar to our own, but were relatively free of these diseases. The first 5 years of life were hazardous but for those who reached that milestone, life expectancy was as good as ours today; and their chances of a healthy old age were far better than ours – without the 'benefits' of modern drugs, surgery and diagnostics (9).

The degenerative diseases are often referred to as lifestyle diseases, or diseases of civilisation. The lifestyles we live today create chronic inflammation; Victorian lifestyles did not.

We now know that the main reason for the Victorians' near freedom from degenerative disease was a diet rich in Omega 3 fatty acids, polyphenols and (1-3), (1-6) beta-glucans (see below), and which was therefore profoundly anti-inflammatory. A few Victorians (probably those with strong genetic risk factors) developed heart disease and cancer, but the vast majority were protected, and attained a healthy and vigorous old age.

The traditional Mediterranean diet, which in terms of its anti-inflammatory content is mid-way between the mid-Victorian diet and our own, used to offer an intermediate degree of protection. Sadly, if you visit any of the Mediterranean cities today, you will see that the traditional diet is being replaced by modern foods. The youth are expanding like balloons, and the internal damage caused by this new diet is already driving an increase in diabetes and other degenerative diseases.

In other words chronic inflammation has always been with us, but never on the scale that we see in the developed nations today. Previous generations lived a very different lifestyle to ours. Not only did they consume far higher levels of natural anti-inflammatory compounds in their diets, they were also not exposed to as many inflammatory compounds as we are today. Tobacco, for example, is a modern vice, and high temperature cooking methods such as deep frying, which produce inflammatory chemicals in our food, are also recent arrivals.

Because our lifestyles condemn so many of us to chronic, sub-clinical inflammation, it is no wonder that the steady accumulation of tissue damage eventually surfaces, in so many of us, as a major degenerative disease. And this is why the degenerative diseases increase in frequency as we get older. It is nothing to do with ageing per se, for if we ate a profoundly anti-inflammatory diet (as the Victorians did, or as the Mediterranean folks used to do) we would not become more prone to disease as we aged. We would age more slowly, as the Victorians did, and in a much healthier way.

So far we have talked about chronic inflammation as the consequence of a failed acute inflammatory response. But there are at least **five** more causes of chronic, sub-clinical inflammation in our bodies.

1. A pro-inflammatory diet

a) Not enough Omega 3, too much Omega 6

The main hormones that control the inflammatory response are called eicosanoids. The body uses fatty acids from the food we eat to make these eicosanoids. Omega 6 fatty acids, found in polyunsaturated plant oils like safflower, sunflower and corn oil, produce eicosanoids that promote inflammation. Omega 3 fatty acids (from oily fish) have the opposite effect – they produce eicosanoids that reduce inflammation (10-11).

Our ancestors ate a diet with a ratio of Omega-6 to Omega-3 of between 1:1 and 2:1, which is a healthy ratio (12-13). The balance today has become very unhealthy. We consume foods containing far too much Omega 6 fatty acids and too few Omega 3 fatty acids. As a result, our current ratio is anywhere between 10:1 and 40:1, with some individuals as high as 100:1. The body is therefore forced to use too many Omega 6 fatty acids to build cells, tissues and hormones, causing the balance in the body to become pro-inflammatory and prone to disease (14).

The prevalence of Omega 6 over Omega 3 in today's diet is because our intake of oily fish, the only significant source of the Omega 3's we need, has fallen, while our intake of plant oils, which provide Omega 6's, has risen dramatically. Plant oils such as soy and corn oil are widely used in cooking and in processed foods because they are cheap and palatable. Food manufacturers do not have a mandate to produce healthy food.

To make matters worse, most animals raised for human consumption are also packed with Omega 6. Grass-fed animals have healthier levels of Omega 3, but today only sheep and lambs are consistently raised this way; most cows and pigs are cereal fed, and have a much higher 6 to 3 ratio as a result. You find the same pattern in chickens and eggs. Battery and barn chickens are fed grains high in Omega 6, and have a high 6/3 ratio as a result; free range chickens consume more Omega 3 fatty acids, and produce meat and eggs with a better Omega 6/3 balance.

Notice the word '**balance**'. Some Omega 6 fatty acids are essential for life, and in any case it is impossible to avoid all of them. But you can easily adopt a lifestyle that tips the balance back towards a lower 6/3 ratio which is anti-inflammatory, and therefore considerably healthier.

b) Not enough fruits and vegetables

Fruits and vegetables are important because they contain inter alia polyphenols, a group of compounds that exert potent anti-inflammatory effects in the body. These compounds can greatly modify the effects of the eicosanoids because they have the ability to block many of the key enzymes involved in eicosanoid synthesis. They block, for example, COX-1 and COX-2, the same enzymes that are blocked by many anti-inflammatory drugs (15-17). They also block a related pair of inflammatory enzymes called LIPOX-5 and LIPOX-8 (18-19). Perhaps even more critically, they block a group of enzymes called the matrix metallo-proteases, known as MMP's) (20).This exerts a more potent protective effect than any pharmaceutical, as the MMP's are directly responsible for the tissue damage that mediates between chronic inflammation and disease.

Because we eat so few fruits and vegetables these critically important enzyme blockers are not present in our bodies in adequate amounts, and this, together with the excess 6/3 ratios, creates the conditions for the perfect fire storm. And here is another part of the problem; our diet – so poor in so many ways – is rich in fast foods, cooked at high temperatures. These provide the matches.

c) Too much salt

This is a bit of a special case, and is – at this time – only relevant to those with autoimmune diseases such as Multiple Sclerosis, rheumatoid arthritis and Grave's Disease. These diseases destroy the nervous system, joints and thyroid respectively, by causing local and intense chronic inflammation. There is evidence that a high-salt diet makes matters worse by increasing the activity of immune cells called TH17 cells, which are active in the disease process [21]. Accordingly, people with autoimmune disease would be well advised to add salt reduction to their anti-inflammatory regime.

2. Pro-inflammatory cooking methods

When foods containing proteins are cooked at high temperatures, the protein binds with glucose or other sugars in the food to produce compounds called Advanced Glycation End Products, or AGE's. Many foods brown at high temperatures and this discolouration is a sign of AGE production. AGE compounds are very pro-inflammatory – and very ageing.

The best known AGE compound is acrylamide. This forms when starchy foods are cooked at high temperatures, and sugar molecules in the starch react with an amino acid called asparagine. It has been found in crisps, french fries, toast, Pringles and other foods. Worryingly, acrylamide has been classified as carcinogenic in humans [22].

AGE's can also be formed within the body. Some glucose molecules are bound by enzymes to proteins in the body, forming glycoproteins which are essential to normal body functioning. But when glucose binds to proteins (or fats) in the body through NON-enzyme action, it creates AGE products. Non-enzymatic binding occurs when levels of glucose are too high for too long, as happens in diabetes. This drives the formation of AGE's, and leads to inflammation – which helps to explain why diabetics suffers from excessive inflammation, and accelerated ageing.

AGE's are ageing because they stimulate inflammation, but this is not the only way they accelerate the ageing process. The binding of glucose to proteins in the body also causes cross-linking between proteins, binding them together in a random and dysfunctional manner. Externally, this shows up as skin ageing, wrinkling and reduced elasticity. Internally, this drives diseases such as cataracts, hypertension, blood clotting and kidney damage.

Dr Levi of the American Journal of Kidney Diseases says: "AGE reactions ... gradually accumulate over the lifetime of the protein. The goal must be to prevent AGE's forming in the first place".

AGE's in the diet can be reduced by adopting different cooking techniques, and the AGE's formed internally in diabetes can be reduced by controlling blood sugar levels. So here are two more ways to shift from an inflammatory to an anti-inflammatory and healthier way of living.

It is not just AGE's we have to be careful of. High temperature cooking also creates ALE's, which might sound friendlier but are just as harmful. Advanced Lipoxidation End products are created when fats and oils are heated, and like the AGE compounds they are highly pro-inflammatory.

Foods containing high levels of both AGE's and ALE's include powdered milk as used in enteral nutrition, numerous industrially produced foods and baby formulae[2]; high temperature fried and grilled meat and poultry, deep fried and shallow fried fish, coffee and colas, soy sauces, balsamic products and smoked and cured foods – in short, fast food staples. Higher intakes of these foods cause chronic inflammation [91] and an increased risk of insulin resistance and metabolic syndrome. [92]. Higher levels of these pro-inflammatory compounds in the blood are linked to higher rates of *many* degenerative diseases, including a large number of cancers [23].

But let us not all become Puritans. The aim is **balance**. Humans (and other omnivores) like high fat, high sugar foods; and life without the occasional dessert, cake, chip or snack would be – well, less enjoyable. But if you consciously balance those foods with anti-inflammatory foods and nutrients, you can indulge occasionally without harm.

3. Getting older ...

Levels of the sex hormones estrogen, progesterone and testosterone fall as we age, and lower hormone levels are implicated in age-related inflammation [24]. Symptoms of chronic inflammation often become more apparent during and after menopause in women and in men as testosterone levels fall with age. Chronic inflammation has been cited as one cause of sarcopenia, the debilitating muscle loss that occurs with ageing. For both sexes therefore the tendency to increased inflammation typically starts to increase after about 45-50.

To make matters worse, there is evidence that our immune systems may become less efficient at dealing with inflammation as we get older. On a positive note this is related, at least in part, to age-related changes in dietary habits – and it can be rectified by broad spectrum micro- and phytonutrient support.

4. Being overweight or obese

Overweight and obesity are major causes of chronic inflammation today. This is because excess adipose (fat) tissue secretes pro-inflammatory compounds [25].

2.. Most dried milks are made in spray driers at 150 to 175 degrees C, and produce significant amounts of AGE's. High grade milk powders such as those used in 1Life are made by freeze drying and are AGE-free.

In a society where almost 30% of people are obese and 62% are officially overweight, the pro-inflammatory role of abdominal fat has become an important cause of ill health and accelerated ageing. There is a mesh of reinforcing factors here; our expanding waistlines are linked to our high intakes of processed and fast foods high in Omega 6 fatty acids, sugar, salt and pro-inflammatory, processed foods; and to our low physical activity levels, which are themselves pro-inflammatory.

(Moderate exercise is anti-inflammatory, due in part to an up-regulation of anti-oxidant defences and a down-regulation of the stress hormones adrenalin and cortisol. Excessive physical exercise, on the other hand, is pro-inflammatory, due to oxidative stress and tissue damage.)

As excess fat is pro-inflammatory, and chronic inflammation is a factor in heart disease, stroke, diabetes, Alzheimer's and even some cancers, it is hardly surprising that being overweight is a risk factor for all these diseases.

The good news is that an anti-inflammatory food regime is often also a weight loss regime.

5. Environmental factors

Exposure to air pollutants such as cigarette smoke triggers chronic inflammation, as can diesel exhaust particulates (26-29). Exposure to certain pesticides may also trigger inflammation (30).

Smoking is universally recognised as a leading cause of illness, accelerated ageing and death, but it is less well known that city dwellers exposed to high levels of diesel exhaust particulates are also at increased risk (31).

ACTION: Stop smoking (but you already know this!) Minimise exposure to air pollution when possible. In heavily polluted areas consider using a mask; and in all the above cases, increase your intake of anti-inflammatory nutrients.

Inflammation and free radicals

Most people have, by now, heard that free radicals can damage your health. In fact it is only an *excess* of free radicals that is damaging, as some level of free radical action is normal and necessary, forming as it does an important part of the immune response to pathogens. However, excess free radical action can indeed cause cell damage and, eventually, major health problems.

Free radicals are minute particles formed during the billions of chemical processes that take place in the human body, and make life possible. We are made of molecules that are in turn made up of atoms, and all atoms (and molecules) have electrons surrounding them. Electrons are generally paired, but during certain reactions one of an electron pair may be detached. The remaining atom (or molecule) is now an unstable free radical, with one unpaired electron.

To become stable again the free radical must grab an electron from another molecule, but now that other molecule becomes a free radical in turn. The chain reaction of molecules stealing electrons from each other continues; it can be thousands of events long and very destructive until the sequence ends. These chain reactions are damped down by antioxidant enzymes (all of which require trace elements, obtained from the diet, to function), and a sequence or ladder of antioxidant nutrients involving, among others, vitamin E, lycopene and finally vitamin C. Vitamin C often forms the base of the ladder because vitamin C radicals are only weakly reactive and can be safely excreted in the urine. Other antioxidant phytonutrients (plant-derived nutrients) such as the polyphenols also play an important role; one reason why broad spectrum nutrition is so critically important for health.

This process of free radical formation and quenching is also called oxidative damage as oxygen molecules and species are often involved.

Excessive free radical (oxidative) damage to the tissues contributes to age-related diseases from heart disease to cancer; and there are a number of well-known factors that increase levels of free radicals in our bodies, and increase the risks of such diseases These include smoking, exposure to radiation (from ultra violet to X-rays and all things radioactive) – and inflammation.

Inflammation-induced cell damage produces toxic compounds which trigger the release of excess free radicals. The resulting 'oxidative stress' further damages those cells, and this process releases a second wave of inflammatory mediators, completing a vicious circle which drives both disease and the ageing process itself – unless sufficient anti-inflammatory and antioxidant defences are in place. And these require a wide range of trace elements, vitamins, Omega 3 fatty acids and phytonutrients.

Some years ago, the Centre for Environmental and Health Science in Australia stated that: *"Evidence is accumulating that most of the degenerative diseases that afflict humanity have their origin in deleterious free radical reactions. These diseases include atherosclerosis, cancer, inflammatory joint disease, asthma, diabetes, senile dementia and degenerative eye disease. The process of biological ageing might also have a free radical basis".*

Their more recent position is that ageing and age-related diseases are driven by the chronic inflammation/free radical feedback loop.

This is why there is a growing consensus among scientists and clinicians that a comprehensive disease preventative and health protective lifestyle should include foods / nutrients with high anti-inflammatory *and* high anti-oxidant capacity. This is less complicated than it sounds, as anti-inflammatory and anti-oxidant foods are often (but not always) the same foods. These foods are listed in Chapter 2.

Inflammation and genes

I don't want to give the impression that all illness and all age related diseases are exclusively caused by lifestyle and dietary factors. Genetic inheritance can be a contributing factor, and a determining factor in single locus diseases such as Huntingdon's disease or Sickle Cell. Strong genetic risk factors have also been implicated in about 5 – 8% of cases of heart disease, cancer, Alzheimer's and the other major diseases. But for most of us, our destiny is not written in genetic code. The developing science of epigenetics shows that our genes can be switched on and off by external influences, including a wide range of nutritional factors. Our genetic inheritance may make us more or less susceptible to lifestyle and dietary influences – but we can control those.

For example, researchers Fredrico **Licastro** and colleagues from the University of Bologna state that: "Alzheimer's disease, atherosclerosis, diabetes and even sarcopenia and cancer, just to mention a few – have an important inflammatory component, though disease progression seems also dependent on the genetic background of individuals"

In other words certain gene types are more susceptible to age related disease – but the same researchers conclude that "controlling inflammatory status may allow a better chance of successful ageing." So whatever your genotype, establishing an anti-inflammatory lifestyle is a priority if you wish to improve your health prospects.

This is amply proven by the mid-Victorians, who shared the same genetic palette as we do today, but not our vulnerability to degenerative disease.

The role of Inflammation in specific diseases

Heart disease

Heart disease has been simplistically described as a 'plumbing' problem – ie, plaque builds up in the walls of blood vessels, clogs and blocks them. But blood vessels are not like pipes; they are composed of living, reactive tissue, and are sensitive to damage and injury.

For example, they are highly sensitive to pro-inflammatory compounds such as AGE's and Advanced Lipoxidation End products or ALE's. These toxic compounds are formed when different types of foods are cooked at high temperatures. They can also be formed in the body; diabetics produce their own AGE's due to their high blood sugar levels, and smokers produce ALE's internally because of the high oxidative stress in their bodies caused by smoking.

Whether eaten or formed in the body, these compounds attack the linings of the blood vessels, causing chronic inflammation and tissue damage. Immune cells then target the damaged site, and migrate into the vessel wall where they attempt to resolve the damage. If the toxins are present in too high amounts the immune cells die, and their remains build up as atheroma; a toxic sludge rich in oxidised cholesterol compounds that came not from circulating cholesterol, but from the dead immune cells.

There are healing mechanisms, but if there are too many pro-inflammatory compounds, too much oxidative stress and inflammation, and insufficient antioxidant and anti-inflammatory compounds in the diet (and this combination is all too common in the developed world), the rate of atheroma formation outstrips the body's ability to remove it; and so over time the atheroma builds, forming plaque inside the artery walls. Eventually the plaque may grow until it bulges out into the space inside the artery, reducing blood flow. If this is an artery supplying the heart, this can cause angina; if it supplies the brain, it can cause confusion, dizziness and other symptoms. If the plaque ruptures, as they often do, this can cause a heart attack or a stroke.

The problem is made worse by the fact that the same chronic inflammation that drives the formation of atheroma in the artery walls also causes them to constrict, so that there is a gradual rise in blood pressure. This forces the heart to work harder and it makes the arteries less elastic, creating a combination of effects which increases shear stresses and shock waves within the arterial system. And that creates more sites of damage, leading to more inflammation and more atheroma.

Statins are not very effective because they attack the wrong target, ie cholesterol levels in the blood. In fact blood cholesterol is a very inaccurate biomarker, as fully half of all heart attacks occur in folks with normal cholesterol levels. There is a growing suspicion that the relatively minor protective effects of statins (and we will not talk about their adverse effects here), are due to the fact that some of them have a mild anti-inflammatory effect as well as a cholesterol-lowering action.

The Mediterranean and similar diets rich in anti-inflammatory compounds, are more cardio-protective than statins (44-45, 87). They are also, of course, a good deal safer.

Alzheimer's Disease

Chronic inflammation is a significant factor in Alzheimer's. It was long ago known that the risk of Alzheimer's was reduced in people who, because they had an inflammatory condition such as arthritis, took certain anti-inflammatory drugs (which are too toxic to be used today, let alone for long term prophylactic use). A diet rich in anti-inflammatory compounds also reduces the risk of developing Alzheimer's (46-47). Conversely, a long term study called the Honolulu-Asia Ageing Study found that men with the highest levels of inflammation, as measured by CRP, were three times as likely to develop dementia as those with the lowest levels (48).

How dementia develops is the focus of intense study, and it is undoubtedly a very complex process. But we do know that chronic inflammation is involved, and that this attacks and kills brain cells. The Omega 3's, of course, are anti-inflammatory. We also know that the brain relies on a continuous supply of fatty acids, and particularly the Omega 3 fatty acid DHA, to build and renew the walls of its brain cells. The evidence is inconsistent; the omega 3 fatty acids undoubtedly have neuro-protective effects (49-51), but when given on their own do not appear to be sufficiently protective (52). This is not surprising, given that so many people are depleted in most if not all of the necessary co-factors. Perhaps the most important of these are the polyphenols, which have complementary neuro-protective properties.

Polyphenols derived from fruits and vegetables reduce inflammation directly by blocking key inflammatory enzymes. They also exert indirect anti-inflammatory effects by binding free iron (which is pro-inflammatory) and by reducing the production of free radicals which would otherwise cause collateral damage (53). There is a strong rationale for combining Omega 3's with the right kinds of polyphenols, which protect the Omega 3's and prevent them from being broken down into pro-inflammatory metabolites. Conversely, it is inappropriate (and often counter-productive) for clinicians to attempt to treat complex conditions like Alzheimer's with single compounds. That kind of pseudo-pharmaceutical approach is singularly unsuited to nutritional programmes; nutrients work *together*.

More evidence on the importance of combining the right nutrients comes from scientists at the University of California, published in the *Journal of Alzheimer's Disease*. They tested a combination of curcumin (a compound derived from the spice turmeric) and vitamin D3 to enhance the activity of two types of immune cell acting in the brain (54). They stated: '*Our findings demonstrate that active forms of vitamin D3 and curcumin may be an important regulator of immune activities of macrophages in helping to clear amyloid plaques.*'

Diabetes

Researchers have noted a connection between obesity, chronic inflammation and insulin resistance, culminating in Metabolic Syndrome and Type 2 diabetes. In obesity the fat cells – especially abdominal fat cells – release pro-inflammatory chemicals. These are implicated in insulin resistance (90), which inhibits the body's ability to regulate blood sugar.

The hormone insulin works by ensuring that muscle cells take up blood sugar after a meal, in a process which lowers blood sugar levels. A combination of excess body fat / chronic inflammation, a carb-rich diet and insufficiently exercised muscle impedes this process, leading to chronically elevated blood sugar levels. This creates AGE products and cross linking damage to tissues, leading over time to accumulated damage in many sites including the blood vessels, eyes, kidneys and brain.

The diet / nutritional regime in this book is anti-inflammatory *and* has a low Glycaemic Index (G.I.). This makes it a particularly suitable defence against diabetes – especially when coupled with exercise and, where appropriate, weight loss.

Cancer

Cancer is not one disease, but many. Inflammation is not currently implicated in them all by any means. However, patients with colon cancer, for example, have consistently raised levels of biomarkers for inflammation; and chronic inflammation is looking more and more like an essential part of the chain of events that leads to disease.

Here's what Scientific American said in a key article in 2008. *'Cancer begins with a series of genetic changes that prompt a group of cells to over-replicate and then invade surrounding tissue, the point at which true malignancy begins. Eventually some tumour cells may break off and establish new growths (metastases) at distant sites'.*

What appears to cause that progression from DNA damage to cancer is chronic inflammation encouraging free radical damage. As the magazine then puts it: *'genetic damage is the match that lights the fire, and inflammation is the fuel that feeds it'.*

The converse is also true. There is good evidence that an anti-inflammatory diet – for example, one rich in Omega 3 fatty acids - slows down cancer growth [55].

Summary

Over the last century or so, levels of anti-inflammatory compounds in our diet have declined and levels of pro-inflammatory factors have increased. As a result we have become much more prone to chronic inflammation and all the degenerative diseases. Pharmaceutical medicine suppresses the symptoms of these diseases but cannot prevent or cure them. A better diet, however, can.

Chapter 2: We're living longer than ever before – surely we must be healthier?

There is overwhelming evidence that as our diet has degenerated and we have become more prone to chronic inflammation, the degenerative diseases have become far more common. But whenever I discuss these ideas with medical colleagues, someone inevitably protests that the story of diet and inflammation cannot be true because we are all living longer lives than before. A powerful argument – if it were true.

According to the crude statistics, we're living longer. According to the Global Burden of Disease Study, an enormously expensive and rather fatuous exercise in number crunching funded by the Gates Foundation and just published in the Lancet (56), global life expectancy has risen from 59 in 1990 to 70 today. According to the medical profession and the pharmaceutical industry all is increasingly for the best in this, the best of all possible worlds. And according to those who really know, this is nothing short of a public health disaster.

World life expectancy map

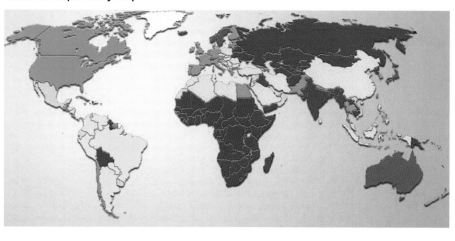

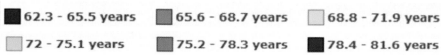

Average life expectancy for males at birth in 2009 (Lancet 2013)

A very large part of the increase in global life expectancy is due to reduced infant mortality in the developing world, which has been achieved with improved sanitation, clean water and immunisation programmes. But what has modern medicine done for life and health expectancy for adults?

The results have been mixed, to say the least. In the UK, for example, and comparing like for like, the situation for men has worsened significantly over the last century and a half. In mid-Victorian England, male children aged 5 could expect to achieve, on average, another 75 years of life (57-58). By 2002-2006, the life expectancy of boys born to 'parents with routine occupations' (formerly 'working class') had *fallen* to 74.6 years (59) – a loss of 5 years.[3]

Women have done better. Mid-Victorian girls aged 5 could expect another 72 years of life (57-58), and in 2002-2006, the life expectancy of girls born to C1-C2 parents was 79.7 years (59) – a gain of nearly 3 years.[4]

Why have men and women fared so differently? The answer is simple; in the 19th century, female life expectancy was dragged down by multiple pregnancies - contraception was rudimentary at best - and the perils of childbirth. Family planning and better obstetrics (such as doctors learning to wash their hands between patients) have given women an average of three more years of life.

Why have men lost life expectancy? The answer again is simple; nutritional standards have fallen hugely since the 19th century, thanks to our low energy lifestyles and the modern food industry. Our appalling nutritional status condemns us to an unnecessarily high risk of acquiring, as we age, one or typically more of the non-communicable degenerative diseases; and thus we spend far more of our old age suffering from the so-called diseases of civilisation than ever before (9, 60-62).

The resulting increased need for medical resources has driven up healthcare spending from circa 1% of GDP in the second half of the 19th century (63) to approximately 18% today (64); and it is getting worse. According to leading oncologist Professor Karol Sikora, *'The incidence of cancer is dramatically increasing ... the last eight cancer drugs approved by the US Food and Drug Administration will cost over £10,000 a month per patient ... no healthcare system can afford this ..'* (65-66).

Unfortunately it's not just cancer. If diabetes, coronary artery disease, dementias and cancer are diseases of civilisation, we are certainly becoming more civilised. But conversely, this is telling us that none of the on-going pandemics of degenerative disease are inevitable. They are not occurring because we are growing older (we are not, much); but are being triggered by our unhealthy lifestyles and sustained, often life-long dysnutrition.

---

3. USA trends have, until recently, been slightly more positive. Men and women aged 60 both gained about 5 years between 1850 and 2004 (88). In the last decade, however, it appears that dietary and lifestyle changes have begun to drive life expectancy down again (89).
4. Ibid

These diseases cannot be cured with drugs, and so increasing numbers of us develop health problems that burden us with many years of pain, disability, mental distress and medical dependency (60-62). This is no 'distressing irony', as the Lancet papers' authors call it, but a direct result of the way in which medicine is practised.

20th century medicine focussed on the curative treatment of bacterial, fungal and protozoal infection with antibiotics; the prevention of infection via immunisation; and the (non-curative) treatment of symptoms of the non-communicable disease, using specific and often hazardous drugs. Taught at medical school to disregard nutrition, 21st century doctors remain fixated on drugs even though the literature linking nutrition and nutrients to health outcomes is growing at a rate of hundreds of papers per week. They ignore the root causes of the flood tides that wash, every day, the victims of poor diets and lifestyles into their surgeries.

And the tides are rising. Overweight, diabetes, hypertension, cardiovascular disease, cancer – *all* of the chronic degenerative diseases - are driven by lifestyle factors. Not enough exercise, Omega 3 fatty acids, fruits and vegetables; too much smoking, alcohol, salt, Omega 6 fatty acids and fast food. *All* of these factors are going in the wrong direction.

Supermarket food prices are rising much faster than incomes and as a result shoppers are buying less healthy food and more of the fatty, filling, salty products that provide both comfort and disease. In the last year there has been a 10% fall in fruit and vegetable purchases, with an even greater fall (22%) in low income homes (67). This study of more than 6,000 households compared actual food consumption to the government recommended 'Eatwell Plate' (itself a very low standard), and concluded that 'neither low income households nor all households are close' to achieving it.

Chris Murray, Professor of Global Health at Washington University and a lead author of the global survey, summarised his team's findings. 'Very few people are walking around with perfect health' he said,' and as people age, they accumulate health conditions. This means we should recalibrate what life will be like for us in our 70s and 80s. It also has profound implications for health systems as they set priorities.'

I agree that very few people have perfect health, but the rest of Professor Murray's statement represents a profound failure of courage and intellect. It implies that a globally ageing population will inevitably become sicker, and that this must be planned for in a framework based on drugs, surgery and expensive medicine. It ignores the fact we cannot afford this future. It ignores the fact that current trends will degrade life and health expectancy way beyond the basic demographics; and it effectively ignores the fact that the only way to prevent these tides of disease is to cut them off at source, by improved nutrition.

Let us hope that the growing evidence base linking good nutrition to better health will eventually overcome the resistance of the pharma lobby and become incorporated into government policy, agricultural practice and food design. The barriers between us and vastly better health are no longer scientific but political; and when it comes to politics, you should ignore the political brands on offer (they're mostly for show), and follow the money.

The emerging consensus that almost all the major diseases have, at their core, chronic inflammation driven by lifestyle factors, is deeply political. This new Grand Unified Theory of disease is transforming modern medicine just as the Grand Unified Theory of forces transformed modern physics – and its implications are staggering. It shows that the tides of chronic illness we see today are unnecessary. It also shows that our apparently unavoidable and increasing risk of acquiring a so-called 'disease of ageing' as we get older is entirely artificial, something that could be neutralised if we could find a way of suppressing the chronic inflammation that sickens and kills so many of us.

But Big Pharma makes a very good living indeed from chronic inflammation. In 2010, global sales of anti-inflammatory drugs amounted to over $100 Billion, with the major disease categories being (in descending order of financial significance) pain management, asthma and chronic obstructive pulmonary disease, rheumatoid arthritis, multiple sclerosis, inflammatory bowel disease and psoriasis (68-71).

This is not the only price we pay. Over 100,000 deaths are caused by adverse drug effects every year in the USA alone (72-73), and another 100,000 die as a result of medical errors and other causes due to the medical treatment of avoidable diseases (74-75). If we add the hundreds of millions of deaths caused by illnesses that we now know are avoidable, but which our doctors insist on treating with drugs (because they are trained to do so in institutions largely funded by Big Pharma money), it is clear that pharmadollars have created an on-going, slow-motion holocaust. This holocaust is so pervasive that we have accepted it as normal, but I hope by now you can see that it is anything but normal.

As the current medical model is so saturated and dominated by Big Pharma, and as public health has suffered so much as a result, the obvious answer is to take matters into your own hands. Beating chronic inflammation via nutrition is cheap, easy, safe and considerably more effective than relying on the tender mercies of the current healthcare model. You could entrust your health to the wisdom and benevolence of our politicians and banksters, and die. Or you could take matters into your own hands, adopt an anti-inflammatory lifestyle, and live.

If that is not enough of an inducement to live a healthier lifestyle, consider this. There is good evidence that our diet is not only making us sick, it is also making us stupid. Visual reaction speeds are a good measure of the functionality of the central nervous system, and correlate highly with IQ; brains that are less efficient at handling information react to stimuli more slowly. A tightly controlled and rather beautiful meta-analysis of 14 age-matched studies carried out between 1884 (the earliest recorded data) and 2004 shows that our brains have indeed slowed down (95).

Compared to the Victorians, our visual reaction speeds have slowed by 81.4 milliseconds or 30%. This corresponds to a fall in average IQ of 14 points – a highly significant decline in our mental health, and very much in step with our declining physical health[5]. We are eating the wrong fuel for our bodies and our brains, and creating a morass of problems that drugs cannot fix.

---

5. Some claim that the recorded decline in average intelligence is due to differential breeding rates in different ethnic groups or social classes, but the evidence base indicates that the fall in IQ is due to our declining nutritional status (103). Sub-optimal intakes of omega 3 and polyphenols increase inflammation in the brain and compromise synaptic and neuronal function and viability (96-102).

The fall of the Roman Empire is considered to have many causes including political corruption, the over-growth of the state and its bureaucratic institutions, and wide-spread lead poisoning due to the use of lead drinking vessels. Chronic lead poisoning damages the brain and reduces intelligence. Substitute junk food for lead and the picture looks eerily familiar ...

Chapter 3: Putting out the Flames – a Basic Guide

For long term health, chronic inflammation and excess free radical activity must be kept in check. There are just seven actions to take which check and neutralise the causes of inflammation. They are surprisingly easy to carry out.

Action 1   Eat an anti-inflammatory diet

The key anti-inflammatory foods include fruits, vegetables and Omega-3-rich oily fish. Together they form a powerful anti-inflammatory combination. The Omega 3 fatty acids produce anti-inflammatory hormones called eicosanoids, and the polyphenols block the key pro-inflammatory enzymes. The combination is logical and, as the Victorian example shows, highly effective in preventing chronic inflammation and the degenerative diseases.

Once ingested, Omega 3 fatty acids are built into the membranes of all the cells in our body, and once there they remain for quite some time. The polyphenols, however, are regarded by the body as foreign. After ingestion, they do not remain in the body for long but are broken down and excreted. For this reason the Omega 3 fatty acids are best regarded as creating an anti-inflammatory climate, whereas a good intake of polyphenols creates anti-inflammatory weather. When both of these elements are in place chronic inflammation is minimised or stopped, and healing processes in the body can once again predominate.

Fish high in Omega 3 fatty acids include **wild salmon** (not farmed salmon), **mackerel, herring, tuna, sardines and pilchards**. Fruits with high anti-inflammatory and anti-oxidant scores include **blueberries, raspberries, blackberries, strawberries, cherries and blackcurrants**. High scoring vegetables include **broccoli, asparagus, beets, olives, mushrooms, chard, spinach and cabbage**. (Mushrooms are actually fungi, but they usually live in the vegetable section).These fruits and vegetables are good sources of polyphenols, carotenoids and other phyto-nutrients with anti-inflammatory and antioxidant properties. Eating a rainbow is sound advice, although don't forget the more traditional apples, pears and citrus. Generally the more (natural) colours there are on your plate, the higher the anti-oxidant and anti-inflammatory content of your diet.

Use Table 1 to increase anti-inflammatory foods in your diet and reduce the levels of pro-inflammatory foods. Although not a weight loss diet in itself, many people find it easier to maintain a healthy weight on this type of food regime and most lose weight.

Table 1   Anti and pro-inflammatory foods

	EAT MORE	EAT LESS
Fruits	All red / black / purple fruits, all berry fruits; strawberries, raspberries, blackcurrants, mulberries, blackcurrants, citrus, blueberries, plums, cherries, grapes, acai, elderberries etc.	
Vegetables	broccoli, chard, spinach, cabbage, collards, kale, onions, carrots, sweet potatoes, garlic, peppers, mushrooms, courgette (zucchini), celery, asparagus	Potatoes and potato products, corn and corn products
Legumes	Beans, peas, pulses	
Herbs and Spices	Turmeric, garlic, ginger, cayenne, chili, curry powder, basil, thyme, black pepper, cinnamon, oregano, rosemary, nutmeg	Salt
Fats and oils	Olive oil – good Canola oil – acceptable	Grapeseed, sunflower, safflower, soy, corn, cottonseed, maize and palm oils. Hard margarines
Dairy products	Cheeses esp. green & blue; unsweetened yoghurt	Sweetened yoghurt, ice cream
Fish	Salmon (if wild), herring, tuna, mackerel, sardines, pilchards, trout, oysters	Deep-fried fish, fish fingers
Meat	Game, grass-fed beef, mutton & lamb, free range chicken	Beef & pork products if intensively farmed. Sausages, burgers, bacon and other cured meats such as hot dogs, salami
Breads	Wholemeal & rye in moderation, although physically active folk can eat more	White (refined) flour products
Cereals	Bran cereals, no added sugar muesli, porridge oats	Cornflakes, all sugared cereals
Biscuits and snacks	Dried fruits	Crisps and chips, pretzels, sweet biscuits and cookies, pies
Pasta, grain and legume products	Tofu, hummus, dal	White rice, pasta, gnocchi
Nuts and seeds	Peanuts , coconut	Most nuts, esp. if salted and roasted
Sweeteners	Intense sweeteners such as stevia, sucralose	Sugar, honey, syrup, molasses

| Desserts and confectionary | dark chocolate | Most sweets and desserts – inc. cakes, pastries |
| Drinks | Fruit and vegetable juices, tea, coffee, milk, red wine | Sugar-sweetened soft drinks, spirits |

Cooking oils	**Olive, peanut, canola**	**Safflower, sunflower**

Action 2   Switch to safer cooking techniques

Use less Omega 6 polyunsaturated plant oils; switch to (monounsaturated) olive oil. Cut down on foods cooked at high temperatures, whether grilled, fried, barbequed or roasted. Meats are best stewed, slow cooked, or stir fried or sautéd quickly in thinner cuts. Steam or microwave vegetables.

Rub joints for roasting with thyme and/or oregano which helps counteract the formation of AGE (Advance Glycation End) products. Do not use honey or sugar to glaze meats, as this encourages AGE formation.

Action 3   Speed Up to Slow Ageing Down

Moderate exercise increases your health prospects, because it has anti-inflammatory effects (32-33). The standard advice is to take 30 minutes of exercise, five times a week at a level that raises your heart rate. People who exercise at around this level have lower rates of heart disease, cancer, diabetes and dementia. If exercise was a drug it would be a 'miracle breakthrough', but like all drugs you can over-dose. Intense exercise can trigger inflammation and excessive free radicals - which is why athletes should be particularly aware of eating an anti-inflammatory diet.

Action 4   Lose weight if you need to

If you carry excess weight, do try to slim down – but do it in a gradual and sustainable way. Crash diets are not recommended as they don't generally work, and there is evidence that yo-yo dieting is intrinsically pro-inflammatory. Since excess fat cells are inflammatory, support your weight-loss regime with a supplement that includes the full range of anti-inflammatory nutrients and phytonutrients listed above. These all tend to be low in calorie restricted diets, which increases the need for broad spectrum micro- and phytonutrient support.

There is a **free** weight loss support site at www.anti-inflammatorydiet.co.uk It provides practical advice, daily motivation, tips, and menus.

Action 5   Prevent acute inflammatory responses from failing

If the body is invaded by a harmful micro-organism (pathogen), and the acute inflammatory response is insufficient to clear that threat, the infectious agent may linger on. The body will then switch over to a chronic inflammatory response, which – as you know by now – is damaging and can lead to serious diseases. This is why, for example, poor oral hygiene and subsequent chronic gingival inflammation are linked to heart disease. And this is why it is important to ensure that your acute immune response to external challenges is effective.

The most effective (and natural) way to boost your immunity is to take (1-3), (1-6) beta-glucans. These are a class of polysaccharides, derived from bakers' yeast, that have been proven to increase the effectiveness of macrophages and neutrophils, your front line defence against bacteria and viruses.

The (1-3), (1-6) beta-glucans (not to be confused with the (1-3), (1-4) beta-glucans in oats and other cereals), have been tested against a wide range of pathogens, from E. coli to flu viruses and the deadly anthrax bacillus (35), and shown to be highly protective against all of them.

When the Canadian Department of Defence was searching for an immune enhancer that could help protect against anthrax, they tested over 300 products – and the (1-3), (1-6) beta-glucans extracted from Baker's yeast gained the highest score.

Action 6   Counteract or avoid harmful environments

Stop smoking (but you already knew that!), and minimise exposure to air pollution where possible. If you live in a city where air quality is an issue, consider an anti-inflammatory supplement at any age.

Action 7   Good Oral Hygiene

Periodontal disease (chronic inflammation of the gums) is the cause of more tooth loss than dental decay. Bleeding when brushing or flossing is a tell-tale sign, an alarm bell that should trigger a visit to the dentist and improved oral hygiene. Periodontal disease and tooth loss have been linked in many studies to an increased risk of heart disease and diabetes (36-37). Conversely, improved oral hygiene leading to reduced periodontal inflammation has been shown to lower levels of a range of blood biomarkers linked to heart disease (38).

Despite many such studies, the American Heart Association's position is that perio does not cause heart disease or stroke (39). They take the view that while there is an association, it may not be causative; for example, an unhealthy diet and lifestyle would be expected to cause both periodontal and heart disease. There must be some truth in this, but the AHA published before it was known that improved oral hygiene reduced cardiotoxic compounds in the blood.

On balance, chronic inflammation in the gums must increase the risk of degenerative disease elsewhere in the body; we already know that other chronic inflammatory conditions such as rheumatoid arthritis or systemic lupus increase the risk of heart attack and stroke (40-42).

Reasons for optimism

A study in a 2004 issue of Metabolism showed that a diet rich in anti-inflammatory fruits, vegetables and whole grains and which reduced refine flours, sugars and saturated fats led to a 45% average reduction in inflammation levels as measured by C-Reactive Protein (CRP) in just two weeks (43).

CRP is produced in the liver and measured in the blood, and is a measure of the presence and intensity of inflammation anywhere in the body. It is a non-specific marker but it is cheap and convenient so it is still used by many doctors and general practitioners. Some doctors test for Fibrinogen which also rises in response to inflammation and which may, at elevated levels, signal a potential blood clot.

These are quite basic tests, and to get a better idea of what is going on one should ideally carry out a more extensive series of tests. There are a number of recognised biomarkers for inflammation. The industry standard biomarkers are: Interleukin 1-β – (IL1-beta), Tumor Necrosis Factor-α (TNF-alpha), Interleukin 6 (IL-6), Interleukin 8 (IL-8), Prostaglandin E2 (PGE2) and Isoprostane 8 (Iso-PGF2-alpha Isoprostan).

1Life, a combination of Omega 3 fatty acids and lipid-soluble polyphenols derived from olive, has been shown to reduce all the above biomarkers in individual cases, and is due to be formally trialled in 2014. It has already been tested against a more user-friendly and equally profound marker, the Omega 6 / 3 ratio. This can be measured using the validated 1Life self-test.

1. You order a self-test from the 1Life website, which then posts a test kit to your home.
2. Use a styret to take a single drop of blood from the fingertip. The drop is placed on a strip of absorbent paper and sealed in a foil envelope which is already addressed and ready for posting.
3. The sample is tested in the labs at St Olave's Clinic, University of Trondheim, Norway.
4. The test results are posted on the 1Life website. Each result is only available to the test subject, and is exclusively accessed by the code in each test kit

This test system has already been used in well over 100,000 subjects, and ILife has been shown to consistently enhance the Omega 6 / 3 ratio.

The evidence indicates that 1Life exerts potent anti-inflammatory effects, and is a bioactive nutraceutical which can be used to help prevent and treat inflammatory disease of any kind.

Omega 3's and/or polyphenols?

We've discussed anti-inflammatory Omega 3 fatty acids from fish, polyphenols from fruit and vegetables, and the 1-3, 1-6 beta-glucans from baker's yeast. Which of these is the most important in keeping chronic inflammation under control?

I travel widely for my work. In 2012 I studied and lectured in Finland, Sweden, the USA, Australia, Greece, Turkey, New Zealand, the UK, Malaysia, Thailand, Taiwan, Japan and India. I always try to eat local food, and am constantly surprised by the variety of dishes that different cultures have to offer. Stinky tofu stewed with clotted pig's blood in Taipei was a high point, a malodorous dish which, like the similarly fermented fish of Northern Norway and Sweden ('surströmming'), is crammed with polyamines. These highly bioactive compounds accelerate the healing process (76-77), which might explain the fabled ability of the Samurai and the Vikings to recover very rapidly from their battle-field injuries. I do not recommend these dishes to everyone, however. They smell awful, and more seriously, in these days when cancer is so prevalent, they speed tumour growth (78).

But I digress ...

A large part of the ageing process as we experience it today is driven by chronic inflammation, and the major dietary and other factors that either slow or accelerate this process are, as we have seen, well characterised. I had often wondered how people manage to live well in such different environments, consuming such different diets. How can an Indian and an Inuit, for example, both maintain an anti-inflammatory internal environment, and thus both achieve healthy old age? And what implications might this have for regional health issues as the Juggernaut of fast food franchising, which combines empty calories with pro-inflammatory toxins (23, 79-80), rolls over the globe?

A few months ago, I gained a little nutritional enlightenment while visiting an IT college in New Delhi. In South East Asia, and in the tropical and sub-tropical regions in general, intakes of the essential Omega 3 fatty acids are very low. There are no cold water fish and the only Omega 3's available are in plant oils, which are notoriously poor sources; so the folks who live in these areas tend to have very high Omega 6 to 3 ratios in their blood (81). However they do consume large amounts of spices, in almost every dish and at every meal, and the spices are excellent sources of polyphenols. In contrast, Northern Europeans eat a diet relatively high in Omega 3's but low in spices - Scandinavian food, for example, tends to be very bland. Polyphenols and the Omega 3 fatty acids have different but equally potent anti-inflammatory effects, and it seems that if you eat enough of at least one of these nutrient groups you gain a reasonable degree of anti-inflammatory health protection.

For maximum protection, however, you need both of these anti-inflammatory nutrients. The mid-Victorians, who consumed large amounts of both, were almost free of degenerative disease. Our increasing burden of ill health is directly linked to fact that we eat less of these important nutrients, thanks in no small measure to the growth of the fast food franchises which have spread like a cancer across the globe. In other parts of the world, the picture looks even bleaker.

Fast foods have had serious public health consequences in the West, but we have a residual degree of protection against chronic inflammation due to our intakes of Omega 3 fatty acids in salmon, sardines, herring and other oily fish. We do not need to eat these foods every day, as the Omega 3's we consume are stored in the body. The Asians do not have this kind of protection, and rely on the anti-inflammatory polyphenols in the spices they consume. These compounds are not stored in the body and have to be consumed every day (ideally at every meal) to confer meaningful anti-inflammatory protection.

The problem is that there is a generation of IT and office workers all across Asia who have left their native cuisine behind, and combine a sedentary lifestyle with cigarettes and a diet consisting mainly of burgers, fries, pasta, pizza and soft drinks. They are consuming virtually no Omega 3's or polyphenols, and thus have no anti-inflammatory protection at all.

The impact of this is just starting to emerge. I believe that the surprisingly high frequency of obesity, Type 2 diabetes and hypertension I saw in the young IT students will soon grow into a tsunami of degenerative disease in urbanised Asians and which will overwhelm their healthcare systems. Their situation may be made even worse by specific metabolic factors linked to the so-called 'thrifty gene' [83].

Modern medicine can do nothing to prevent or cure these problems, and 're-setting healthcare priorities', as envisaged by the Professor Murray / Bill Gates cabal, is tantamount to re-arranging the deckchairs on the Titanic. Nutritional, dietary and lifestyle re-programming is the only way to ensure that India, China and their neighbours do not sink under the burden of bad Western dietary habits and unnecessary disease.

And the beta-glucans?

The (1-3), (1-6) beta-glucans have direct anti-inflammatory effects [83-85]. They also reduce the burden of chronic inflammation by helping the immune system deal with infections effectively, thus reducing the risk of chronic infections which cause chronic inflammation. This complements the anti-inflammatory effects of Omega 3's and polyphenols, but there's more …

If you consume excessive amounts of Omega 3's and polyphenols, there is at least a theoretical risk that an excessive inhibition of the inflammatory responses might reduce the immune system's ability to fight infection and cancer. This means that if you decide to eat a high-octane anti-inflammatory diet, it makes sense to add (1-3), (1-6) beta-glucans to the regime to enhance your innate immune system.

This brings us back to the mid-Victorians, who enjoyed fabulous personal and public health thanks in large measure to their high intakes of Omega 3's, polyphenols **and** yeast-derived beta-glucans.

Beta-glucans are essential trace nutrients

Humans evolved in an environment without soap, fungicides, or food sterilization technology; in short, in a highly microbiologically contaminated environment. We survived in such an environment partly because our innate immune systems were constantly exposed to (1-3), (1-6) beta-glucans. Since our species emerged we have consumed significant amounts of these compounds as contaminants in almost all foods, and since circa 10,000 BC we have eaten them in larger amounts in fermented drinks and leavened breads.

In the last half-century, however, our food chain has been sanitized to near sterility thanks to the introduction of the synthetic fungicides after WW2, and modern food technology. Consumption of yeast in fermented foods has declined also. The beta-glucan content of beers and wines was effectively eliminated by the introduction of microfiltration in the 1950s, and consumption of bread has fallen dramatically in the last century (9). These changes have left our immune systems compromised, resulting in impaired innate immune function and increasing the risk of antibiotic resistance. In this context, replacing (1-3), (1-6) beta-glucans in the food chain restores an element that was present historically, and restores normal immune function.

The best source of (1-3), (1-6) beta-glucans is Baker's or Brewer's yeast, formally known as Saccharomyces cerevisiae. Until very recently, this yeast was a major player in the personal ecosystem of microbes that live on and inside us.

Trillions of bacteria, yeasts and viruses live in our gut, mouth and nose, on our skin and in each crevice and orifice. Collectively they form an organ called the microbiome, which has evolved to become critically important for our health – it is as important as the liver, kidneys or endocrine system.

Microbial species within the microbiome that contribute to our health are called symbionts. Saccharomyces cerevisiae is not a classical symbiont as it does not -- under normal circumstances – live on or inside us. However, its universal presence in the food chain prior to 1950 meant that (1-3), (1-6) beta-glucans were constantly passing through the gut and entering the bloodstream, acting as key immuno-modulatory compounds. Saccharomyces cerevisiae may, therefore, be regarded as an atypical symbiont (86) and essential to our long-term health.

The (1-3), (1-6) beta-glucans fulfil all the key characteristics of an essential, if atypical, micro-nutrient. They cannot be synthesised in the body, but must be obtained in trace amounts from the diet if our immune systems are to work effectively. Given the beta-glucans' actions in the body, their absence from the diet inevitably leads to a decreased resistance to infection and to an increased risk of allergy and cancer. Restoring them to the diet corrects these disease risks. This strategy enhances innate immunity, which in turn reduces the risk of clinical infections, allergy and cancer.

Anyone who looks back at medical textbooks over the last century can see that the list of vitamins and trace elements waxes and wanes over time, as science has proven or disproven each candidate. There is a strong case for adding 'vitamin Y' (for Yeast) to the list of essential dietary components, and a trial is currently underway which should resolve this issue. Groups of mice have been allocated to two different diets, identical to each other save that one contains beta glucans and the other does not[6]. The animals are being allowed to live out their life-spans and the researchers involved are measuring cumulative mortality, ie the rates at which the different groups of animals die. I hope to be able to report on the findings in the next edition of this book.

End Note

The science is still under construction, but most scientists now believe that chronic inflammation is at the core of most diseases. As a result, chronic inflammation is being targeted by the pharmaceutical industry, and industrial teams are trying to develop new synthetic anti-inflammatory drugs. Our view is that this is a dead-end. Drugs have an overwhelming tendency to produce adverse effects, and more of these emerge the longer the drugs are used. Very few drugs are safe enough to be used for long-term prevention.

In any case, why wait for the next crop of drugs when you could be eating the latest and freshest crop of fruits, vegetables and – to strain a point – oily fish? The diet / supplement route is inherently safer, and far more effective.

Evidence for this comes, yet again, from the mid-Victorians. These folk, who had a life expectancy very similar to our own, ate a diet containing levels of anti-inflammatory compounds roughly ten times higher than we do. As a result, they were almost immune to degenerative disease. Heart attacks and cancer were known but rare, occurring at less than 10% of the levels we think of as normal today.

Chronic inflammation is like a series of slow, smouldering fires that gradually burn away healthy tissue and drive us towards illness, disability and premature death. CRP and the other lab tests that doctors use are fire alarms, and the right diet and lifestyle provide you with a set of powerful fire retardants and extinguishers.

6. We had to have beta glucan-free mouse chow specially made for this trial. Animal feed producers have long known that if beta glucans are not in their feed the animals die young, and so they include it in all chows as standard. In other words, 1-3, 1-6 beta glucans are already recognised to have all the characteristics of a vitamin. It only remains to convince the medical profession of this!

Now it's up to you. You can put this book down, go out and make these simple lifestyle changes, and get healthy. Alternatively, if you want to know more about the science, have a look at Section 3.

Section 3: Putting out the Flames of Disease – An Advanced Course

Chapter 4. Why have we become so unhealthy?

Our society is very sick and very fat, and it is getting sicker and fatter. The way we live, combining junk diets with the kind of sedentary lifestyle that modern technology makes possible, has created a situation where today's adults are so unhealthy that they are, in almost every sense, 15 years 'older' than their parents and grandparents were at the same age (1). The fact that we are ageing more rapidly than our recent ancestors did tells us that there is something seriously wrong with today's lifestyles – and it is showing through in our terrible health statistics.

An authoritative and depressing study recently predicted, on the basis of current trends, another 76 million obese adults by 2030 with an additional 6–8.5 million cases of diabetes, 6–7 million cases of cardiovascular disease and 492,000–669,000 cases of cancer in the UK and USA alone (2). This huge burden of disease will cause dramatic and unaffordable increases in health care costs, already out of control at around a fifth of GNP. Things do not get any better after 2030; leaders in these fields forecast that by 2050 the incidence of diabetes will double (3), while Alzheimer's disease (4) and cancer (5) will triple[7].

In technical terms, we are going to hell in a handcart – and it is getting worse (1). To the 20% of GDP we must add the costs of lost productivity caused by absenteeism due to illness. In the USA, the total yearly bill for lost productivity due to workers being above normal weight or having a history of chronic conditions is an astonishing $84 billion (6) and rising.

We cannot afford to continue like this. Given the growing mis-match between our spiralling healthcare costs and the wider economic environment, we will soon arrive (many would say we have already arrived) at an inflection point. We cannot blindly continue, as we have been doing for the last century, to medicalise and medicate our lives. Developing new drugs to treat the symptoms of these rising tides of disease is like applying new coats of paint to crumbling plaster while the foundations of the house rot. We must return to basics and rebuild the foundations – and this means re-designing our lifestyles and our diets. Fortunately, the science we need to do this is already in place.

Large and growing numbers of pre-clinical studies show that when animals are fed diets containing higher levels of the key anti-inflammatory nutrients, their risk of developing signs and symptoms of the degenerative diseases linked with ageing diminishes dramatically (7-17). There is little doubt that humans react in the same way; similar findings have emerged

---

7. The dogs and cats that share our homes and unhealthy lifestyles are experiencing the same catastrophic rise in obesity, diabetes, heart disease and cancer (36).

in a range of multi-national epidemiological and prospective studies. A Mediterranean Diet, for example, which contains higher levels of anti-inflammatory compounds than occur in the depleted Western diet, reduces the risk of many diseases by around 50% (18-23).

This has lead to calls for changes in the regulatory framework to encourage the marketing and consumption of anti-inflammatory foods and supplements which are currently so heavily censored that it is impossible for responsible manufacturers in this sector to say anything meaningful about their products. The laws around supplements and foods, which were originally drafted to protect consumers from unscrupulous pill peddlers, are now actively blocking the flow of information to consumers which they should be able to use to improve their health.

The only people to gain from the current laws are the drug and medical insurance companies; and the constant exchange of personnel between the regulatory agencies and the pharma / insurance complex has led many to conclude that a collusion is taking place which is doing great damage to individual and public health. Very senior regulators have admitted to me (off the record) that their decisions are frequently based more on political and financial criteria than on science.

Some of the more progressive regulators agree privately that we must liberalise the current laws but are out-voted by their colleagues who say that as we only have two data points (ie Western and Mediterranean diets), we cannot derive a dose-response curve. In layman's terms, we do not know whether supra-Mediterranean intakes of anti-inflammatory compounds would be even more protective, or whether adverse effects might emerge at high doses. This is known as the hormetic argument.

In toxicology, hormesis refers to a biphasic dose response to a substance or activity, characterized by a beneficial effect at low doses and a toxic effect at high doses. In biology, hormesis is defined as an adaptive and positive response of cells and organisms to low-level (and usually intermittent) stressors. These same stressors at high doses are harmful our health.

Stress is a two-edged blade, operating within an evolutionary dialectic that is red in tooth, claw and – if we could only see it – leaf and root. Polyphenols, for example, are phytochemicals that plants produce both as anti-stress compounds for themselves, and as stressors for other hostile organisms. They protect the plants from stresses such as UV, but at the same time they act as stressors against microbes and animals that might attack the plant. Specifically, the polyphenols have anti-nutrient and anti-microbial properties which reduce the nutritional gains a predator might make from eating the plant, and the risk of the plant acquiring an infection.

The Omega-3 fatty acids are also anti-stress compounds, produced by marine algae to defend themselves aginst the thermal stresses they encounter in conditions of extreme cold. Omega-3 fatty acids are more flexible than saturated fatty acids and have a lower freezing point; algae that contained mostly saturated fat would solidify in the cold Polar waters, as would the rest of the Polar marine food chain. Cold water krill which eat the algae that contain Omega-3 fatty acids, and the cold water fish and mammals that eat those krill, gain the same defence against thermal stress. (Psychrophilic or cold-tolerant bacteria utilise an analagous anti-freeze defence involving proteins which, like omega-3's, have a structure which makes them more flexible and lowers their effective freezing point[8]).

From our perspective, however, polyphenols and Omega-3 fatty acids are important anti-inflammatory nutrients we use to defend ourselves against chronic inflammatory stress. When we consume low doses of these compounds they elicit adaptive cellular stress responses (24-25), such as the production of sirtuins and anti-inflammatory lipid mediators and enzymes, which confer significant health benefits. These benefits go a long way to explaining the positive effects of the Mediteranean diet. But if we were to eat polyphenols or Omega-3's in excessive amounts, they would damage our health. They would do this by binding essential trace elements and thus creating nutritional stress (the polyphenols); or by oxidising and exerting oxidative stresss (the Omega-3's).

This, in a nutshell, is what the regulatory bodies say they are concerned about. If we ate too much of these normally health-promoting nutrients, say these regulators, we would suffer toxic consequences – and they have a statutory concern for our health. (It is fair to say that some of these bureaucrats are more concerned by the considerable damage that better nutrition would do to the profit margins of the pharmaceutical industry).

I understand their argument but it is obsolete. A recent, detailed study of 19th century public health in Britain showed that a diet which contained roughly 10 times more of the key anti-inflammatory compounds than the Mediterranean diet does today, is even more protective in humans; the mid-Victorian diet reduced the incidence of the major degenerative diseases to 10% of contemporary levels (26). The research behind the mid-Victorian story is presented in detail in the next chapter.

Given today's appalling health statistics, it is a public health tragedy that no prospective randomised clinical trials have yet been done to 'prove' the protective effects of an anti-inflammatory diet to the stipulated, quasi-pharmaceutical standards. This failure is largely due to the pharmaceutical perspective of the current regulators.

When deciding what levels of nutrients can be put into supplements or added to foods, they use the wrong risk / benefit assessment models. These models attempt to balance the risk of the toxicity that could occur at high doses of a nutrient, against the risk of deficiency, when intakes are so low that they cause deficiency disease[9]. With vitamin C for example, excessive doses increase the risk of oxalate kidney stones, whereas a diet deficient in vitamin C quickly leads to scurvy.

The public health problem is not deficiency, however, which is rare - when was the last time you heard of a case of scurvy? - but depletion. Depletion refers to a level of intake not low

---

8. Many of these bacteria also utilise the fascinating anti-freeze sugar, trehalose.
9. Deficiency of this sort is also known as Type A malnutrition.

enough to cause deficiency but low enough to skew metabolic and physiological processes in the body; and multiple micronutrient depletion (a.k.a. Type B malnutrition) is rife, due to a combination of our low energy needs and poor food choices.

Type B malnutrition creates a pro-inflammatory environment in the body, and this is the most important cause of illness and death in our time. A diet chronically depleted in anti-inflammatory nutrients does not cause acute problems but it will, by encouraging chronic and tissue-destroying inflammation, eventually lead to the emergence of symptoms of degenerative disease.

Our diet is more depleted than ever before because we are eating so little, and making such poor food choices. Our calorie and nutrient intakes have fallen by over half since 1890 (26) and by a fifth since 1980 (27), due to our increasingly sedentary active lifestyles. But over that same period we have gained weight, due to the universality of cheap, high calorie food and the slight excess of generally empty calories so many of us snack on every day (26, 27). The average 20-year old man weighs 7kg more today than a man in his twenties did three decades ago, while the average 50-year old has gained 14kg (27, 35). This has created a nutritional paradox. We are increasingly overweight and obese, and on the surface look over-nourished - yet under the surface we are suffering from chronic malnutrition. It is a lethal combination.

The regulators do not yet understand any of this. Fortunately we do not have to wait for the bureaucrat and Eurocrat generals to move their Maginot Line. If we wish for better health, we can take matters into our own hands. We can increase our intakes of natural anti-inflammatory compounds, and improve our own chances of a longer and healthier life. And we can do this in two ways.

1. Change your lifestyle. There is overwhelming evidence that if you eat a diet rich in fruits, vegetables and oily fish, take moderate exercise, maintain a healthy body weight and don't smoke, you can dramatically reduce your risk of an early death. Different studies have measured this in slightly different ways (21, 28-29), but the average reduction of risk is 66% (30). Unfortunately, in the generally urban environment that we have created for ourselves, fewer than 4% of the population are able or willing to eat healthily (31) or take enough exercise (32).

2. If you are unable or unwilling to change your lifestyle, take the right nutritional supplements. These MUST include the key anti-inflammatory nutrients, ie the 1-3, 1-6 beta glucans, the omega-3 essential fatty acids, the polyphenols and vitamin D and the other fat-soluble nutrients. These are all detailed in following chapters. I have also written about damulin and other phytonutrients which mimic the effects of exercise (33-34), and appear to provide the same spectrum of health benefits. These nutrients form a health-promoting baseline, to which other nutrients can be added if needed.

Chapter 5. What we can learn from the (Victorian) past

We used to be far healthier than we are today and we lived healthier lives for longer, because we ate an anti-inflammatory diet. The evidence to prove this was presented in a series of scientific papers I co-wrote with the eminent historian Dr Judith Rowbotham, which were published in the Journal of the Royal Society of Medicine and the International Journal of Environmental Health and Public Health.

We were able to show that contrary to received opinion, modern medicine has not made our lives healthier. Our findings demonstrated that life expectancy today has, in some groups, fallen back from its high point in the late 19th century; and our health expectancy – the number of years we can expect to live in good health - has fallen even further.

Our papers caused consternation in the medical profession because they showed just how ineffective modern medicine has been. Senior scientists and doctors told us that our conclusions were wrong because our history was wrong. But scientists and doctors are not historians; they tend to focus on the latest science and the newest publications as they struggle to keep up to date with their peers. Many of them know something of their illustrious scientific forebears, but few have the time or the inclination to study the history of medicine.

That is hardly surprising. Our species has a dark and bloody history, and the history of medicine is particularly neuralgic. Many brilliant men and women have contributed to the medical sciences, but much of the history of medicine is a history of cruelty, prejudice, stupidity, charlatanry and outright fraud. No wonder we prefer to look forwards! And no wonder we are so susceptible to the pernicious error of thought known as modernism, in which we bind our anxiety by telling ourselves that things are getting better, and that we are the best, the brightest and the rightest there have ever been.

Our papers on 19th Century public health threw a very harsh light on modern medicine, and it is unsurprising that they were initially damned by the clinicians. Our science must be wrong, they argued, because our history was wrong. But then the historians rode into the lists. They accepted our reading of medical and dietary history and destroyed the clinicians' argument. At that point most doctors withdrew from the field of battle, unwilling to debate our case and too uncomfortable with its implications to re-examine their own deepest held and most uncritical assumptions. After all, we had proved that almost the entirety of 20th century medicine – with all of its new drugs, screening methods, diagnostics and surgical techniques – had done little to improve personal or public health.

In order for science and scientific practice to progress new ideas must be contested and tested, whenever possible, to destruction. We have sought debate but the silence from our medical colleagues has been deafening. Our position is uncontested but it is also largely ignored, even though new scientific papers have appeared which support our arguments.

The great physicist Max Planck famously said, 'Science progresses funeral by funeral'. This aphorism can be read in different ways. One reading is that the social prejudices embedded in all scientific models cannot die until their most devoted proponents have passed away. A bleaker reading is that new ideas cannot emerge until too many victims have died to allow the old, destructive regime to continue.

That is where the pharmaceutical model of medicine stands today. J'accuse. Disasterously ineffective in stemming the ongoing pandemics of degenerative disease, ruinously expensive (total health care costs now at 12% of GDP in the UK and 20% in the USA) and needlessly cruel (fatalities caused by medical intervention are a leading cause of death), the system is not fit for purpose. The model has long outlived its original rationale. Its zombie institutions only survive because they are too stuffed with cash and influence to know that it is time for them to die and be replaced by something more effective, more cost-effective and very much kinder.

The regulatory system is an equal part of the problem. EFSA and FDA, the bodies that regulate supplements and functional foods in Europe and the USA respectively, are desperately dysfunctional. Originally created to defend consumers from hucksters and snake oil salesmen, they have become – perhaps unintentionally – the pharmaceutical industy's last best defence. Their screening methods, largely inherited from the pharma model, are inappropriate when dealing with nutritional issues and prevent almost all progress. Health claims are routinely and unreasonably rejected; EFSA recently ruled, for example, that no one should claim that regular water consumption is the best way to rehydrate the body. This is scientific nonsense, born purely out of unnecessary and overly complex commercial and legislative bureaucracy. It might seem comical, but rulings like this have stifled the development of functional, health-promoting foods. More seriously, they harm public health by preventing the food and drink industry from passing information (and selling products) to the general public that the public could use to improve their own health. At the same time, the regulators are perfectly happy to allow unscrupulous fast food companies to continue to sell foods that are hugely pro-inflammatory, and responsible for many millions of cases of avoidable disease and premature deaths.

In fact, the food industry is as culpable as the pharma industry and the regulators. I recently chaired an international conference in Geneva on regulatory issues and had the good fortune to share a platform with Professor Ambroise Martin, new head of health claims at EFSA. A formidable and open-minded scientist, he clearly understood the vast capacity of an improved diet to improve public health; but as he pointed out, he and his colleagues are constrained both by the bureaucratic system they inherited and the food industry's inability to produce (so far) anything that might really exploit that capacity.

And there's the rub. The food industry is unwilling to develop anything really meaningful because they know that they will not be allowed to talk meaningfully about it. The regulators fail almost every application, as their screening system is inappropriate. The pharma companies are delighted with this impasse. They do everything they can to prevent regulatory progress, and are continually inventing new 'diseases' such as 'social anxiety disorder' and 'night eating syndrome' (two new uses for SSRI antidepressant drugs) in order to swell their market and grow their profits. And all the while, imprisoned within this infernal triangle of vested interests, we grow fatter and sicker.

The barriers that keep us from better individual and public health are no longer scientific but political. We know how to support good health and a longer life, and it is not by medicine but by nutrition. If you wait for your doctor to tell you this you'll have to wait a long time – maybe too long. In the meantime your health is in your own hands, and on your plate.

Our Key Findings

Analysis of the mid-Victorian period in the U.K. revealed that healthy life expectancy at age 5 was better than exists today, and the incidence of degenerative disease was 10% of ours. Their levels of physical activity and hence calorific intakes were approximately twice ours. They had relatively little access to alcohol and tobacco; and due to their correspondingly high intake of fruits, whole grains, oily fish and vegetables, they consumed levels of micro- and phytonutrients at approximately ten times the levels considered normal today. This diet provided high levels of anti-inflammatory compounds, which contributed to the Victorians' freedom from degenerative disease; and provides a blueprint for nutritional and health improvement today (1-3).

The mid-Victorian period is usually defined as the years between 1850 and 1870, but in nutritional terms we identified a slightly longer period, lasting until around 1880. During these 30 years, a generation grew up with probably the best standards of health ever enjoyed by a modern state. The British population had risen significantly and had become increasingly urbanised, but the great public health movement had not yet been established and Britain's towns and cities were still notoriously unhealthy environments (4,5). Despite this, and contrary to historical tradition, we found, using a range of historical evidence, that Britain and its world-dominating empire were supported by a workforce, an army and a navy comprised of individuals who were healthier, fitter and stronger than we are today. They were almost entirely free of the degenerative diseases which maim and kill so many of us, and although it is commonly stated that this is because they all died young, the reverse is true; public records reveal that they lived as long – or longer – than we do in the 21st century.

These findings are remarkable, as this brief period of great good health predates not only the public health movement but also the great 20th century medical advances in surgery, infection control and drugs (6-8). They are also in marked contrast to popular views about Victorian squalor and disease, views that have long obscured the realities of life and death during that 'period of equipoise' (9).

Our recent research indicates that the mid-Victorians' good health was entirely due to their superior diet. This period was, nutritionally speaking, an island in time; one that was created and subsequently squandered by economic and political forces. This begs a series of questions. How did this brief nutritional 'golden age' come about? How was it lost? And could we recreate it?

One key contributory factor was what used to be called the Agricultural Revolution; a series of developments in agricultural practice that massively improved crop and livestock yields. This slow green revolution started in the late seventeenth century, gradually accelerated into the mid-19th century, and underpinned both modern urbanisation and the associated Industrial Revolution (10). Arguably the most critical agricultural development was a more complex system of crop rotation, which greatly improved both arable output and animal husbandry. In the 1730's a new breed of innovative land-owner epitomised by Marquis 'Turnip' Townshend introduced new systems of crop rotation from Sweden and the Netherlands, and new crops like the swede (Brassica napus napobrassica). The new crop rotation systems avoided the need to let land lie fallow one year in three, and instead used a four or five year cycle in which turnips and clover were used as two of the crops because of their ability to replenish the soil.

These new systems created immense gains in food productivity. Between 1705 and 1765 English wheat exports increased ten-fold, while the increased availability of animal feed meant that most livestock no longer had to be slaughtered at the onset of winter so that fresh (instead of salted) meat became cheaper and more widely available throughout the year (11).

Population shifts also played a key contributory role. The bulk of the population had always lived on the land but by 1850, as revealed by the 1851 census, more Britons were living and working in towns than in the countryside (4). The agricultural improvements of the previous 150 years meant that agriculture produced far more than before, but used far fewer people to achieve this. As a result, people moved to towns to find work: Britain was the first modern consumer society and there was real demand for workers in an increasing number of urban industries (12). Traditionally, urban life expectancy was significantly lower than rural life expectancy, but from the mid-Victorian period on this difference disappears.

Victorian society was very different to traditional society. It was a class society as we understand it today rather than the older, more deferential model, and this created enormous social tensions though it is important not to exaggerate these (13). For the very poor, towns remained deeply unpleasant places to live, and it can be argued that for many, the social structure of towns even got worse. As more of the working classes moved into towns, more of the middle classes moved out to create the beginnings of suburbia (14). The great Victorian commentator Thomas Carlyle claimed that in cities, little tied one human being to another except for the 'Cash Nexus', where employer and employee met in an uncomfortable wage and profit-driven relationship *(15)*, as Mrs Gaskell revealed in books like North and South (16).

In many ways, however, urban socio-economic conditions were getting better by the mid-century. Trades unions and philanthropists were slowly but surely improving urban working conditions and wages throughout the last half of the century (17). The threats of political instability which had seemed most threatening in towns up to the late 1840s were largely dispersed during the mid-Victorian era, as a result of changes in the political and legal systems. For example, the Great Reform Act of 1832 was followed by the 1867 Reform Act, which meant that most male urban heads of households were now able to vote. In 1845 the notorious Corn Laws were finally repealed, ushering in the era of cheap food for the urban masses.

One of the most important results of these changes was that the interests of the landed classes were no longer protected. Traditionally, parliament had always sought to protect the income of farmers and landowners, and after the end of the Napoleonic Wars, this stance had seen the introduction of the highly unpopular Corn Laws from 1815. These kept the price of grain at a level that ensured agricultural prosperity, but they had a disastrous effect on the price of food. This particularly affected the new urban, industrial workforce, which was heavily dependent on bread as a staple food. The Corn Laws kept the price of bread artificially high, even during economic depressions such as the 1840s, a decade which became notorious as the 'Hungry 40's' (18).

The post-Great Reform Act parliament, however, was susceptible to pressure from groups such as the Anti-Corn Law League led by Richard Cobden and Joseph Bright. When the situation was exacerbated by the Irish Great Potato Famine, Prime Minister Sir Robert Peel, the grandson of a mill-owner, forced through the repeal of the Corn Laws (18). From that time on farming interests were under pressure to produce cheap food because it had become clear that the prosperity of the country depended on industrial rather than on agricultural output (19). As the Great Exhibition of 1851 underlined, Britain had become the Workshop of the World (20).

Improved agricultural output and a political climate dedicated to ensuring cheap food led to a dramatic increase in the production of affordable foodstuffs; but it was the development of the railway network that actually brought the fruits of the agricultural and political changes into the towns and cities, and made them available to the mid-Victorian working classes (21).

The start of the modern railway age is usually marked by the opening of the Stockton & Darlington line in 1825. From the late 1830s on, progress was impressively rapid. Important long-distance lines came first, followed by smaller local lines criss-crossing the country. The London and Birmingham line opened in 1838, part of Brunel's London to Bristol route the same year and the London and Southampton line in 1840. By the mid-century the key lines were already operational. The railway system grew exponentially, reaching 2500 miles by 1845, and continued to expand, carrying goods as well as passengers. Thanks to trains, producers were now supplying the urban markets with more, fresher and cheaper food than was previously possible[10]. This boosted urban demand for fresh foodstuffs, and pushed up agricultural output still further (22). A survey of food availability in the 1860s through sources such as Henry Mayhew's survey of the London poor shows substantial quantities of affordable vegetables and fruits now pouring into the urban markets (23).

This fortunate combination of factors produced a sea change in the nation, and in the nation's health. By 1850 Britain's increasing domestic productivity and foreign power had created a national mood of confidence and optimism which affected all levels of society. Driven far more by better nutrition than the new schemes of clean air and water (which were only beginning to have an effect from the 1870s on), adult life expectancy increased from the 1850s until by 1875 it matched our own (24). The health and vitality of the British population during this period was reflected in the workforces and armed forces that powered the transformation of the urban

---

10. There were, for instance, the water cress trains, bringing that commodity in from as far afield as Hampshire.

landscape at home, and drove the great expansion of the British Empire abroad (20). Per capita numbers of significant innovations in science and technology and the per capita numbers of scientific geniuses peaked in the Victorian era (91).

Unfortunately, negative changes that would undermine these nutritional gains were already taking shape. Thanks to her dominant global position, and developments in shipping technology, Britain had created a global market drawing in the products of colonial and US agriculture, to provide ever-cheaper food for the growing urban masses. From 1875 on and especially after 1885, rising imports of cheap food basics were increasingly affecting the food chain at home. Imported North American wheat and new milling techniques reduced the prices of white flour and the nutritional value of bread. Tinned meat arrived from the Argentine, Australia and New Zealand, which was cheaper than either home-produced or refrigerated fresh meat also arriving from these sources. Canned fruit and condensed milk became widely available (25).

This expansion in the range of foods was advertised by most contemporaries, and by subsequent historians, as representing a significant 'improvement' in the working class diet. The reality was very different. These changes undoubtedly increased the variety and quantity of the working class diet, but its quality deteriorated markedly. The imported canned meats were fatty and usually 'corned' or salted. Cheaper sugar promoted a huge increase in sugar consumption in confectionery, now mass-produced for the first time, and in the new processed foods such as sugar-laden condensed milk, and canned fruits bathed in heavy syrup.

The increased sugar consumption caused such damage to the nation's teeth that by 1900 it was commonly noted that people could no longer chew tough foods and were unable to eat many vegetables, fruits and nuts (26). For all these reasons the late-Victorian diet actually damaged the health of the nation, and the health of the working classes in particular. The decline was astonishingly rapid, particularly amongst men who 'benefitted' most from the new foodstuffs because wives and mothers would give them first to their menfolk, often continuing to consume a more traditional diet themselves.

At one extreme end of the scale, per capita numbers of significant innovations in science and technology and the per capita numbers of recognised scientific geniuses went into a sustained decline (92-95). At the other extreme were the mid-Victorian navvies. These seasonal workers, who were towards the bottom end of the economic scale, could routinely shovel up to 20 tons of earth per day from below their feet to above their heads (27). This was an enormous physical effort that required great strength, stamina and robust good health. Within two generations, however, male health nationally had deteriorated to such an extent that in 1900, five out of 10 young men volunteering for the second Boer War had to be rejected because they were so malnourished. They were not starved, but had been consuming the wrong foods (28,29). This reality is underlined by considering army recruitment earlier. The recruiting sergeants had reported no such problems during previous high profile campaigns such as the Asante (1873–4) and Zulu (1877–8) Wars (30).

The fall in nutritional standards between 1880 and 1900 was so marked that the generations were visibly and progressively shrinking. In 1883 the infantry were forced to lower the minimum height for recruits from 5ft 6 inches to 5ft 3 inches. This was because most new recruits were now coming from an urban background instead of the traditional rural background; the 1881 census showed that over three-quarters of the population now lived in towns and cities. Factors such as a lack of sunlight in urban slums (which led to rickets due to Vitamin D deficiency) had already reduced the height of young male volunteers. Lack of sunlight, however, could not have been the sole critical factor in the next height reduction, a mere 18 years later. By this time, clean air legislation had markedly improved urban sunlight levels; but unfortunately, the supposed 'improvements' in dietary intake resulting from imported foods had had time to take effect on the 16–18 year old cohort.

It might be expected that the infantry would be able to raise the minimum height requirement back to 5ft. 6 inches. Instead, they were forced to reduce it still further, to a mere 5ft. British officers, who were from the middle and upper classes and not yet exposed to more than the occasional treats of canned produce, were far better fed in terms of their intake of fresh foods and were now on average a full head taller than their malnourished and sickly men.

In 1904, and as a direct result of the Boer disaster, the government set up the Committee on Physical Deterioration. Its report, emphasising the need to provide school meals for working class children, reinforced the idea that the urban working classes were not only malnourished at the start of the twentieth century but also (in an unjustified leap of the imagination, reinforced by folk memories of the 'Hungry 40's) that they had been so since the start of nineteenth century industrial urbanisation [28,31]. This profound error of thought was incorporated into subsequent models of public health, and is distorting and damaging healthcare to this day.

The crude average figures often used to depict the brevity of Victorian lives mislead because they include infant mortality, which was tragically high. If we strip out peri-natal mortality, however, and look at the life expectancy of those who survived the first five years, a very different picture emerges. Victorian contemporary sources reveal that life expectancy for adults in the mid-Victorian period was almost exactly what it is today. At 65, men could expect another ten years of life and women another eight [24,32,33]: the lower figure for women reflects the high danger of death in childbirth, mainly from causes unrelated to malnutrition. This compares surprisingly favourably with today's figures: life expectancy at birth (reflecting our improved standards of neo-natal care) averages 75.9 years (men) and 81.3 years (women); though recent work has suggested that for working class men and women this is lower, at around 72 for men and 76 for women [34].

If we accept the working class figures, which are probably more directly comparable with the Victorian data, women have gained three years of life expectancy since the mid-Victorian period while men have actually fallen back by 3 years. The decline in male life expectancy implicates several causal factors; including the introduction of industrialised cigarette production in 1883, a sustained fall in the relative cost of alcohol and a severe decline in nutritional standards, as outlined below. The improvement in female life expectancy can be partly linked to family planning developments but also to other factors promoting women's health such as improvements in dress. Until widespread accessible family planning facilities arrived after the First World War, women's health could be substantially undermined by up to 30 years of successive pregnancies and births (35–37). These figures suggest that if twentieth century women had not also experienced the negative impacts of tobacco consumption becoming respectable, along with an increased alcohol intake and worsening nutrition as they began to consume the imported delicacies originally preserved mainly for the men (all those things which had cost their menfolk three years), they would have gained six years.

Given that modern pharmaceutical, surgical, anaesthetic, scanning and other diagnostic technologies were self-evidently unavailable to the mid-Victorians, their high life expectancy is very striking, and can only have been due to their health-promoting lifestyle. But the implications of this new understanding of the mid-Victorian period are rather more profound. It shows that medical advances allied to the pharmaceutical industry's output have done little more than change the manner of our dying.

The Victorians died rapidly of infection and/or trauma, whereas we die slowly of degenerative disease. It reveals that with the exception of family planning, the vast edifice of twentieth century healthcare has not enabled us to live longer but has in the main merely supplied methods of suppressing the symptoms of degenerative diseases which have emerged due to our failure to maintain mid-Victorian nutritional standards (38).

Above all, it refutes the Panglossian optimism of the contemporary anti-ageing movement whose protagonists use 1900 – a nadir in health and life expectancy trends - as their starting point to promote the idea of endlessly increasing life span. These are the equivalent of the share pushers who insisted, during the dot.com, municipal bond and sovereign debt booms, that we had at last escaped the constraints of normal economics. A few believed their own message of eternal growth; most used it to sell junk bonds they knew were worthless. The parallels with today's vitamin pill market are obvious, but this also echoes the way in which Big Pharma trumpets the arrival of each new miracle drug.

In short, the majority of even the poorest mid-Victorians lived well, despite all their disadvantages and what we would now consider physical discomforts. Their healthy life span was better than ours in an era when being defined as 'old' depended more on the decline in your ability to work than on chronological milestones. Their prolonged good health was due to their high levels of physical activity, and as a consequence, how and what they ate. We could learn a good deal from them.

How the Mid-Victorians Worked

Due to the high levels of physical activity routinely undertaken by the Victorian working classes, calorific requirements ranged between 150 and 200% of today's historically low values. Almost all work involved moderate to heavy physical labour, and often included that involved in getting to work. Seasonal and other low-paid workers often had to walk up to six miles per day (39). While some Victorian working class women worked from home (seamstressing for instance) more went out to work in shops, factories and workshops, necessitating long days on their feet, plus the additional burden of housework (39,40). Many single women were domestics, either live-in servants or daily workers. This was particularly physically demanding, as very few households had male servants, so women did all the heavy household work from scrubbing floors to heaving coals upstairs. Men worked on average 9–10 hours/day, for 5.5 to 6 days a week, giving a range from 50 to 60 hours of physical activity per week (40). For those working outside their homes, factoring in the walk to and from work increased the range of total hours of work-related physical activity up to 55 to 70 hours per week. Women's expenditure of effort was similarly large (41). Married women also had domestic chores to perform in their own homes after work, and in addition, their daily dress up to the 1890s at least (when the development of the tailor-made costume reduced both corseting and the weight of numerous layers of fabric) involved real physical effort just in moving around. Male leisure activities such as gardening and informal football also involved substantial physical effort.

Using average figures for work-related calorie consumption, men required between 280 (walking) and 440 calories (heavy yard work) per hour; with women requiring between 260 and 350 calories per hour. This gives calorific expenditure ranges during the working week of between 3,000 to 4,500 calories /day (men) and 2,750 to 3,500 (women).

Total calorific requirements were likely to have been even higher during the winter months; with less insulated and less warmed homes, working class Victorians used more calories to keep warm than we do. The same held true for workplaces, unless the work (certain factory operations, blacksmithing, etc) heated the environment to unhealthy levels. At the top end of the physical activity range were the 'navigators', the labourers who built, largely without machinery, the roads and railways that enabled the expansion of the British economy. These men were expending 5,000 calories or more per day.

In short, working class mid-Victorians ate twice as much as we do, but due to their high levels of physical activity remained slim; overweight and obesity were relatively rare, and (unless associated with ill-health) were generally identified as phenomena associated with the numerically smaller middle and upper-middle class. But it is not just the amount of food the mid-Victorians consumed that is so unfamiliar; the composition of their diet was also very different from our own.

What the Mid-Victorians Ate

Vegetables
Onions were amongst the cheapest vegetables, widely available all year around at a cost so negligible that few housewives budgeted what cost them around a halfpenny (even cheaper if bruised) for a bunch containing at least a dozen. They might become slightly more expensive in the late spring, when leeks could be substituted (41). Watercress was another cheap staple in the working class diet, available at a halfpenny for four bunches in the period April to February (41). The Jerusalem artichoke was consumed from September through to March, often home-

grown as it was one of the easiest vegetables to grow in urban allotments (42). Carrots and turnips were inexpensive staples, especially during the winter months. Cabbage was also cheap and readily available, along with broccoli. Fresh peas were available and affordable from June to July, with beans from July to September (41).

Fruit
Apples were the cheapest and most commonly available urban fruits from August through to May; with cherries taking over in the May– July period, followed by gooseberries in June, up to August, then plums and greengages in July through to September (41). Dried fruits and candied peel were always cheaply available, and used to sweeten desserts such as bread puddings and for cakes and mincemeat. They were also consumed as an afternoon snack, particularly by children, according to Victorian cookery books (42,43) and many other sources from Dickens to Mayhew. All fruits and vegetables were organically grown, and therefore had higher levels of phytonutrients than the intensively grown crops we eat today (44).

Legumes, Nuts and Seeds
Dried legumes were available all year round and widely used in dishes such as pease pudding. The chestnut was the most commonly consumed nut and one of the most commonly eaten street snacks in the chestnut season, running from September through to January. Filberts or hazelnuts were available from October through to May; walnuts were another regularly bought seasonal nut. Imported almonds and Brazil nuts were more expensive, but widely consumed around Christmas as a 'treat'. Coconuts were also imported, often given as presents or won at fairs; commonly grated for use in cakes and desserts (23). Cocoa was consumed in large amounts, achieving 5.7lb per capita per annum by 1891 (89, 90).

Fish and seafood
The herring was one of the most important fish in the Victorian urban working class diet; fresh in the autumn, winter and spring; dried and salted (red herring) or pickled/soused all year round. Red herrings were a staple throughout the year because they were easily cooked (e.g. Idylls of the Poor). Other favourites were cheap and easily obtainable varieties with better keeping qualities than the more vulnerable white fish, including sprats, eels, and shellfish (oysters, mussels, cockles, whelks). Of the white fish consumed, cod, haddock and John Dory were preferred. Typically, and unlike today, the whole fish was consumed including heads and roes (22). Fish was available from Monday evening to Friday evening; with broken and day old fish or eels and shoreline shellfish available on Saturdays, as fishermen did not go out over the weekends (45).

Meats
Consumption of meat was considered a mark of a good diet and its complete absence was rare: consuming only limited amounts was a poverty diet (23). Joints of meat were, for the poor, likely to be an occasional treat. Yet only those with the least secure incomes and most limited housing, and so without either the cooking facilities or the funds, would be unlikely to have a weekly Sunday joint; even they might achieve that three or four times a year, cooked in a local cookhouse or bakery oven. Otherwise, meat on the bone (shin or cheek), stewed or fried, was

the most economical form of meat, generally eked out with offal meats including brains, heart, sweetbreads, liver, kidneys and 'pluck', (the lungs and intestines of sheep). Pork was the most commonly consumed meat. All meats were from free-range animals, and contained a more favourable Omega 6:3 ration than intensively raised meats today.

Eggs and Dairy Products
Many East End households kept hens in their backyards, and Robert's study of Lancashire suggests similar patterns (36). Keeping a couple of hens could produce up to a dozen eggs per household per week. There were fears about adulteration of milk (frequently watered-down). Butter did not feature largely in the working-class diet. Dripping was a preferred substitute in the days before cheap margarine. Hard cheeses, as opposed to soft cheeses, were favoured by the working classes as a regular part of their diet, partly because even when the heel of the cheese was too hard to eat, the ends could be toasted.

Alcohol
Beer was the most commonly consumed form of alcohol, but it had an alcohol content significantly lower than today's beers. Careful reading of contemporary sources including cookery and domestic economy books suggest that the alcohol percent of beer consumed in the home was probably only 1% to 2%; often less as it was watered down, especially for consumption by women and children (43,46,47). In pubs, the alcohol content of beer was more regulated and generally higher, ranging from 2% to 3%. These are still weak beers, compared to today's average of around 5%. Spirits were more intermittently consumed by men and rarely by women: respectability and gin did not go together (48). Working class men and women seldom drank wine, except for port or sherry. A third or more of households were temperate or teetotal, partly due to the sustained efforts of the anti-alcohol movement (49,50).

Tobacco
Pipe smoking was widespread but intermittent amongst working class males, and a cigar or cheroot might be smoked on special occasions. Snuff had largely fallen out of favour, as had chewing tobacco. The big expansion in mass tobacco consumption by the working classes did not take place until after 1883, when industrial cigarette production was introduced (51). It was not until the twentieth century that women of all classes became major consumers of tobacco, under the pressure of heavy advertising.

Adulterants
Some adulterants commonly used in Victorian foods were well-known to be toxic even then: lead chromate in mustard, mercury and arsenic compounds as colourants in confectionery and picrotoxin in beer all undoubtedly contributed to ill health. In contrast, modern nutritional biochemistry reveals that some of the other common 'adulterants' have potentially significant health benefits. The hawthorne used to extend tea, for example, contained vaso- and cardio-protective flavonoids (52–57). The coriander in beer may have had some anthelmintic activity (58), and the watering down of beer and spirits was – from a health perspective – a generally good thing!

Dietary Summary

Mid-Victorian working class men and women consumed between 50% and 100% more calories than we do, but because they were so much more physically active than we are today, overweight and obesity hardly existed at the working class level. The working class diet was rich in seasonal vegetables and fruits; with consumption of fruits and vegetables amounting to eight to 10 portions per day. This far exceeds the current national average of around three portions, and the government-recommended five-a-day. The mid-Victorian diet also contained significantly more nuts, legumes, whole grains and omega three fatty acids than the modern diet. Much meat consumed was offal, which has a significantly higher micronutrient density than the skeletal muscle we largely eat today (59). Prior to the introduction of margarine in the late Victorian period, dietary intakes of trans fats were very low.

There were very few processed foods and therefore little hidden salt, other than in bread (Recipes suggest that significantly less salt was then added to meals. At table, salt was not usually sprinkled on a serving but piled at the side of the plate, allowing consumers to regulate consumption in a more controlled way). The mid-Victorian diet had a lower calorific density and a higher nutrient density than ours. It had a higher content of fibre (including fermentable fibre), and a lower sodium/potassium ratio. In short, the mid-Victorians ate a diet that was not only considerably better than our own, but also far in advance of current government recommendations. It more closely resembles the Mediterranean diet, proven in many studies to promote health and longevity; or even the 'Paleolithic diet' recommended by some nutritionists (60).

In terms of alcohol consumption, the comparisons with today are also revealing. Many contemporary reports suggest that around a fifth of Victorian working class men might, when employed, spend up to a fifth of their income on beer (61). Assuming an average urban income ranging from £1 to £4 per week, and given mid-century pub prices of 3d to 8d per pint for beer, the reported expenditure would account for around 16 pints to 20 per week maximum or between three and four pints per night.

As Victorian beer generally had an alcohol content ranging between 1 and 3.5% (62), this is equivalent to one and a half to two pints of beer per day in contemporary terms. Seen in this light, the huge Victorian concerns about drunkenness in the Victorian working classes appear to be more a reflection of respectable morality than a real public health issue (63). Cost implications ensured that for most, the Victorian 'alcohol problem' was certainly less significant than it is in our time, when the frequency of public drunkenness and levels of injury and illness have become a serious public health concern (64). Finally, mid-Victorian tobacco consumption was very much lower than today.

These new findings reveal that, contrary to received wisdom, the mid-Victorians ate a healthier diet than we do today. This had dramatic effects on their health and life expectancy.

How the Mid-Victorians Died

Public Health Patterns
The overall pattern of Victorian causes of death broadly resembles that found in developing countries today, with infection, trauma and infant/mother mortality in the pole positions, and non-communicable degenerative disease being relatively insignificant.

Common causes of death (65,66)

1. Infection including TB and other lung infections such as pneumonia; epidemics (scarlet fever, smallpox, influenza, typhoid, cholera etc), with spread often linked to poor sanitation: and the sexually transmitted diseases.

2. Accidents/trauma linked to work place and domestic conditions. Death from burns was an important cause of death among women, due largely to a combination of open hearth cooking, fashions in dress, and the use of highly flammable fabrics.

3. Infant/mother mortality (66). This was generally due to infection, although maternal haemorrhage was another significant causative factor.

4. Heart failure. This was generally due to damage to the heart valves caused by rheumatic fever, and was not a degenerative disease. Angina pectoris does not appear in the registrar general's records as a cause of death until 1857 – and then as a disease of old age - although the diagnosis and its causes were recognised (67–70).

Uncommon causes of death

5. Coronary artery disease (see above)

6. Paralytic fits (strokes, see Webster's Dictionary). Stroke was mainly associated with the middle and upper classes who ate a diet in which animal derived foods had a more significant role, and who consumed as a result rather less fruits and vegetables. Strokes were generally non-fatal, at least the first time; although mortality rates increased with each subsequent stroke (65).

7. Cancers were relatively rare (65). While the Victorians did not possess sophisticated diagnostic or screening technology, they were as able to diagnose late stage cancer as we are today; but this was an uncommon finding. In that period, cancer carried none of the stigma that it has recently acquired, and was diagnosed without bias. For example, in 1869 the Physician to Charing Cross Hospital describes lung cancer as '... one of the rarer forms of a rare disease. You may probably pass the rest of your students life without seeing another example of it.' (71).

Not only were cancers very uncommon compared to today, they appear to have differed in other key respects. James Paget (of Paget's Disease) built a large practice on the strength of diagnosing breast cancer, which he did by sight and palpation – that is at Stages 3 and 4. In this group he describes a life expectancy of 4 years after diagnosis, extending to eight or more with surgery (72). We say 'eight years or more' because so many of Paget's patients were still alive when he died, so the figures are, if anything, under-estimates. The corresponding figures today are Stage 3: 50% survival at 10 years if given surgery, chemo- and radio-therapy, and Stage 4: overall survival about 15 months. These data suggest that breast cancer during the Victorian period was significantly less rapidly progressive than is the case today, probably due to the Victorians' significantly higher intakes of a range of micro- and phytonutrients which slow cancer growth.

In short, although the mid-Victorians lived as long as we do, they were relatively immune to the chronic degenerative diseases that are the most important causes of ill health and death today.

Figure 1.Causes of Death in England and Wales: 1880 and 1997. Reprinted from Charlton (24), vol. 2, p. 9.

Cause of Death in England and Wales: 1880 and 1997

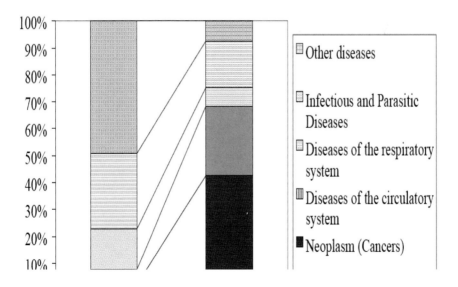

Chapter 6. The case for supplements

The implications of the mid-Victorian story are far-reaching because, unlike the Paleolithic scenario, details of the mid-Victorian lifestyle and its impact on public health are extensively documented. Thus, the mid-Victorian experience clearly shows that:

Degenerative diseases are not caused by old age (the 'wear and tear' hypothesis), but are largely driven by chronic malnutrition. Our low energy lifestyles leave us depleted in anabolic and anti-catabolic co-factors, and this imbalance is compounded by excessive intakes of inflammatory compounds. The current epidemic of degenerative disease is caused by the widespread problem of multiple micro- and phyto-nutrient depletion (Type B malnutrition.) This leaves us riddled with chronic inflammation, and at the same time unable to repair our progressively disintegrating tissues.

With the exception of family planning and antibiotics, the vast edifice of twentieth century healthcare has generated little more than palliatives that can only suppress symptoms of the many degenerative diseases which have emerged due to our failure to maintain mid-Victorian nutritional standards.

The only way to combat the adverse effects of Type B malnutrition, and to prevent and / or cure degenerative disease, is to enhance the nutrient density of the modern diet.

The Case for Supplements

Our levels of physical activity and therefore our food intakes are at an historic low. To make matters worse, when compared to the mid-Victorian diet, the modern diet is rich in processed foods. It has a higher sodium/potassium ratio, and contains far less fruit, vegetables, whole grains and omega 3 fatty acids. It is lower in fibre and phytonutrients in both proportional and absolute terms; and, because of our high intakes of potato products, breakfast cereals, confectionery and refined baked goods, may have a higher glycemic load. Given all this, it follows that we are far more likely to suffer from dysnutrition (multiple micro- and phytonutrient depletion) than our mid-Victorian forebears.

This is supported by survey findings on both sides of the Atlantic; the U.S.D.A.'s 1994 to 1996 Continuing Survey of Food Intakes by Individuals (73,74), and the National Diet and Nutrition Surveys (75) both show that many individuals today are unable to obtain RNI values of a variety of vitamins and minerals. But the reality is even worse, as some current RNI values are very obviously too low to sustain health; which means that the numbers of individuals consuming the optimal (higher) levels of many micronutrients are even lower (see chapter 23). Nutritionists bleat about getting everything you need from a well-balanced diet, but this is self-evident nonsense. It is impossible to derive all the micro- and phyto-nutrients needed for good health from less than about 3,500 calories / day – and that is when consuming nutrient-rich foods such as liver. (This is detailed in the next chapter). If you are living at 2 to 2.5 thousand calories / day, you are malnourished. If you make poor food choices, your dysnutrition will be even more severe.

Malnutrition in the U.K. is now reckoned to contribute to illness-related costs in excess of £7.3 billion per annum (76). Since it would be unacceptable and impractical to recreate the mid-Victorian working class 4,000 calorie/day diet, this constitutes a persuasive argument for a more widespread use of food fortification and/or properly designed food supplements.[11]

To insist, as conservative nutritionists and dieticians do, that only whole fruit and vegetables contain the magical ingredients needed for health represents little more than the last gasp of the discredited and anti-scientific theory of vitalism. 'Vitalism—the insistence that there is some big, mysterious extra ingredient in all living things—turns out to have been not a deep insight but a failure of imagination' (78). Even EFSA concedes that fruit juices count towards your five-a-day, as do freeze-dried powdered extracts of fruits and vegetables. As our knowledge of phytochemistry and phytopharmacology increases, it has become perfectly acceptable to use rational combinations of the key plant constituents in pill or capsule form.

These arguments are developed in 'Pharmageddon'[12] (79), a medical textbook which illustrates how micro- and phyto-nutrients can be specifically combined in order to prevent and treat disease. It also shows how they could be integrated into our food chain in order to reduce the contemporary and excessively high risks of the degenerative diseases to the far lower mid-Victorian levels.

The medical profession is finally beginning to take an interest. In light of the huge body of evidence linking diet to health, many researchers are now studying the dietary intakes of different groups of people and attempting to tease out such esoteric factors as, for example, just how much omega 3 fish oil is necessary to reduce the risk of Alzheimer's; or how what dose of flavonoids should be consumed to reduce the risk of stomach cancer.

Most of this research is patently a waste of time. Current generations are, from an historical point of view, anomalous. Our historically low levels of physical activity and consequently food intakes mean that even those groups consuming the highest levels of berry fruits, green leaf vegetables or oily fish, are still well below optimal (mid-Victorian) levels of consumption.

For example, scientists working with dietary elements thought to reduce the risk of cancer have commented that although 'pharmacological levels' of compounds such as flavonoids or salicylates have strong anti-cancer properties in vitro, there is little evidence that dietary (or 'physiological') levels of intake have any protective effects in humans.

The mid-Victorians, with their far greater intakes of fruits and vegetables, which were organic and in many cases contained significantly higher concentrations of phytonutrients than our intensively grown crops do (80–85) *were* consuming 'pharmacological' levels of these valuable and protective compounds. This explains why they were so effectively protected against

---

11. Unfortunately, most supplements are not well designed; they are assembled by companies which do not understand the nutritional issues that confront us today, and sell us pills containing irrational combinations and doses that can do more harm than good (77). Most of the high street brands are worthless.
12. Pharmageddon is due to be published in 2016

cancer, and heart disease, and all the other degenerative, non-communicable disorders. And it also explains why, with our very low 'physiological' intakes, we are so terribly prone to these largely avoidable diseases.

I believe also that the on-going search for disease susceptibility genes is ahistorical and therefore largely misinformed. The mid-Victorian gene pool was not significantly different to our own, yet their incidence of degenerative disease was approximately 90% less (24). In the high-nutrient mid-Victorian environment, the vast majority of the population was protected; and the combination of high levels of physical activity and an excellent diet enhanced the expression of a coordinated array of health-promoting genes (86,87). As the nutrient tide has receded, increasing numbers of genetic polymorphisms have become exposed (88), making current genome-wide association studies (GWAS) largely redundant. If we take this argument to an extreme, and progress to a diet totally devoid of micronutrients, all polymorphisms become disease-associated. It follows that the pharmaceutical industry's attempts to develop genomically derived and individualized treatments such as RNA interference and ISPC are unlikely to impact on public health. The steel vessel of Public Health is rent asunder, and the drug companies are selling us high-priced pots of caulk.

Do not, therefore, look to the drug companies to provide remedies for the appalling state of our health; nor to our politicians who seem largely unable to see beyond the brims of their parliamentary troughs. Look instead to the food and beverage industries, and perhaps the supplement companies, who will hopefully step up to the plate with better designed foods and nutritional programmes once the currently profoundly counter-productive regulatory system has been reconstructed on more scientific lines.

Chapter 7. Why You Cannot Get Everything You Need from a 'Well-Balanced' Diet

Thanks to cheap energy, the internal combustion engine and other labour-saving technologies, we are much less physically active than the mid-Victorians. Indeed, we are the least physically active generation of humans that has ever slouched (or driven) across the face of the earth. Our levels of physical activity, calorific needs and appetites, have shrunk to the point where we have all become malnourished, and this in turn has created a 'new normal' where we think it is entirely natural to spend the last 10% or more of our lives dying.

It is very simple. If you are a sedentary urbanite you are not eating enough, and it is very likely that you do not always eat all the right foods. Even if you did make all the right food choices, you still could not obtain all the nutrients you need for good health. This chapter provides a list of all the micro- and phyto-nutrients essential for your health, showing how much of each you need and how much of which foods are need to supply all of them. All of these are derived from official sources / nutritional tables. The results show that if you are living at a typical 2 to 2.5 thousand calories / day, you canot get everything you need even from a well-balanced diet.

Essential Fatty Acids

α-linolenic Acid (*ALA*)
Dietary sources: flaxseed and rapeseed oil
Biological functions: *ALA* is an essential *omega-3* fatty acid, which is converted into *DHA* in the body. This conversion is generally insufficient, which is why DHA and EPA are critically important dietary constituents.
Deficiency: Deficiency of *omega-3 fatty acids* has been linked to attentional and mood disorders. Depletion is linked to an increase risk of chronic inflammation.
Excess: Excessive fatty acid supplementation has been linked to mild gastrointestinal disturbance.
Essential? Yes
Recommended Daily Intake (males): 5.21 (females): 4.158 kcal
On your plate: ¼ tsp flax seed oil

Docosahexaenoic Acid (*DHA*)
Dietary sources: oily fish
Biological functions: *DHA* is a major component of the brain and the retina. It also has important anti-inflammatory effects.
Deficiency: Deficiency of *omega-3 fatty acids* has been linked to a variety of attentional and mood disorders. Depletion is linked to an increase risk of chronic inflammation.
Excess: Excessive fatty acid supplementation has been linked to mild gastrointestinal disturbance.
Essential: Effectively, yes.
Recommended dose: NIH Workshop recommends 650 mg/day; optimal dose is higher.
On your plate: 200 g herring

Eicosapentanoic Acid (*EPA*)
Dietary sources: oily fish
Biological functions: *EPA* is a major component of brain cell membranes. It also has important anti-inflammatory effects.
Deficiency: Deficiency of *omega-3 fatty acids* has been linked to a variety of attentional and mood disorders. Depletion is linked to an increase risk of chronic inflammation.
Excess: Excessive fatty acid supplementation has been linked to mild gastrointestinal disturbance.
Essential? Effectively, yes..
Recommended Daily Intake: No official recommendation but 200 – 250 mg has been suggested
On your plate: 200 g herring

Linoleic Acid (*LA*)
Dietary sources: sunflower and rapeseed oil
Biological functions: *LA* is an essential *omega-6* fatty acid, from which *arachidonic acid (AA)* is made. *AA* in turn is the source of numerous molecules important in inflammatory immune responses.
Deficiency: rare to non-existent
Excess: Excessive fatty acid supplementation has been linked to mild gastrointestinal disturbance.
Essential? Yes.
Recommended Daily Intake (males): 26.05 (females): 20.79 kcal. This official figure is increasingly considered to be excessive; to obtain a healthier omega 3/6 ratio, it probably should not be more than 15 kcal.
On your plate: approx. 2.5 g or about 2/3 tsp safflower oil

Essential Trace Elements

Boron (B)
Dietary sources: fruits, vegetables, legumes and nuts
Biological functions: Boron is thought to be involved in brain, immune and bone function
Deficiency: May increase urinary losses of calcium and magnesium, and therefore the risk of osteoporosis.
Excess (>100 mg): A red rash with weeping skin, vomiting, diarrhoea.
Essential? Yes
Recommended Daily Dose: no official recommendation, some experts suggest 1-2 mg / day
On your plate: 40 g raisins

Calcium (Ca)
Dietary sources: milk, cheese, green leafy vegetables
Biological functions: Calcium has many functions, including in the nervous system and in bone development.

Deficiency: Osteoporosis and rickets, but these are rare. Depletion is common and is linked to an increased risk of heart disease and cancer
Excess (> 2500 mg): nausea, vomiting, muscle weakness. If long term, kidney stones
Essential? Yes.
Recommended Daily Intake (adults): 700 mg
On your plate: 100 g cheddar cheese or 300 g tofu

Chloride (Cl-)
Dietary sources: table salt
Biological functions: Chloride ions play a key role in cellular functions including *neurotransmission*, and are needed for making hydrochloric acid in the stomach.
Deficiency: rare, but can occur after prolonged vomiting or diarrhoea. Symptoms include low blood pressure, feelings of weakness and eventually loss of muscle control and function.
Excess: In practice, unlikely to occur without a parallel excess of sodium (in table salt). Nausea, dry mouth, dehydration, lethargy, stupor, coma
Essential? Yes.
Recommended Daily Intake (adults): 800 mg
On your plate: 1.2 g table salt

Chromium (Cr)
Dietary sources: meat, nuts, legumes, wholegrain cereals
Biological functions: Chromium is thought to boost insulin's action, thus helping to regulate blood sugar levels. It may also participate in the *metabolism* of fat, protein and carbohydrate.
Deficiency: Rare. Depletion is linked to insulin resistance.
Excess (>0.8 g): Can irritate the stomach and cause rapid heartbeat, light-headedness and skin rashes. Hexavalent chromium, a form used in industry, has been identified as a *carcinogen*.
Essential? Yes. The trivalent chromium is essential.
Recommended Daily Intake (adults): 0.04 mg
On your plate: 150 g broccoli

Cobalt (Co)
Dietary sources: nuts, green leafy vegetables, fish, cereals
Biological functions: Cobalt forms part of *Vitamin B١٢*, and is involved in the oxygen-carrying function of red blood cells. Cobalt salts have been used to treat anaemia.
Deficiency: Human dietary deficiency 'has never been described'.
Excess (>0.5 g single dose or long-term > 0.25 g approx): Angina, panic-anxiety attacks, shortness of breath, asthma, cardiomyopathy, congestive heart failure, other.
Essential? Yes.
Recommended Daily Intake (adults): 0.012 mg:
On your plate: 1 kg fish

Copper (Cu)
Dietary sources: nuts, pulses, meat, potatoes
Biological functions: Copper is important for oxygen *metabolism* and for connective tissues
Deficiency: Rare. Severe cases are caused by the genetic condition Menke's Syndrome.
Excess: Mild effects are not clear; severe cases are caused by the genetic condition Wilson's syndrome.
Essential? Yes.
Recommended Daily Intake (adults): 1 mg
On your plate: 10 g calves liver or 120 g cocoa powder

Fluoride (F)
Dietary sources: drinking water (esp. if fluoridated), seafood
Biological functions: Fluoride is important for preventing tooth decay, but its roles within the body are not clearly understood.
Deficiency: rare, may be linked to increased risk of caries and weakness of bone.
Excess (levels in water > 1mg/l): mottled teeth, skeletal deformity, weakening of bones, IBS, joint pain
Essential? Maybe.
Recommended Daily Intake (adults): 1.5 mg
On your plate: In your water if you live in a fluoridated area. Tea contains up to 20 mg / cup.

Iodine (I)
Dietary sources: seafood, meat, milk, cereals
Biological functions: Iodine is a key constituent of thyroid hormones.
Deficiency: Deficiency causes hypothyroidism, goitre. Depletion is common, and may be linked to weight gain.
Excess: High levels of iodine can affect thyroid function and may increase the risk of Grave's Disease.
Essential? Yes.
Recommended Daily Intake (adults): 0.15 mg, but this may be sub-optimal.
On your plate: 125 g cod or 2 g iodised salt

Iron (Fe)
Dietary sources: wheat flour (except wholemeal), fortified cereals, meat, vegetables
Biological functions: Iron is essential for making haemoglobin, the key oxygen-carrying molecule in blood.
Deficiency: Anaemia, weakness, low resistance to infection.
Excess: High dose supplements have been linked to vomiting, diarrhoea and constipation.
Essential? Yes.
Recommended Daily Intake (males): 8.7 (females): 14.8 mg
On your plate: 50 g cockles or 100 g lamb's kidneys

Magnesium (*Mg*)
Dietary sources: widespread, especially plant sources
Biological functions: Magnesium has many roles in the body, including in *neurotransmission*, and bone growth and health.
Deficiency: Deficiency has been associated with seizures, heart problems and sudden death. Alcoholism and diabetes are risk factors for deficiency. Depletion is common, and is linked to an increased risk of cardiac arrhythmias and heart disease.
Excess: The effects of high magnesium levels have been described as a result of renal failure; *neurotransmission* at the *neuromuscular junction* is suppressed impairing function.
Essential? Yes.
Recommended Daily Intake (adults): 375 mg
On your plate: 120 g sesame seeds or 500 g spinach

Manganese (Mn)
Dietary sources: bread, nuts, tea, vegetables
Biological functions: Manganese is thought to have numerous roles in human *metabolism*, including in the brain's glial cells, where it is a co-factor for the synthesis of the amino acid glutamine.
Deficiency: disruption of normal growth, reproductive problems, painful joints, memory loss
Excess: impotency and nervous system disorders similar to Parkinson's disease. Excessive long term intakes can cause "manganese madness", characterized by irritability, hallucinations, and violent acts
Essential? Yes.
Recommended Daily Intake (adults): 2 mg
On your plate: 10 g wheatgerm or 50 g hazelnuts

Molybdenum (Mo)
Dietary sources: leafy vegetables, nuts, oats
Biological functions: Molybdenum serves as a co-factor in the *metabolism* of the amino acids methionine and cysteine. Without it toxic sulphites build up in the body.
Deficiency: Rare, may be associated with impotency.
Excess: Almost unknown, may be linked to increased risk of gout.
Essential? Yes.
Recommended Daily Intake (adults): 0.05 mg
On your plate: 150 g lentils

Nickel (Ni)
Dietary sources: nuts, preserves, chocolate
Biological functions: Nickel may be involved in maintaining healthy liver function, but its biological functions are unclear.
Deficiency: not seen.

Excess (> 100mg, or via exposure to nickel fumes): nausea, vomiting, thyroid disease, cancers?
Essential? Probably.
US Tolerable Upper Intake (adults): 1 mg. No official recommended dose. .....
On your plate: 1 kg mussels

Phosphorus (P)
Dietary sources: cheese, eggs, meat, marmite, wholemeal bread
Biological functions: In the form of phosphate, phosphorus is a component of many molecules, including the phospholipids of which cell membranes are made.
Deficiency: Rare.
Excess: Tetanus (muscular convulsions) as well as high levels of phosphorus early in life can reduce blood calcium levels.
Essential? Yes.
Recommended Daily Intake (adults): 700 mg
On your plate: 125 g parmesan or 75 g rice bran

Potassium (K)
Dietary sources: raisins, marmite, crisps and much else
Biological functions: Potassium ions play a key role in cellular functions including neurotransmission.
Deficiency: Rare, severe cases can cause heart failure.
Excess: nausea, fatigue, muscle weakness, and tingling, eventually cardiac arrest.
Essential? Yes.
Recommended Daily Intake (adults): 2000 – 300 mg
On your plate: 200 g apricots or 500 g white beans

Selenium (Se)
Dietary sources: brazil nuts, meat, fish, eggs, cereals
Biological functions: In the body, selenium is incorporated into anti-oxidant and other enzymes.
Deficiency: Has been linked to hypothyroidism and increased susceptibility to infection and cancer.
Excess: Upset stomach, nail deformities, garlic-smelling breath, fatigue, irritability, cardiac arrest
Essential? Yes.
Recommended Daily Intake (adults): 0.055 –0.1mg
On your plate: 200 – 400 g brazil nuts or 75 g lambs liver

Silicon (Si)
Dietary sources: beer, cereals
Biological functions: Silicon compounds bind to and neutralise toxic aluminium ions
Deficiency: Has been linked to skeletal deformities
Excess: None known

Essential? Probably, but depends on exposure to soluble and bioactive aluminium
Recommended Daily Intake: no official recommendation, but 10 mg seems reasonable
On your plate: 1 pint of beer, 50 g whole grains

Sodium (Na)
Dietary sources: salt
Biological functions: Sodium ions play a key role in cellular functions including *neurotransmission.*
Deficiency: very rare. Hypotension, salt craving.
Excess: High blood pressure, probable increased risk of stomach cancer.
Essential? Yes.
Recommended Daily Intake (adults): 1600 mg
On your plate: 4g table salt

Sulphur (S)
Dietary sources: eggs, onions, high protein foods
Biological functions: Sulphur has numerous roles in human *metabolism*, for example in oxidation – reduction reactions and certain detoxification reactions.
Deficiency: very rare, tends to occur in conjunction with protein deficiency. Symptoms may include joint pain, reduced immunity, muscle pain and dry skin
Excess: very rare. No toxicity has been noted.
Essential? Yes.
Recommended dose: No official recommendation but about 850 mg / day is reasonable.
On your plate: 12 scallops

Zinc (Zn)
Dietary sources: meat, milk, shellfish, dairy products, wholegrain cereals
Biological functions: Zinc has many roles in human *metabolism*, including in *DNA* synthesis, immune function and the development of taste and smell.
Deficiency: retarded growth, slowed healing of wounds, hair loss, impaired immune system
Excess: Nausea, vomiting, headache, fatigue
Essential? Yes
Recommended Daily Intake (males): 9. (females): 7 mg
On your plate: 10 – 100 g oysters (depending on type) or 100 g wheat germ

Vitamins

Vitamin A (retinol, retinoic acid)
Dietary sources: oily fish, cheese, eggs, milk, liver, reduced-fat spreads, red and yellow vegetables
Biological functions: *Vitamin* A, a fat-soluble compound, is best-known for its importance in vision, especially in low light. It is also important for healthy skin and immunity.
Deficiency: Deficiency can lead to night blindness, eye lesions and eventually to complete blindness.

Excess: Nausea and vomiting; skin dryness and peeling, liver damage and osteoporosis. Excess taken during pregnancy may cause birth defects.
Essential? Yes
Recommended Daily Intake (males): 0.7 (females): 0.6 mg
On your plate: 100 g pork, beef or lambs liver

Vitamin **B1 (thiamine, thiamin)**
Dietary sources: pork, milk, cheese, eggs, fruit and vegetables
Biological functions: *Vitamin B¹*, which is water-soluble, is required for the release of energy from carbohydrates.
Deficiency: Beriberi, a disease whose symptoms include loss of sensation and muscle function, pain, vomiting, shortness of breath and heart problems. Deficiency may also be associated with alcoholism (Korsakoff's syndrome).
Excess: No ill effects are known.
Essential? Yes
Recommended Daily Intake (males): 1 (females): 0.8 mg
On your plate: 15 g marmite or 200 g tuna

Vitamin **B2 (riboflavin,'***vitamin* **G')**
Dietary sources: milk, eggs, mushrooms, rice, fortified cereals
Biological functions: Riboflavin is a water-soluble compound which contributes to the body's processing of fat, carbohydrate, protein and oxygen.
Deficiency: Signs are rare, but may include sores and cracks in the lips and tongue, *inflammation.*
Excess: No ill effects are known.
Essential? Yes.
Recommended Daily Intake (adults): 1.4 mg
On your plate: one tsp coffee

Vitamin **B3 (niacin,** *vitamin* **P,** *vitamin* **PP)**
Dietary sources: beef, pork, eggs, milk, wheat flour
Biological functions: *Vitamin Bʳ* is a water-soluble compound which regulates *cholesterol metabolism,* increasing plasma HDL and decreasing LDL.
Deficiency: Pellagra is characterised by patches of dark, scaly skin. In severe forms, pellagra is associated with insomnia, mental confusion, physical weakness, diarrhoea and dementia.
Excess: Excess *Vitamin Bʳ* may cause nausea and vomiting, also the 'niacin flush' as blood vessels dilate.
Essential? Yes.
Recommended Daily Intake (adults): 16 mg
On your plate: 3 tsp's marmite. If you hate marmite, 150g wheat bran.

Vitamin **B5 (pantothenic acid)**
Dietary sources: chicken, potatoes, porridge, brown rice, wholemeal bread, broccoli, tomatoes, beef, liver

Biological functions: *Vitamin B* is a water-soluble compound required in order for energy to be released from carbohydrate and fat.
Deficiency: Deficiency can cause acne.
Excess: No ill effects are known.
Essential? Yes.
Recommended Daily Intake (adults): 6 mg
On your plate: 125 g chicken liver

Vitamin B6 (pyridoxine, pyridoxamine, or pyridoxal)

Dietary sources: chicken, fish, pork, eggs, peanuts, brown rice, oatmeal
Biological functions: *Vitamin B*, which is water-soluble, participates in many biochemical reactions and is involved in the synthesis of *neurotransmitters*.
Deficiency: Deficiency symptoms include itchy, peeling skin (dermatitis), cracked and sore lips, inflamed tongue and mouth (skin disorders similar to vitamin B2 and vitamin B3deficiencies),and peripheral neuropathy. This presents with poor coordination, staggering and numbness in the hands and feet.
Excess: gross overdose, as with deficiency, may be associated with peripheral neuropathy;
Essential? Yes.
Recommended Daily Intake (males): 1.4 (females): 1.2 mg
On your plate: 120 g raw pistachios or 25 g rice bran

Vitamin B7 (biotin, '*vitamin* H')

Dietary sources: liver, egg yolk, dried mixed fruit, some vegetables
Biological functions: *Vitamin B7* is a water-soluble compound required for the *metabolism of fatty acids*.
Deficiency: In infants, lack of biotin may lead to neurological disorders. Signs in adults are rare.
Excess: No ill effects are known.
Essential? Yes.
Recommended Daily Intake (adults): 0.05 mg
On your plate: 20 g chicken liver or 200 g mushroom

Vitamin B9 (folic acid, folate, '*vitamin* M')

Dietary sources: fortified cereals and bread, green leafy vegetables, oranges, bananas, marmite, brown rice
Biological functions: *Vitamin B9* is a water-soluble compound involved in *DNA* synthesis and maintenance.
Deficiency: Deficiency can cause birth defects if pregnant women are deficient, so supplementation in pregnancy is recommended. Depletion is linked to an increased risk of cancer.
Excess: Taking folate supplements can mask the early effects of *vitamin* B12 deficiency.
Essential? Yes.
Recommended Daily Intake (adults): 0.2 mg
On your plate: 75 g marmite, or 80 g liver

Vitamin B12 (cobalamin)
Dietary sources: liver, meat, cheese, fish, fortified cereals
Biological functions: Vitamin B12 is a water-soluble compound required for DNA synthesis.
Deficiency: Lack of cobalamin can cause peripheral neuropathy and cognitive deficits resulting from neurological damage. It is more common among the elderly.
Excess: Excessive Vitamin B12 may be associated with skin problems, but ill effects are rare.
Essential? Yes.
Recommended Daily Intake (adults): 0.0025 mg
On your plate: 20 g mussels or oysters

'Vitamin Bp' (choline)
Dietary sources: eggs, fish, chicken, milk, liver, vegetables
Biological functions: Choline is a water-soluble compound required for DNA maintenance. It is also an important part of some phospholipids, and the chemical precursor to the neurotransmitter acetylcholine.
Deficiency: Choline deficiency is associated with fatty liver and kidney problems, high blood pressure and infertility.
Essential? Yes, although choline is not officially recognised as a vitamin.
Recommended Daily Intake (males): 550 (females): 425 mg
On your plate: 200 g whole eggs (= 4 large eggs)

Vitamin C (ascorbic acid)
Dietary sources: potatoes, vegetables, fruit (especially citrus fruit)
Biological functions: Vitamin C is a potent, water-soluble antioxidant. It is necessary for the synthesis of collagen, which confers elasticity to skin.
Deficiency: Bleeding, scurvy, eventually death. Depletion is common, and may be linked to an increased risk of cardiovascular disease.
Excess: High dose supplements have been linked to vomiting, diarrhoea and kidney stones.
Essential? Yes.
Recommended Daily Intake (adults): 40 mg
On your plate: 50 g red chilies or 100 g kale

Vitamin D (ergocalciferol, cholecalciferol)
Dietary sources: sunlight, oily fish, eggs, liver, fortified cereals, spreads
Biological functions: Vitamin D, a fat-soluble compound, has many roles, including in the immune system, blood sugar and blood pressure regulation, and cardiovascular function.
Deficiency: Vitamin D deficiency affects the bones, causing rickets in children and osteomalacia in adults. Depletion is very common, and is associated with an increased risk of a very large number of diseases.
Excess: Vitamin D excess may be linked to weight loss and nausea, and in severe and chronic cases to calcification of soft tissues and kidney damage
Essential? Provisionally, yes. It is made in the body, in sunlight-exposed skin, but most people do not get enough D in this way.
Recommended Daily Intake (adults): 0.005 mg. See RNI guidelines.
On your plate: 1 tsp cod liver oil or 50g herring

Vitamin E (tocopherols and tocotrienols)

Dietary sources: olive oil, nuts, seeds, fat spreads, biscuits and cakes
Biological functions: The various forms of Vitamin E are potent, fat-soluble antioxidants, and are important for healthy neurological function.
Deficiency: *Vitamin* E deficiency has been associated with infertility and with hemolytic anaemia, in which red blood cells break down faster than usual. Deficiency may also increase the risk of cancer and neuro-degenerative disease.
Excess: Large doses may cause headaches and nausea, and worsen the effects of *vitamin* K deficiency, thus imparing blood coagulation.
Essential? Yes.
Recommended Daily Intake (adults): 12mg. Se RNI guidelines.
On your plate: 50 g sunflower seeds or 200 g peanuts

Vitamin K (naphthoquinoids)

Dietary sources: green leaf vegetables (K1) and fermented cheeses (K2).
Biological functions: *Vitamins* K1 and K2 are fat-soluble compounds important in blood clotting and calcification.K2 is the more important of the two for long term health.
Deficiency: Deficiency is rarely seen, and mostly in new-borns. It's characterised by excessive bleeding. Depletion is common, and is linked to an increased risk of osteoporosis and calcification of soft tissues.
Excess: No ill effects are known.
Essential? Yes.
Recommended Daily Intake (adults): 0.075 mg. See RNI guidelines.
On your plate: K1 - 10 g kale or 50 g spring onions, **K2 –** 150 g blue cheese or 250 g natto

Phytonutrients

'Vitamin P' (polyphenols)

Dietary sources: fruits, vegetables, nuts, coffee, tea
Biological functions: polyphenols are anti-inflammatory agents and have cardio-protective, neuro-protective and anti-cancer properties
Deficiency: Deficiency is rarely seen, although depletion is common and is associated with an increased risk of chronic inflammation, and degenerative disease
Excess: Some polyphenols bind iron, so very high doses reduce iron absorption.
Essential? Not yet officially recognised, but Yes.
Recommended Daily Intake (adults): *there are no officially recommended levels of intake.* Dietary intake today is around 1g/day, but this is probably insufficient for good health. The mid-Victorians, who enjoyed near-immunity to conditions caused by chronic inflammation, consumed 5 g or more / day.
On your plate: 1 g is contained in approximately 5 portions fruit and vegetables. To obtain 5 g, 10 portions or more with the emphasis on berry fruits.

Carotenoids & xanthophylls (beta carotene, alpha carotene, lycopene, lutein, zeaxanthin, meso-zeaxanthin)
Dietary sources: fruits, vegetables, grains
Biological functions: some of these compounds (lutein, zeaxanthin, meso-zeaxanthin) are essential for the health of the retina, and many of them have anti-cancer properties.
Deficiency: Deficiency is unrecognised, and is probably rare. Depletion leads to an increased risk of blindness and cancer.
Excess: No ill effects are known, although skin colouration may occur. Beta carotene supplements are not recommended for smokers as they may increase the risk of lung cancer.
Essential? For long-term health, Yes.
Recommended Daily Intake (adults): *There are no officially recognised levels of intake.* A total dose of 25 mg / day is considered by many to be essential for good health, spread across the whole group.
On your plate: Eat your colours! 1 sweet potato (beta carotene), 300-400 mls tomato juice (lycopene), 200 g prunes (lutein / zeaxanthin)

Cyanogens (glucosinolates, cyanogenic glycosides)
Dietary sources: vegetables esp brassica, beans and cereals
Biological functions: These compounds are substrates for the enzyme lactoperoxidase, an essential part of the innate immune system.
Deficiency: Deficiency is unrecognised and probably rare. Depletion is more common, and will reduce resistance to infection.
Excess: Chronic excess can cause goitre if diet is low in iodine. Acute overdose - weakness, vertigo and difficulty with breathing. Fatal at over 0.5g/kg bodyweight..
Essential? Not yet officially recognised, but Yes.
Recommended Daily Intake (adults): No official recommendation but science supports ١٠ mg of thiocyanate equivalents / day
On your plate: 200 g broccoli, 300 g brussels sprouts

Non-digestible carbohydrates (dietary fibres)
Dietary sources: fruits, vegetables, legumes, pulses and cereals
Biological functions: Required for gut function and a healthy microbiome.
Deficiency: Deficiency is rare but depletion is common. In the short term this manifests as constipation and over the longer term as an increased risk of gastro-intestinal diseases and other inflammatory diseases.
Excess: Flatulence, diarrhoea.
Essential? Not yet officially recognised, but Yes.
Recommended Daily Intake (adults): No official recommendation, but science supports 20 g of mixed fibres or more / day
On your plate: Approximately 1 kilo of mixed fruits, vegetables, legumes and whole grains

Other

1-3, 1-6 beta glucans
Dietary sources: baker's or brewer's yeast
Biological functions: immune-modulation, ie enhanced innate cellular immune function and (in the adaptive immune system), TH1 dominance.
Deficiency: impaired resistance to infection, increased allergy, increased gastrontestinal inflammation, increased risk of cancer
Excess: no adverse effects known
Essential? In the long term, Yes.
Recommended Daily Intake: 2.5 mg / kg body weight / day
On your plate: yeast tablets / capsules; 500 ml unfiltered beer or wine; 500 g yeast-leavened bread

A la Carte: A Good Day's Menu.

Obtaining the recommended amounts of all the above essential nutrients from foods is quite complicated, and not for the faint-hearted. A minimal day's menu is listed below; it is shorter than the preceding list because most foods contain more than one nutrient. You don't need to worry about proteins, fats and carbohydrates as these are all contained in the same menu.

200 g herring (provides the DHA and EPA, vitamin D, some Iodine). **320 Kcals**
300 g other fish (provides Cu, Fe and the rest of the Iodine). Would be 800 g, but can be reduced due to the liver in the menu (below). **300 Kcals**

The fish also contains, in addition to the Cu and Fe, some Se and Zn; but not enough of any of these hence:

100 g wheat germ (Zn) **350 Kcals**
150 g lambs liver (Se) **200 Kcals**

The wheat germ will also provide enough Mn. The liver and wheat germ will get you up to enough Cu, Zn, Fe and Si, and provide sufficient vitamins A, B3, B5, B7 and B9. They also provides some choline, but not enough so:

3 large eggs get you up to a sufficient intake of choline. These also provide enough beta carotene, vitamin A and B2 and B12. **230 Kcals**

150 g broccoli provides enough Co; and some vitamin C and cyanogens, but not enough of either of these so .. **50 Kcals**

100 g kale will bring you up to speed with vitamin C and the cyanogens. It also provides the right amount of vitamin K1, but no vitamin K2 so ... **35 Kcals**

150 g blue cheese or quark.for the K2. This will also be enough to top up your Co intake. Blue cheese **Kcals 380** or quark **Kcals 150**

50 g lentils. It takes 150 g of these to provide the right amount of Mo, but this is in many other foods so we can reduce the amount to 50g. **Kcals 60**

50 g apricots. This only contains 25% of the needed potassium, but the other 75% is provided in the other foods listed above and below. **Kcals 100**

200 g peanuts will top up your B6 and provide sufficient vitamin E **Kcals 1200**

300 mls tomato juice (lycopene) **Kcals 50**
200 g prunes (lutein) **Kcals 400**

250 g more fruits, vegetables and whole grains: to top up on polyphenols and fibers: **Kcals 200**

The above day's menu will also provide sufficient LA, ALA, sulphur, sodium, chloride, nickel, phosphorus, magnesium, boron and B1.

Calories.

The above day's menu contains between 3,250 and 3,500 Kcalories. This seems – and is – excessive for today's urban-dwelling office workers; in the 21st century, cheap energy and labour-saving technology allow or encourage most of us live a low energy lifestyle of 2,000 and 2,500 Kcalories / day. If we were to consume 3,500 Kcalories / day, most of us would quickly gain weight and move rapidly towards overweight and obesity[13].

In 19th century Britain, however, adults routinely consumed 3,500 Kcalories / day or more, and remained slim due to their far more physically active lifestyle. Processed foods were limited to simple items such as bread, butter and cheese. The mid-Victorian diet was replete with the sorts of basic food items listed above (they consumed an average of 10 portions of fruit and vegetables per day), and there were few foods or beverages that contained the large amounts of empty calories that so many products do today.

Although our great grand-parents ate what might seem to us to be a very limited diet, it was a very healthy diet. The medical records show that these folk lived as long as we do today, but were almost immune to the degenerative diseases that affect and kill so many of us.

---

13. Whenever I make this point in public there is always some hero who insists that he (it is inevitably a he) has no problem with consuming 4,000 Kcalories / day because he is such an athlete. Yes, there are those who still run at a high rate of calorific expenditure, and can therefore get all they need from their food IF they make the right food choices; but this is no longer typical.

If we are to gain their considerably better health prospects, we have to find ways of shoe-horning the nutritional content of the Victorians 3,500 Kcalorie diet, into today's 2,000 (for women) to 2,500 (for men) Kcalorie diet. Simply telling people to eat more fruits, vegetables oily fish and liver does not work. Many people will not eat oily fish or liver. Offal meats, for example, which contain highr levels of many nutrients than skeletal muscle, are now mostly sold for pet food.

There are only two ways of increasing the nutrient density of today's diet, and improving our appallingly bad public health. These are food fortification and/or supplementation.

In the light of our new understanding of the role of chronic inflammation in causing disease, either of these strategies must focus on the anti-inflamatory nutrients.

Chapter 8. How we lost the nutritional wisdom of our ancestors

The mid-Victorian diet combined a potent cocktail of all of the anti-inflammatory nutrients listed above with very low levels of the pro-inflammatory compounds, in a diet which contained very few processed foods. These eating habits, together with their significantly higher levels of physical activity, made overweight and diabetes rare; creating a total lifestyle which protected the Victorians against chronic inflammation and gave them near-immunity to the degenerative diseases.

We squandered the Victorian virtues in the name of progress and easier lives, and we are paying a very heavy price for that. We don't, however, have to recreate Victorian conditions to radically improve our health. We have to untangle the skein of factors that, taken together, make us so sick. We have to accentuate the positive, eliminate the negative, and look after Mr (and Mrs) In-Between. It's a simple question of identifying the things we got wrong, and putting them right. This starts with the beta glucans, Omega 3 fatty acids and polyphenols; and includes vitamins D and E, and the trace element selenium.

Our intake of (1-3), (1-6) beta-glucans has been very significantly reduced, for a range of reasons which include the introduction of the synthetic fungicides circa 1950, micro-filtration in brewing in the 1960's, and our historically low consumption of bread. The uncontrollable increase in asthma and allergy since 1950 (1-2) is indirect but clear evidence of inadequate intakes of the (1-3), (1-6) beta-glucans and widespread beta- glucan depletion (3).

Intakes of Omega 3 fatty acids and polyphenols have also declined, although these changes started rather earlier than the decline in (1-3), (1-6) beta-glucans and can be traced back as far as the early 20th century (4). This is due to a progressive shift from basic to processed foods and to our physically inactive lifestyles, which have reduced our calorific requirements.

It is likely that average levels of 'vitamin' D have also fallen. In the 19th century rickets was common in the great cities, where coal smoke darkened the skies for weeks at a time; but according to a survey undertaken by the British Medical Association during the 1880's, the disease hardly existed in small towns with populations of less than 5000, villages, and in the countryside (5). Rural Victorians spent far more time out of doors than we do, ensuring a good vitamin D status, and some urban workers did as well. They walked to and from work every day and spent much of their leisure time on outdoors pursuits due to an acute shortage of TV's, smart phones and i-Pads.

Today we have a major problem with D. Data from the U.S. National Health and Nutrition Examination Survey found that a staggering 61% (50.8 million!) were depleted in D, and 9% of children were clinically deficient (6). The situation in Europe is as bad, and rickets is re-appearing in some subgroups of the population in the UK, predominantly in those of African–Caribbean and South Asian origins (7-8).

The Victorians consumed large amounts of seafood which provided selenium, and nuts and wholegrain foods which provided vitamin E. The fact that we eat less than the Victorians, together with our preference for processed and often nutritionally-depleted foods and our fear of sunlight, has left many of us substantially depleted in these nutrients (9-11) and increasingly vulnerable to inflammatory and auto-immune diseases (12-17).

At the same time, in an apparent paradox, our sheer lack of physicality has made it very difficult for us to maintain healthy body weight. At our current and historically low levels of physical activity, the satiety mechanisms that keep animals in the wild lean (and which used to work well in humans too, overweight and obesity were rare among the Victorians) break down. Surrounded by convenience foods and bombarded with messages to consume, many of us eat a few hundred calories too many per day; and this, over time, is enough to create the weight problems that affect so many. Excess adipose tissue is pro-inflammatory unless it is protected with lipophile nutrients (see chapter 17), as are the high levels of blood glucose in diabetes caused by the interlinked factors of physical inactivity and obesity (see chapter 18).

The decline in anti-inflammatory nutrients and the increase in obesity and diabetes provide two of the elements needed for a perfect inflammatory storm. The third exacerbating factor, which makes the storm inevitable, is our hugely increased intake of pro-inflammatory toxins.

The proliferation of fast food franchises with their rapid, high temperature cooking methods has made a very significant contribution to our public ill health; but so has the modern food processing and manufacturing industry, which uses high temperature technologies such as spray drying to speed up production.

In short, the way we live today conspires in many ways against good health. From a health perspective everything that could go wrong, has gone wrong; and the idea touted by Big Pharma that there are simple pills to cure all of our modern ills, makes little sense. (Although it makes good financial sense for the drug companies.)

There is a good deal of science behind all the anti-inflammatory nutrients, and an overwhelming public health case to adding them as fortificants to the major food items in our diet. However, until our politicians start to take public health more seriously than their expense claims, you would be well advised to take matters into your own hands and add the key anti-inflammatory nutrients to your own diet. The same goes for reducing your intake of pro-inflammatory toxins, taking more exercise and maintaining healthy weight and blood sugar.

Chapter 9. Putting out the flames: an advanced course

19th century Victorians were almost immune to the degenerative diseases that damage and kill so many of us in the 20th and 21st centuries. What made us so much more prone to chronic inflammation, degenerative disease and unhealthy ageing was the emergence of Type B malnutrition, the progressive removal of immuno-modulating and anti-inflammatory nutrients from the diet and a huge increase in our intake of pro-inflammatory toxins. This has been exaccerbated by living ever more sedentary lifestyles, eating more refined foods and consequently becoming fatter and more diabetic. If we wish to protect ourselves from the 'diseases of civilisation', we have to put at least some of these changes into reverse. This is the basis of a 3-step program to prolonged good health.

3 Steps to Health

*The first and easiest step to better health involves increasing the nutrient density of the foods we eat, putting the key anti-inflammatory nutrients back into our diet. These are detailed in Chapters 12 to 17.

* The second step is taking more exercise, eating fewer carbohydrates (if we wish to keep our sedentary lifestyles), and getting our weight and blood sugar under control. This is detailed in Chapter 18.

* The third step involves changing our cooking and eating habits in order to reduce our intake of pro-inflammatory toxins. This is detailed in Chapter 19.

1. Increase your intake of anti-inflammatory nutrients

The most critical anti-inflammatory nutrients are the (1-3), (1-6) beta-glucans, the Omega-3 polyunsaturated fatty acids and the polyphenols. These all have different but mutually reinforcing mechanisms of action. The (1-3), (1-6) beta-glucans enhance innate immune activity, reduce the risk of chronic inflammation caused by lingering infections, and exert intrinsic anti-inflammatory efects. Omega 3 fatty acids create anti-inflammatory mediators, and the polyphenols inhibit key inflammatory and tissue-damaging enzymes.

Other nutrients play ancillary anti-inflammatory roles. The most important of these appear to be the trace element selenium (1-3), and a group of lipophilic (fat-soluble) micronutrients which includes vitamins A, D and E, and the carotenoids (4).

2. Take more exercise, eat fewer carbohydrates, get your weight and blood sugar under control

Probably the hardest step to take, but it pays many dividends. Taking more exercise improves muscle tone, body shape, general fitness and self-confidence, and is extremely positive in terms of improving blood sugar control. If combined with a low-carb diet and less processed and fast foods, Type 2 diabetes can be forced to regress back to Metabolic Syndrome (a pre-clinical form of diabetes), and this in turn can be completely normalised. This not only reduces chronic inflammation, it also switches on 'housekeeping' genes which help to re-build and restore healthy cells and tissues.

3. Reduce your intake of pro-inflammatory toxins

When foods containing proteins are cooked at high temperatures, the protein binds with glucose or other sugars in the food to produce compounds called Advanced Glycation End Products, or AGEs. Many foods brown at high temperatures and this discolouration is a sign of AGE production. AGE compounds are very pro-inflammatory, as are the Advanced Lipoperoxidation End Products, known as ALE's, which form when oils and fats are heated.

Foods processed at high temperatures and which contain high levels of both AGEs and ALEs include powdered milk as used in enteral nutrition, numerous industrially produced foods and baby formulae (!), high temperature fried and grilled meats and poultry, deep fried and shallow fried fish, coffee and colas, smoked and cured foods – in short, fast food staples (5-6). Higher levels of these pro-inflammatory toxins in the blood are linked to higher rates of *many* degenerative diseases, including a large number of cancers. Processed meats such as bacon and sausages seem to be particularly harmful, and have been linked to as many as 3 in every 100 deaths (8).

Chapter 10. Key Anti-Inflammatory Nutrients #1: Yeast-Derived (1-3), (1-6) Beta-Glucans

Yeast-derived (1-3), (1-6) beta-glucans increase the effectiveness of acute inflammation. The resulting improvement in the body's ability to deal with pathogens (1) and repair tissue damage (2-3) means that there is less likelihood of a progression to chronic inflammation. These nutrients restore the immune system to its normal and optimal state.

Your Immune System

The immune system is your body's natural defence system, patrolling and defending your body 24 hours a day, every day of your life. It protects against invasion by bacteria, viruses, parasites and fungi and, on the relatively few occasions that these gain entry to the body, it fights the resulting infection. It is also one of the body's defences against cancer.

A weakened immune system, therefore, leaves your body vulnerable to disease. The immune system is degraded by factors such as chronic stress, a poor diet, and long-haul flights which expose air travellers to significant levels of ionising radiation. Certain medications such as steroids and the drugs used to treat cancer, and HIV, degrade the immune system. The immune system is also in the winter months when vitamin D levels fall, very inconveniently just when adverse weather conditions keep many indoors and in closer contact with others.

The dangers of inadequate immune function are very real. In the United States and in the United Kingdom, more people die each year from severe and systemic bacterial infections than from breast, colorectal and pancreatic cancer combined. Nor can we continue to rely on antibiotics to save us. The rise of 'super-bugs' such as MRSA and VRSA (methicillin- and vancomycin- resistant Staphylococcus aureus), C. Difficile, and the progression through MDR- and XDR- to TDR-TB (Multi-, Extensively and Totally Drug Resistant Tuberculosis) (4), indicates that antibiotics are increasingly losing their effectiveness. The arrival in 2010 of the New Delhi Metallo-Lactamase plasmid, which confers resistance to almost everything in the armoury, tells us that the antibiotic game is nearly over.

As the drugs fail, it becomes more important than ever to ensure that your immune system is working as effectively as possible.

Your two immune systems

We talk of 'an' immune system, but in fact there are two distinct but inter-connected immune sub-systems; the innate immune system and the acquired immune system.

The **adaptive immune system** is that part of the immune system with 'memory'. It is involved (positively) in immunisation, and (negatively) in allergy and auto-immunity. Once the acquired immune system has learned to recognise an enemy, after an initial infection or after a vaccination, it remembers the enemy's characteristics. On second exposure to the threat, the memory cells recognise it, and generate an immune response involving highly specific weapons such as antibodies. That's why it is highly unusual to catch measles or the same cold twice.

The adaptive immune system is powerful, sophisticated and highly specific, but it is initially slow to respond and often insufficient to protect the host against the first onslaught of a virulent bacterium or virus. It is only able to respond rapidly and at peak effectiveness if you have already encountered the threat previously. Even small mutations in a virus may be enough to 'fool' the adaptive immune system. These are some of the reasons why the adaptive immune system is only our <u>second</u> line of defence.

Our first line of defence, the **innate immune system,** is rather more basic. In evolutionary terms, it is much older than the more sophisticated and more recently adaptive immune system. It is faster to respond to a threat but it is less specific; it can only recognise a limited number of compounds ¾ around a dozen or so ¾ that commonly occur on the surface of bacteria and yeasts. Its key cellular components are macrophages, neutrophils and Natural Killer (NK) cells.

These 'front line defensive troops' constantly patrol the body and look out for anything that doesn't belong there. If macrophages and neutrophils spot a bacterium they swallow it and try to digest it. If NK cells recognise a virally infected cell they will kill it to prevent further viral replication, and if they encounter a cancer cell (and recognise it as cancerous) they will kill it to prevent tumour growth and spread. **(Figure 1)**

Figure 1

Immunology 101

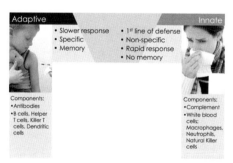

Illustration 1: The human immune system has two major subsystems: innate immunity and adaptive (acquired) immunity. Both must work together to clear the body of an infection.

All this makes the innate immune system very important indeed. Insects and other invertebrates – a group that constitutes the majority of animal species – rely solely on an innate immune system. They have no acquired immune system, and manage very well without one. Another sign of the importance of the innate immune system is that while people born without a functional acquired immune system may live into their 30's, mutations that delete the innate immune system invariably cause death *in utero.*

As the numbers of antibiotic resistant bacteria in our environment continue to increase, and flu and other viral pandemics keep on coming, it makes good sense to ensure that your innate immune system is working as effectively as it should.

Modern immune systems are less effective than they used to be

Despite, indeed ironically partly because of, modern medicine, your immune system is less effective than that of your recent ancestors – for two reasons.

1. We live in an unnaturally sterile environment

Humans evolved in a dirty environment. We have been on the planet for hundreds of thousands of years but soap, antiseptics, disinfectants, canned and frozen foods have only been with us for a few generations, and antibiotics arrived less than a century ago.

During most of our time on this planet, therefore, our environment was replete with microbial hazards, and our immune systems were constantly challenged. And as we had strong immune systems, which mostly worked very well, we survived and multiplied.

Indeed, recent studies have shown that the innate immune system adapts to facing constant challenges and responds to these by up-regulating its state of readiness and effectiveness. In particular, the innate immune system learned to recognise and respond to molecules called (1-3), (1-6) beta-glucans. These compounds are present in the cell walls of fungi, a family which includes moulds and yeasts; and the innate immune system responds to their presence by mounting a strong counter-attack. In an age before fungicides were routinely sprayed onto every food crop, almost everything we ate would have been contaminated with yeasts and moulds. This was, paradoxically, one of the factors that kept our innate immune systems at peak capacity – and it explains why, when we still lived in caves, we were able to eat foods that, far from being kept in the sanitised conditions of today's food chain, were heavily contaminated with micro-organisms.

Until quite recently it was thought that today's over-sanitised environment left our immune systems with relatively little to contend with, rendering them less active and less able to neutralise new and unexpected threats. This is the so-called 'hygiene hypothesis', and it was used to explain why, when we travel to parts of the world where sanitation standards are lower than ours, we routinely fall victim to pathogens that locals have no problems with. Our vulnerability to Montezuma's Revenge, Delhi belly and other travellers' ills is, according to the hygiene hypothesis, largely due to our under-stimulated immune systems; which at the same time are left unbalanced and more prone to react to normally harmless substances such as pollen or peanuts. This is thought to have contributed to the explosion that we have seen in the numbers of people with asthma and allergy. According to this hypothesis, children who live on farms or with pets and who are known to have a reduced risk of asthma and allergy, are protected because they are exposed to more pathogens; city dwellers who supposedly live in a cleaner environment have a higher risk.

Nice theory, but it doesn't make any sense. Farmhands and city brokers alike are constantly exposed to microorganisms. We ingest them with every mouthful of food, we inhale them with every lungful of breath, they live on and inside us – and no amount of soap or antiseptics can reduce this exposure. This is why the old hygiene hypothesis has been replaced with a new version which focusses on yeast and the (1-3), (1-6) beta-glucans in yeast cell walls.

When Joni Mitchell sang 'Give me spots on my apples, but leave me the birds and the bees, please![14]' it looks as if she was more right than she, or we, knew. The spots on our apples – and indeed, the traces of fungi, yeast and moulds that used to be on almost all our foods – now appear to be as important for our health as the apples themselves. The removal of beta-glucans from our food chain is deeply implicated in the dramatic increases in allergy that have occurred since 1950, and the equally significant increases in cancer. The problems are exacerbated by an increasingly pro-inflammatory environment in the body, due to wide-spread Type B malnutrition.

2. 'Type B' malnutrition

Health researchers are increasingly referring to 'Type B' malnutrition. This is not the sort of malnutrition associated with starving people in developing countries, but people in fully developed societies who have adequate calories - often more than adequate - but an inadequate intake of vitamins, minerals and other vital nutrients. They suffer from multiple micronutrient depletion, including beta glucan depletion. This impairs the immune system, leaving it less able to resist infection and less able to monitor cancer but more likely, when it over-reacts to harmless things such as peanuts, pollen or animal dander, to generate excessive inflammation.

In the population at large, the average person has an intake of vitamin D and selenium that is only about **half** of the Recommended Daily Amount, or RDA (5-7). These are just two of the nutrients that are critical to the proper functioning of the immune system.

Moreover, the RDA was not established to give an optimum level of nutritional intake, but only enough to prevent deficiency. The optimum levels of many nutrients are almost certainly higher than the RDA's (see chapter 23). This means that almost everyone has intakes of many nutrients below the level needed for proper 'base line' support of the immune system.

Recent studies of hospital patients found that a staggering 60% were malnourished on admission (8). In 30 to 40% of patients, the malnutrition was sufficiently severe to cause lymphopenia (9-10), a condition in which numbers of white blood cells are significantly sub-normal. This indicates substantial immuno-suppression, and a significantly increased risk of acquiring an infection while in hospital. This is one reason why infection control in hospitals is so difficult; immuno-compromised patients are being brought into an environment full of resistant bacteria - a situation rather like introducing petrol to flames.

---

14. (From Big Yellow Taxi by Joni Mitchell, 1970).

Fortunately this kind of immuno-suppression is easy to treat, and responds promptly to improved nutrition. Well-designed nutritional supplements have been shown to improve immune function in these patients, and to reduce the incidence of infections and other complications during and after their hospital treatment (11-13).

Hospital admissions are by definition unhealthy people, and the criticism has been raised that the findings of malnutrition in this group do not reflect the situation in the community.

However, similar findings have been reported in the wider community. Sub-optimal immune function is now common in elderly (14) and in middle-aged subjects. As with the hospital patients, however, their impaired immune systems can be improved and brought back to normal with well-designed supplement programmes; both elderly and middle-aged subjects respond positively to supplementation (15-17).

Stress

When we experience stress our adrenal glands secrete the hormone cortisol, and when cortisol levels are too high for too long, the immune system is suppressed.

Stress has always been part of the human condition, but our political and financial masters have lately conspired to making life very stressful indeed. Job insecurity, unemployment and economic hardship all cause chronic stress, leaving more and more of us immuno-compromised. As herd immunity (the general level of resistance to infection in a population) falls, the herd – human or otherwise – becomes more vulnerable to infections, both individually and collectively. The economic down-turn is also causing a drop in nutritional standards (18), which makes the immuno-suppression worse. This is a truly worrying scenario.

Antibiotics and the rise of the 'Super Bugs'

If we ever needed strong immune systems it is now. Since the introduction of the sulpha drugs in the late 1930's we have relied on antibiotics to cure bacterial infections; but the time of antibiotics is nearly over due to wide-spread antibiotic resistance.

Too many visits to the doctor end with a prescription for an antibiotic. That may be perfectly valid for a severe bacterial infection, but coughs and colds, for example, are usually caused by viruses, which cannot be treated with antibiotics. Nevertheless, nearly a half of children with common colds are treated with antibiotics (19).
Because children catch an average of three to eight colds each year, they may be given many courses of unnecessary antibiotics. And although doctors know that antibiotics will not help, they often find themselves pressurised to prescribe them, if only to reassure demanding parents that something – anything – is being done (20). In fact children with colds, ear infections, sinus infections, bronchitis and sore throats account for a staggering three quarters of all antibiotic prescriptions.

This is just one example of the over-use of antibiotics; a potentially dangerous and ultimately self-defeating activity, as antibiotic use inevitably induces antibiotic resistance. It's natural selection in action.

Bugs breed faster than we do

Bacteria have a shorter life cycle than ours and DNA that is somewhat less stable, so they continually and rapidly produce variants on a genetic theme. Take one patient with a thriving bacterial infection. Impose an antibiotic on this genetically unruly mass of micro-organisms and if the right antibiotic was chosen, the vast majority of the bacteria die; leaving a few that the patient's immune system, if all goes well, can finish off.

However, if the antibiotic is given improperly (for example at too low a dose, or too infrequently), or the course is not finished by the patient, those bacteria which were slightly more resistant to the antibiotic survive in larger numbers. Among their descendants, those with the strongest resistance survive preferentially; and within a surprisingly short period of time, full-blown resistance can emerge.

Increasingly, however, the primary infection is caused by the resistant strains now prevalent in hospitals and in the community. The rising tide of 'superbugs' is a warning of bad times to come. Leading bacteriologists now believe that the world is running out of effective antibiotics, and it will be five years or more before new categories of drugs can be developed. There is exciting research going on into Quorum Sensor Blockers and Fluid Shear Sensor Blockers, fascinating strategies which may be less likely to engender resistance than the classical antibiotics, but these are still a long way from the market.

The warning that the age of infectious disease control is coming to an end was issued in early 2005 by the eminent Professor George Poste. Poste is Director of the Biodesign Institute at Arizona State University and an advisor to several US presidents. "Frankly, most governments are asleep at the switch," he said in a recent interview, "even though we are facing a relentless increase in antibiotic resistance across all classes of drug."

Poste's timing was pretty good. 2009 saw the first reports of the New Delhi Metallolactamase plasmid, a gene set that confers resistance to almost all antibiotics. It was initially discovered in minor bacterial species, but within months it made the jump to the major pathogen Klebsiella pneumoniae [21], which has already spread to many countries [22]. 2012 saw the first reports of Totally Drug-Resistant TB [24]. It is very nearly Game Over.

Mass Transport and the Spread of Pathogens

Millions of us commute on local transport systems that are over-crowded, and provide ideal conditions for the transmission of bacteria and viruses. Moreover, rapid global travel means that on any one day, a single passenger can contract a virus or bacterium on one continent and arrive in another before the first symptoms of illness emerge, thus avoiding early detection. And that passenger can be importing more pathogens than there are humans on the planet.

Which brings us to the topic of pandemics ....

The Flu Scare(s)

In the last decade we have seen outbreaks of H1N1 ('swine flu') and H5N1 ('bird flu'). We were lucky. Swine flu spread rapidly but was not very virulent; bird flu killed the majority of humans who contracted it but it did not spread easily between humans. Sooner or later, however, a flu strain will emerge which is both lethal and readily transmitted[15]. At the end of 2004 the World Health Organization (WHO) issued a stark warning of the pending flu global epidemic. According to Klaus Stohr of the WHO Global Influenza Programme, "There will be another pandemic. In the best case we expect billions to fall ill, with 2 to 7 million deaths – but it could be far worse."

Stohr and his colleagues are convinced that there will be a serious pandemic because history shows that flu pandemics occur every 30 years or so. After this time, the genetic makeup of a flu virus has changed so much that people have little or no immunity built up from previous strains.

There were three pandemics in the 20th century, all spread worldwide within a year of being detected. In 1918-19 the so-called Spanish Flu killed up to 50 million people. In the '50s the Asian Flu pandemic killed a million, and in 1968 Hong Kong Flu killed another million or so. That was 45 years ago.

Antibiotics are no use in treating viral infections, and the right vaccines to protect us against the new strain of flu will take up to 6 months to produce in large amounts – which will inevitably be too late for many. Anti-viral drugs such as Tamiflu are barely effective (23), and have done little more than stimulate the development of Tamiflu-resistant flu strains (24).

Flu is just one example of a class of diseases termed 'Zoonotic'. Zoonotic diseases are caused by infectious agents that can be transmitted between (or are shared by) animals and humans; in the case of flu the other main hosts are birds and pigs. Over 400 zoonotic diseases are known, and they are increasing in number; 45 new infections have been identified since 1990, an alarming rate of increase caused by human population and environmental pressures bringing people into contact with previously remote pockets of animals and their pathogens (25). Many of these are viral, and while we have specific drugs for HIV there are none for Crimean-Congo, Ebola, Lassa, Marburg, Nipah, SARS, West Nile, Novel Coronavirus ...

---

15. At the time of writing H7N9 is showing roughly 30% mortality and appears to be spreading.

It's time to take care of our immune systems

Of all the natural compounds known to enhance and activate the innate immune system, the best documented and most effective are the yeast-derived (1-3), (1-6) beta-glucans, technically a special class of carbohydrate [26-31]. When the Department of Defence of a senior NATO member state recently evaluated over 300 potential immuno-boosters, the highest score went to a proprietary (1-3), (1-6) beta-glucan produced by Biothera, a pharmaceutical company based in Minnesota and a leading research player in this field.

(1-3), (1-6) beta-glucans are complex molecules found in the cell walls of fungi and yeasts. These micro-organisms have always been a threat to animal species, and so the innate immune system long ago developed the ability to recognise beta-glucans and react to them by mounting an immune response.

But it went further than that. As yeasts are so universal, the innate immune system became acclimatised to their presence, and finally dependent on them to function at peak effectiveness. All immune cells possess CR3 receptors, which specifically recognise beta-glucans; and activation of the CR3 receptors by beta-glucans is essential for full and effective innate immune function [32].

In the second half of the 20th century, modern technology effectively sterilised the food chain. Levels of yeast and other fungi in our foods and in our immediate environment dropped away; and the lack of beta-glucans left the innate immune system weaker and out of balance. This is the more sophisticated version of the 'hygiene hypothesis' referred to previously. Adding beta-glucan back into the diet restores the effectiveness of the innate immune system, with considerable health benefits.

Not all beta-glucans are equal. Glucans are found in a variety of sources, including not only yeasts, moulds and fungi, but also cereal grains and bacteria. Each beta-glucan type has a distinct molecular structure that translates into unique biological activity; for example, the (1-3), (1-4) beta-glucans in cereal grains have little direct effect on the immune systems, but are good prebiotics. Extensive research shows that yeast-derived beta-glucans possess the greatest immune-enhancing characteristics. Interestingly, critical differences in the purity and sources of yeast beta-glucans can result in substantial differences in efficacy and safety. Impure yeast extracts containing mannoproteins may be ineffective or trigger an allergic reaction.

The following sequence explains how (1-3), (1-6) beta-glucans prime the immune system to work at a higher level of activity. It is provided by Biothera, a US company who use the term gluco-polysaccharides rather than (1-3), (1-6) beta glucans.

How (1-3), (1-6) beta-glucans work

Figure 1

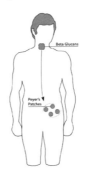

Im-
1. Once swallowed, whole gluco-polysaccharide particles pass through the stomach into the small intestine where they are taken up by M cells in specialised regions called Peyer's Patches **Fig. 1**).

Figure 2

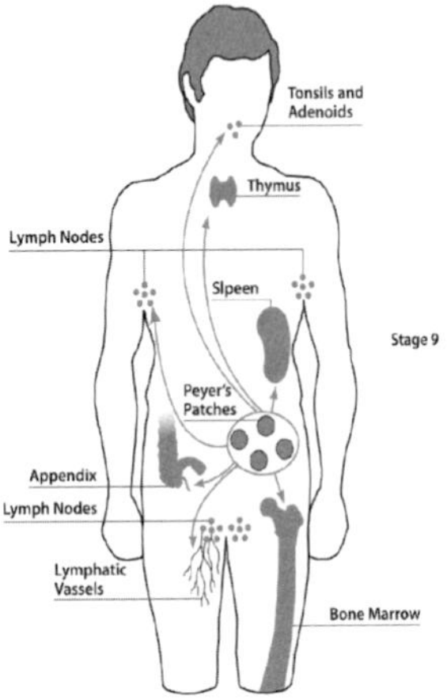

2. In the Peyer's patches, the gluco-polysaccharides are presented to circulating macrophages, immune cells whose function is to engulf and digest foreign invaders such as yeasts.

Macrophages have receptors which specifically recognise and bind gluco-polysaccharides (32). They convey the gluco-polysacharides to various regions of the immune system including the lymph nodes, bone marrow and thymus (**Fig 2**).

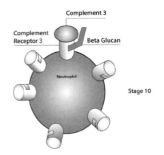

The macrophages break down the gluco-polysaccharides into smaller particles, and release them over a period of 24 to 36 hours. These active fragments bind or lock onto the surface of neutrophils, the most abundant immune cells in the body.

They lock on to a receptor called CR3 – Complement Receptor 3 (**Fig 3**).

Figure 3

The neutrophil is now activated or 'primed' and ready to react to foreign challenges or pathogens. The innate immune system is now fully activated, and resistance to infection is greatly enhanced (26, 33-34).

4. For a neutrophil to kill a pathogen or cancer cell with maximum effectiveness, the complement receptor must be occupied by complement (a blood protein), and the neighbouring CR3 receptor must be occupied by a gluco-polysaccharide.

The CR3 receptor is occupied naturally by gluco-polysaccharide in a fungal infection; but there are other threats including bacteria, viruses and cancer, where, in our over-sterile environment, beta-glucans are not present in sufficient amounts.

By taking gluco-polysaccharides in a food or supplement, the neutrophils are provided with the missing element they need to trigger their full natural killing mechanism.

4. A fully primed neutrophil now migrates to its target via a process called chemotaxis. Fig 4

Fig 4

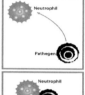

The neutrophil then binds to the surface of this pathogen or cancer cell and recognises it as 'non-self' i.e. foreign. It is now able to destroy the pathogen by releasing toxic chemicals.

6.   At the same time, other killer cells retain fragments of the pathogens that they have destroyed and 'present' them on their surface. These fragments – called antigens – send signals to other members of the immune system family, which become memory cells.

Next time the same pathogen is encountered these newly programmed memory cells will recognise it and produce antibodies. These antibodies stick to the surface of the pathogen and may destroy it, or prevent it from infecting healthy cells.
(See www.drpaulclayton.com for an animated explanation of the immune system.)

The Evidence: Reduced Infection

The beta-glucans' ability to activate macrophages and prime neutrophils has been extensively tested (35-41); and shown to protect animals against otherwise fatal infections (42-48).
In a pre-clinical trial conducted by Dr. Myra Patchen of Biothera, 90% of laboratory animals exposed to very high levels of E-coli survived when their innate immune systems were primed by the proprietary gluco-polysaccharide Wellmune WGP, as opposed to 0% survival in the control group.**(Figure 5)**

**Wellmune WGP Increases Survival
Against Deadly Bacteria**

% Survival

	CONTROL	Wellmune (5 mg/kg)	p-value
Escherichia coli 1.0 X 10⁶ CFU I.P.	0	90	<0.01
Staphylococcus aureus 1.0 X 10⁶ CFU I.P.	0	80	<0.03

Patchen, Alpha Beta Technology

Figure 4: In this animal experiment, subjects were injected
with a lethal dose of the gram-negative pathogen *Escherichia
coli* or the gram-positive pathogen *Staphylococcus aureus.*
In comparing the control group to animals treated with WGP
3-6, there was significant enhancement in survival from 0 to
80 to 90 percent.

In a further test, 80% of test animals survived
exposure to high levels of Staphylococcus aureus as opposed to 0% in the control group.

Studies like these obviously cannot be conducted with humans. However, clinical trials where
the (1-3), (1-6) beta-glucans have been shown to reduce the risk of post-operative sepsis, are
very much in line with the animal findings (49-52).

Synnergy with Antibiotics

In a petri dish, the right antibiotic at the right concentration will kill off all the bacteria present.
The clinical situation is more complex, and when antibiotics are given to treat an infection they
rarely if ever kill all of the pathogens; these may be hiding in different tissues, for example,
where the antibiotics do not penetrate well. In general, when an antibiotic is given to a sick
patient it works together with the immune system in the sense that it brings the numbers of
pathogens down to a level where the immune system can finish the job. If the immune system
is working well, the chances of success are greater. This is the rationale for co-prescribing beta
glucans with antibiotics.

In one experiment, when gluco-polysaccharides were administered in combination with antibiotics after exposure to bacteria, the number of bacteria needed to create infection was increased by up to 2,000 fold. **(Fig 6)**

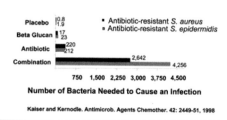

Synergistic with Drug Against Antibiotic-Resistant Bacterial Infections

Placebo |0.8 |1.9
Beta Glucan |17 |23
Antibiotic 220 212
Combination 2,642 4,256

- Antibiotic-resistant S. aureus
- Antibiotic-resistant S. epidermidis

750 1,500 2,250 3,000 3,750 4,500

Number of Bacteria Needed to Cause an Infection

Kaiser and Kernodle. Antimicrob. Agents Chemother. 42: 2449-51, 1998

Illustration 5: Biothera glucopolysaccharide synergizes with antibiotics against methicillin-resistant bacterial strains.

Given that so many people today are malnourished and immune-compromised, I believe that all elective surgery patients should take beta glucans before they enter hospital. The evidence (26, 53-54) also indicates that beta glucans should routinely be co-prescribed with antibiotics.

Effective Against Anthrax, Flu Viruses ...

Biothera conducted a particularly impressive series of experiments with the Canadian Department of Defence.

In the first study mice were given a daily dose of gluco-polysaccharides prophylactically before being exposed to a high dose of anthrax bacilli. Half of the control animals died within seven days, whereas 100% of the gluco-polysaccharide-treated group survived. In a second study beta-glucans were administered as a treatment *after* exposure to a lower dose of anthrax. This is a less effective way to take gluco-polysaccharides, but it models more accurately the situation where an individual or group might be accidentally exposed. In this trial there was 70% mortality in the control group, while in the group that received the gluco-polysaccharides mortality was reduced to under 20% (1, 3).

Studies on influenza showed a similar pattern. The LD50 is a dose that kills 50% of test animals, and the test rodents were exposed to a very high dose, ie 10 times the LD50. As predicted, all the control animals died; but in the group that received gluco-polysaccharides prophylactically, over 50% survived – a stunning result, and a degree of protection far in advance of any immunisation program (50).

Even more persuasively, the (1-3), (1-6) beta-glucans protect pigs. They reduce the harm done to the lungs after infection with swine flu virus, and reduce replication of the virus itself (56). As pigs and people have a good deal in common (metabolically and physiologically speaking), the pig model is very relevant to our own situation.

Radiation Protection, Chemo-Protection

The (1-3), (1-6) beta-glucans stimulate the regeneration of white blood cells after the bone marrow has been suppressed, either by exposure to radiation or chemotherapy. These treatments can be hazardous as they cause bone marrow suppression, leaving the patient vulnerable to overwhelming infection.

When Biothera's gluco-polysacharides were given at the same time as a normally lethal dose of radiation over 50% of the sample survived, in contrast to 100% mortality in control mice (57-58). The protective effects of the gluco-polysaccharides were mediated by accelerated regeneration of the bone marrow, and a faster restoration of white blood cell counts.

The US army was taking careful note of this. Starting in the late '80's, the Armed Forces Radiobiology Research Institute ran an exhaustive test programme to measure the immuno-protective effects of (1-3), (1-6) beta-glucans. As this confers protection against radiation injury bacteria and viruses, it has obvious defence applications. Given that soldiers may at any time face an unpredictable range of biological weapons and even, in the worst case, radiation, the US may begin to stock-pile these valuable and important nutrients.

Outside military and intensive medicine scenarios, bone marrow protection is also relevant to long haul air travellers who are exposed to much higher levels of cosmic radiation than at sea level, due to the absence of atmospheric shielding.

Immuno-Chemo Cancer Therapy

The immune system is only partially successful in fighting cancer, as cancer cells may not 'look' very different to normal cells, and the immune system does not always recognize them as non-self, and harmful. In fact it has been estimated that only 1 in 5 cancers triggers any sort of immune response at all.

It is only when the cancer cells become recognizably abnormal, that the immune system will attack them. The monoclonal antibody (MAb) anti-cancer drugs work by 'painting' cancer cells to make them recognizable as foreign by the immune system.

When beta-glucans are present – together with the blood protein Complement – on the CR3 receptor sites of neutrophils, those neutrophil cells are primed and, once they recognise the cancer cell as non-self, are far more likely to attack it effectively (59). (Illustration 6: CR3)

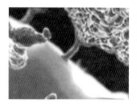

In this way gluco-polysaccharides enhance the effect of mono-clonal antibody anti-cancer drugs such as Herceptin and Avastin. This new form of cancer treatment, called immuno-chemotherapy, is currently showing stunning results. You will find data at www. biotherapharma.com

Ilustration 6: Neutrophils, the most abundant immune cell in the body, have special receptors called CR3 that bind to gluco polysaccharide. Once primed with gluco-polysaccharide, neutrophils are able to recognize and kill cancer cells that are marked with antibody and complement.

SUMMARY

Exposure to:	Survival rate with gluco-polysaccharide	Survival rate control group
E. coli	90%	0%
Staphylococcus aureus	80%	0%
Anthrax	100%	47%
Influenza	50%	0%
Radiation	55%	0%

Safety

Beta-glucans / gluco-polysaccharides are supplements, and the safety of any supplement is a priority.

Because they have always been in our environment and in our food, we can be confident that these yeast derivatives are non-toxic (60-61). This was accepted by the FDA. European regulatory authorities permit the sale of a range of these products and declared them safe for adults and children. They have been incorporated into a premium Mead Johnson baby formula that is available in Thailand, Taiwan and Mexico and will be launched more widely.

While the chronic use of so-called immuno-stimulants such as Echinacea may occasionally cause problems, the (1-3), (1-6) beta-glucans are not stimulants but immune-primers and essential for effective immune function. We evolved in a 'dirty' environment with high background levels of yeast and fungal contamination. Our innate immune systems are designed to cope with constant priming, and depend on it to function properly.

Pure beta-glucans do not trigger allergic symptoms, which involve the adaptive immune system. Indeed, by tricking the acquired immune system into 'thinking' that there is an on-going infection, they trigger changes in the adaptive immune system in a way which makes it more effective against many pathogens, and less likely to develop allergy symptoms (62-64).

CAUTION

Transplant patients should only use beta-glucans cautiously and under medical guidance. As the (1-3), (1-6) beta-glucans can enhance general immune function, they could theoretically increase the risk of graft rejection. Tests to date indicate that this does not occur in practice (65) but graft recipients should approach beta-glucans with caution.

Alternative Sources

Beta-glucans occur in several plants with a history of medicinal use such as aloe vera and Echinacea, and fungi such as Maitake and Shiitake mushrooms. These glucans have a different structure to those in yeast, and are not as effective in occupying the critical CR3 receptor. That is why they are not as good or as consistent immuno-primers as the beta-glucans or gluco-polysaccharides derived from yeast (66).

A recent animal study at the James Brown Cancer Centre showed Echinacea to have only a very minor effect on immune function when combined with Monoclonal Antibody cancer therapy. The 100 day survival rate was 10% with Echinacea and over 90% with Wellmune WGP. (Illustration 7)

Wellmune WGP is far superior to other immune supplements

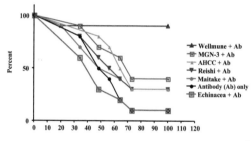

J. Yan, James Graham Brown Cancer Center, University of Louisville. 2006

The Adaptive Immune System

This is called the Adaptive Immune System because, after a first exposure to a pathogen it 'adapts' itself so that it can destroy the same germ the next time it encounters it. Its 'heroes' are lymphocytes (white blood cells) called B cells and T cells. Both B and T cells are made in the bone marrow. B cells grow in the marrow but T cells move out and mature in the Thymus (hence T cells). When mature, both cells travel via the blood stream to the lymphoid tissues – the lymph node, spleen, tonsils, adenoids, Peyer's patches, appendix etc. Some of these cells are relatively sedentary while others travel from site to site.

There are thousands of different B and T cells, each created to recognize one particular antigen – the little piece of pathogen displayed on the surface of a phagocyte. The antigens in turn stimulate the release of chemical messengers called cytokines which tell B and T cells to ramp up their attack on the foreign virus or bacteria. They do this by multiplying into a whole army of cloned cells, some of which become memory cells that ensure your immune system remembers each pathogen and can deal with it effectively should it ever encounter it again.

Much of the time you are unaware of all this drama acting out in your body. At other times swelling, heat and inflammation tell you that B and T cells are multiplying in the area of infection.

Vaccines stimulate the Adaptive Immune System and give you immunity in the same way as a 'real' bacterial or viral attack. By inoculating you with a pathogen that has been inactivated, your B cells are stimulated to produce antibodies as if the attack were real. In this way they create the memory of that yet-to-be encountered threat. The process of vaccination was first developed by Edward Jenner in the late 18th Century when he noticed that milk maids – who were exposed to cow pox – rarely contracted the closely-related small pox. (The word vaccination comes from vacca, the Latin for cow.)

Allergy and Auto-Immunity

Allergies are disorders where the immune system over-reacts to a normally harmless antigen like pollen. That can typically cause a runny nose or sneezing, since many allergies are inhalation-related, but in extreme cases the reaction can be anaphylactic shock – for example to peanuts.

An allergic reaction is essentially a cascade of interlinked cell-to-cell communications. Initially an allergen will bind to an IgE antibody which in turn binds to a type of immune cell called a mast cell, triggering it to release compounds called histamines. It is histamines that cause the symptoms of swelling, itching, runny eyes etc. These symptoms cause more inflammatory cells to mass at the site, a vicious circle that can damage tissue and lead to chronic illness like asthma.

The (1-3), (1-6) beta-glucans / gluco-polysacharides have an important role to play here. They do not act directly on the adaptive immune system. But they do influence it indirectly via a group of cells called mucosal dendrocytes, which act to coordinate innate and adaptive immune function. Elegant work at the University of Oslo and other sites has shown that when beta glucans are present, the mucosal dendrocytes instruct naïve T-Helper cells in the adaptive immune system to become TH1 cells; whereas when beta glucans are absent, naïve T-Helper cells tend to transform into TH2 cells.

Occasionally the immune system will turn on the body it is supposed to protect, resulting in an auto-immune disease. It does this when T cells and B cells – which normally ignore the body's own cells – malfunction and begin to attack the cells as if they were foreign. This is the case with diseases like lupus, Type 1 diabetes and rheumatoid arthritis. Since women are three times more likely to suffer from auto-immune disease, it is thought that hormones may play a role. Genes can be an important factor, and bacteria, viruses and exposure to certain toxic substances may also be involved.

Today's drugs designed to treat auto-immune disease are generally aimed at reducing inflammation. Some of these suppress the overall immune response and are associated with an increased risk of infection and cancer.

Nutrients which act in harness with the beta glucans

There is a small group of micronutrients which are particularly important for immune function but which are too often lacking. This group includes 'vitamin' D, the trace element selenium, iron and the cyanogens.

Vitamin D

In the temperate zones, most people are depleted in vitamin D for most of the year. In most cases this is not bad enough to cause rickets, but it is a key contributory factor to the common problems of osteopenia and osteoporosis.

D depletion also reduces the effectiveness of the innate immune system. A gene called Vitamin D3-Upregulated Protein 1 (VDUP1) plays a crucial role in directing stem cells to diversify into natural killer cells, key elements in the innate immune system. One of their functions is to eliminate virus-infected cells. If you are low in vitamin D fewer NK-cells are formed, and your innate immune defences against viruses become impaired. As another function of NK-cells is to kill tumour cells, D-depletion probably increases our risk of cancer, and is linked to increased mortality from all causes (67).

Adequate vitamin D is extremely important for your health. Leading experts in this area now state that as much as 4000 IU's a day, which is the amount you make in your own body by walking around in the sun without a shirt on for an hour or so (68) is the safe and effective dose (69-70). I absolutely agree - but you should note that the current RDA for vitamin D is only 200 IU's, with the US advising 400 IU's for the over 50's. The current UK official upper safe limit is a ludicrously low 1,000 IU's. However, there is active current discussion about increasing this upper safe limit and it is already assessed as 2,000 IU's in the USA. (See chapter 23).

Selenium

Selenium deficiency allows invading viruses to mutate and remain for a longer period in the host (71-72). Researchers at the University of North Carolina in Chapel Hill compared mice that received a selenium-deficient diet with non-deficient animals, all of which were exposed to the human influenza virus. The deficient mice had more severe cases of the flu that lasted for a longer period of time than the non-deficient mice.

Selenium depletion is prevalent in large parts of the world, including the UK (5-6). Accordingly, here is another dietary factor contributing to an increased risk of infection.
The current RDA is under question, and is also considered further in chapter 23.

Iron

Iron depletion and deficiency is one of the most commonly recognised nutritional problems world-wide. Iron is essential to many immune functions, and iron deficiency is linked to an increased risk of infections. Too much iron, however, may be counter-productive, as iron is also essential for many bacteria. Immune cells fight against bacteria in many ways, including the sequestration (removal) of iron which the microbes need (73). This is probably why chronic infections often present with anaemia; giving iron in this situation may actually assist the pathogens.

Cyanogens and iodine

One of the key elements in the innate immune system is an enzyme called lactoperoxidase (LPO), which defends the gut, lungs and mammary glands against pathogens. This is a ferro-protein (ie it requires iron), and it also requires thiocyanate groups, derived from the diet, to kill and disable bacteria and viruses. Dietary sources of thiocyanates include glucosinolates (typically from brassica) and cyanogenic glycosides (typically from sweet potatoes). Our intakes of vegetables are at an historical low. Consider eating more of these! LPO also utilises iodine, and here too there is evidence of wide-spread depletion (74-76) due to such issues as cutting down on salt and switching from table salt to (non-iodinated) sea salt. Consider an iodine supplement, or an iodine-rich snacks such as Nori.

Frequently Asked Questions

1. **Can (1-3), (1-6) beta glucans trigger yeast allergy?**
   Some people have concerns about yeast because they have been told to avoid brewer's or baker's yeast as it somehow increases the risk of Candida infections. Others believe, rightly or wrongly, that they are allergic to it. These concerns are misplaced. The Candida story was popularised by untrained persons who mistakenly believed that brewer's yeast and Candida were closely related species, which is not the case. Although allergy to yeast can occur, the reaction is to manno-proteins which occur in yeast cell walls. Properly purified beta-glucan / gluco-polysaccharide preparations are free of manno-protein, and are anti-allergenic.

2. **Can antibiotics be counter-productive?**
   Antibiotics have their place. However, the over-enthusiastic use of antibiotics has caused substantial problems of antibiotic resistance. Antibiotics kill both the bad *and* the good intestinal flora, which can disturb the complex bacterial ecosystem and allow harmful bacteria to flourish. This kind of bacterial imbalance, known as dysbiosis, is coming under suspicion as a cause of chronic inflammation of the gastro-intestinal tract and intestinal cancers, and a contributory factor for Alzheimer's, Parkinson's, multiple sclerosis and autism.

3. **When should I give children antibiotics?**
   Broadly, children with sore throats should not be given antibiotics UNLESS lab tests show a strep or other bacterial infection. Bronchitis or non-specific coughs rarely warrant antibiotics, UNLESS the symptoms last more than 10 days, and a particular bacterium is suspected; and in cases where there is an underlying lung disease such as cystic fibrosis - but not asthma.
   Antibiotics should not be given for the common cold, even when there is a nasal discharge (this is fairly normal); and whereas short courses of antibiotics should be given for acute middle ear infections (otitis media), they are not indicated for otitis media with effusion. This is a subtle but vital distinction which the doctor makes when he/she first sees the child. If an antibiotic is going to do the job properly it must be taken for the duration of the recommended course. Antibiotics don't work right away. Most children take a couple of days to start to feel better, yet some parents assume that the drugs aren't working and stop after the first dose. Others stop once the child has started to improve, and do not finish the course. These strategies greatly increase the risk of resistance developing; as does the practice of re-using antibiotics that may have been lying around at home from a previous bout, or even belonged to someone else.

   The problems of drug resistance are too important to be left to specialist infection control teams. We all have a responsibility to ensure antibiotics are used properly, and an important role to play if we want to be able to continue to rely on antibiotics when we really need them.

Chapter 11. Key Anti-Inflammatory Nutrients #2: Omega-3 Fatty Acids

The **Omega-3 fatty acids** have a critically important anti-inflammatory mode of action, which complements and extends the beneficial effects of the (1-3), (1-6) beta-glucans. The fatty acids in cell membranes are substrates for two groups of enzymes called COX and LOX. When these enzymes break down saturated fatty acids and Omega-6 fatty acids in our cell membranes they generate pro-inflammatory metabolites such as IL-1 beta, IL-2, IL-6 and TNF-alpha; when they break down Omega-3 fatty acids they form anti-inflammatory metabolites (1-2). If Omega-3 fatty acids predominate in cell membranes we tend not to suffer from chronic inflammation, and are protected against degenerative disease. If Omega-3 fatty acids are in the minority, and our cell membranes are dominated by saturated and Omega-6 fatty acids, we are more likely to suffer from chronic inflammation and degenerative disease. This is particularly true in individuals with specific genetic vulnerabilities, such as variants of the enzymes delta-6-desaturase and delta-5-desaturase (3).

The relative amounts of the different fatty acids in our cell membranes are determined by the relative amounts of the different fatty acids in our diet. This has changed dramatically over the last century or so (4-5). Between 1909 and 1999 the estimated per capita consumption of soybean oil increased more than 1000-fold, whereas consumption of oily fish declined (5). Accordingly, intakes of the Omega-6 fatty acid Linoleic acid (LA) increased from 2.79% to 7.21% of energy. At the same time there were substantial declines in intakes (as a percentage of energy) of the essential Omega-3 PUFA's eicosapentaenoic acid (EPA), and docosahexaenoic acid (DHA).

In the typical Western diet the ratio of Omega-6 to Omega-3 essential fatty acids in the diet (and therefore in cell membranes) is now as high as 20, 40 or 100 to 1. These abnormal and excessive Omega-3/Omega-6 ratios drive the pathogenesis of all the chronic inflammatory diseases including cardiovascular disease, cancer, depressive illness and the auto-immune diseases (1-2, 6). Conversely, a lower ratio enhances tissue functions, reduces or stops chronic inflammation, and improves or prevents many disease states. For example, whereas an Omega-6/Omega-3 ratio of 10:1 or higher exacerbates asthma, a ratio of 5:1 reduces asthmatic patients' symptoms, and a ratio between 3:1 and 2:1 suppresses inflammation and its related symptoms in patients with rheumatoid arthritis (7-8).

Both Omega-3 and Omega-6 fatty acids are referred to as Polyunsaturated Fatty Acids or PUFA's. Despite all the evidence, some governments still recommend increased intakes of all PUFA's, including the Omega-6 fatty acids from plant oils. This advice is ignorant and dangerous. A recent 7 year study of 458 Australian men who had already had one heart attack (the Sydney Diet Heart Study), substituting the Omega-6 PUFA linoleic acid in place of saturated fats *increased* the rates of death from all causes, coronary heart disease, and cardiovascular disease (9).

To optimise immune and inflammatory function, and reduce our terrible and unnecessary burden of disease, we should increase our intakes of beta-glucans, polyphenols and Omega-3 fatty acids. But while producing (and eating) more beta-glucans and polyphenols is relatively easy, there is a limit to the amount of Omega-3 fatty acids we can haul out of the seas. In fact, if you do the math, there is not enough fish in the sea to feed every human even the minimum 250 mg intake that many countries are recommending, and not nearly enough to provide the 5 grams or more that science now indicates is needed for optimal health (10).

In order to provide enough EPA and DHA to support the human population, we will need to find alternative sources. Fortunately, new sources have been identified. Seaweeds are being commercially developed in Spain and Japan, and on land there is the flowering plant Echium vulgare, also known as Purple Viper's Bugloss or Blueweed.

Echium vulgare is a weed native to most of Europe, and western and central Asia. It is also common in North America. It grows wild and free, but in future you will be seeing this plant being grown intensively in fields near you – because it is an excellent source of an Omega-3 fatty acid called stearidonic acid (SDA. Stearidonic acid is a minor Omega 3 component in fish, making up no more than 2% of their total fatty acids (11); but it occurs in echium seed at around 12.5% of total fatty acids.

This makes echium oil unique because in most plant oils, the predominant Omega-3 fatty acid is alpha-linolenic acid (ALA). When we consume the common plant oils we can convert some of the ALA they contain to the essential Omega-3 fatty acids EPA and DHA, but this is a complex and inefficient process.

And now we have to look (briefly!) at some basic biochemistry.

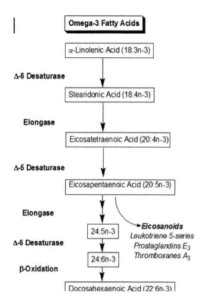

This figure shows why alpha-linolenic acid (ALA) is such a poor source of the essential Omega-3 fatty acids EPA and DHA. The conversion of ALA to EPA requires a chain of three different enzyme-catalysed reactions (above), and is very inefficient. In women conversion is generally around 5% and in men it is far less (12). This is because of the rate-limiting first step in the reaction chain; the enzyme delta-6-desaturase, which converts ALA to SDA, is very ineffective.

This is why so-called 'healthy oils' such as flaxseed or evening primrose oils, which are crammed with ALA, are not worth bothering with. They offer no protection whatever against heart disease (13-14) and are unlikely to offer any health benefits (15).

The next two steps in the chain, involving the enzymes elongase and delta-5-desaturase, are much more efficient. The body converts about 30% of SDA to EPA (16), making SDA six times more effective as a source of the essential Omega-3 fatty acids than the more common ALA.

The high conversion rate of SDA means that it would be possible to use echium and similar oils as a good substitute for fish oils (if fish oils become too expensive or disappear altogether), to optimise our cell membranes and thus protect us from excessive inflammation. Human studies have confirmed this. SDA supplements can be given to increase the EPA content of human tissues and cell membranes, and are roughly five times more effective at doing this than ALA (16, 17-18).

SDA not only offers us an inexpensive and natural way to achieve better health (19), but it is also clean-tasting and eminently suitable for vegetarians and vegans. What is more, there is emerging evidence that SDA has anti-inflammatory (18, 20-21), cardio-protective (22-23) and cancer-protective (15, 24) benefits of its own, as well as its ability to act as a precursor for EPA and DHA.

The agri-biotech company Monsanto has developed an even richer source of SDA, from genetically modified soy beans. This new soy oil, called Soymega SDA, has been shown to increase levels of EPA and DHA when consumed by humans (25-26). Alternatively it can be used to improve the nutritional profile of foods we eat, as it boosts EPA and DHA levels when fed to fish (427-28), chickens (29) and cows (30), which then produce Omega-3 enriched milk. Soy is an entirely inappropriate platform due to its high content of Omega 6's, but Monsanto owns soy and IS more interested in promoting soy than health.

Canola is a much smarter starting point as its levels of Omega 6 are far lower, and a GM canola project is underway in Canada. For those who fear GM there is a new natural source of SDA on the market which is derived from Buglossoides arvensis aka Sheepweed. This plant is related to Purple Viper's Bugloss, but provides higher levels of SDA. Marketed as Ahiflower oil (who would buy Sheepweed oil?), this may well win the commercial stakes.

Chapter 12. Oily Fish or Fish Oil?

There is little doubt that regularly consuming oily fish used to be healthy. In the late '70's, pioneering Danish researchers Hans Olaf Bang and Jørn Dyerberg discovered that the Eskimos, whose diet consisted mainly of meat and blubber of seal and whale and relatively small amounts of oily fish, were substantially protected against cardiovascular disease and had very low rates of the diseases now known to be caused by chronic inflammation, such as cancer and heart disease. The Danes soon worked out that this protection was related to the Omega-3 fatty acids in their food (1-4). A number of studies subsequently confirmed Bang and Dyerberg's ideas, and Omega-3 fatty acids became the poster child for improved health through nutrition. A recent Harvard study which calculated that Omega 3's deficiency was killing 96,000 Americans per year (5) drove Omega 3 awareness even higher.

Today, millions of health-conscious consumers swallow purified fish oil, some in the old-fashioned bottled format but mostly in capsules, in the belief that these supplements encapsulate the Eskimo diet and will help to keep them healthy. This faith in fish oil, however, appears to be largely misplaced.

One little-known aspect of the Eskimo diet is that Eskimos traditionally consumed the bulk of their food raw or dried; it was seldom cooked or exposed to excessive heat. (Fuel was scarce in the Far North until Western companies started to deliver bulk fuel oils in the '80's.) Most sophisticated urbanites would reather swallow purified, de-odorised fish oil capsules than spend their evenings chowing down on whale meat and seal blubber, but highly processed fish oil capsules are a long way from the real Eskimo diet and may do more harm than good[16].

Whale oil is hard to find today, and detailed chemical analyses of unprocessed whale oil are scarce. What we do know, however, is that unprocessed and unrefined whale oil was mid to dark brown in colour, and – despite its content of Omega-3 faty acids, exceptionally stable. This can only mean that the unprocessed oil, as it occurred in the Inuit diet, was rich in ancillary compounds that protected it against oxidation. The dietary carotenoids do not match this colour, and it is far more likely that the dark brown coloration of unprocessed whale oil is due to polyphenols derived originally from brown algae, via krill.

Most polyphenols are water-soluble, but a few of them are oil-soluble. The phlorotannins, a sub-class of polyphenols found in the cold water marine algae that produce the Omega 3 fatty acids, belong to the oil-soluble category. They are extremely effective in preventing the oxidation of Omega-3 fatty acids; so much so that they are being developed for use in industrial fish processing to prevent spoilage (6). Equally importantly they are potent anti-inflammatory, anti-ageing agents (7) with additional properties that should reduce the risk of Alzheimer's (8) and cancer (9). They are also dark brown.

16. Like all PUFA's the Omega-3 faty acids are vulnerable to oxidation which is why, in nature, they are always protected by antioxidants. At the base of the marine food chain, the algae which produce EPA and DHA are protected by multiple antioxidants including the polyphenol phlorotannins; as are the krill which eat the algae, the fish and whales that eat the krill, and the seals which eat\ the fish. Only humans consume purified Omega-3 fatty acids – and most humans today are depleted in antioxidants. This is a recipe for trouble, as oxidised omega 3 fatty acids are pro-inflammatory.

This is only circumstantial evidence, and I am still waiting for some bright chemist to do the requisite analytical work on whale oil, but it looks very much as if the Inuit diet contained high levels of both Omega-3's *and* oil-soluble polyphenols. If the scientists and companies that rushed to commercialise purified fish oils had been more holistic, and less pharmaceutical, we might not have fallen into the current fish oil trap.

The nature of this trap is only now becoming evident. Studies at the University of Tromso in Norway recently found that the industrial processes used to extract fish oil destroy or remove the trace ingredients in fish (such as the polyphenols) that played a critical role in conferring their original health benefits, and greatly reduce the anti-inflammatory effects of the oil (10). In fact, the removal of antioxidants and other trace compounds creates a situation where the purified fish oils can become pro-oxidative (11-15), pro-inflammatory (16-17), and cause increased DNA damage (15). Worryingly, there is evidence that older subjects – ie the bulk of those who take Omega-3 supplements – are intrinsically more vulnerable to its pro-oxidative effects (18), probably because they are not eating enough antioxidants to compensate for the Omega-3's (13).

This matters. A series of Norwegian studies have shown multiple negative effects of purified fish oils; ranging from biochemical markers such as increased inflammatory cytokines and oxidative stress (19-20, 28-29) to clinical end-points including increased angina and atheroma (21). The DART 2 trial, the only clinical trial lasting more than four years, showed that fish oil capsules actually *increase* the risk of heart disease and sudden death (22). And to close the debate, a recent and very large meta-analysis (which reviewed 20 studies involving 68,680 patients) showed that supplementing with purified omega-3 PUFA's was *not* associated with a lower risk of all-cause mortality, cardiac death, sudden death, myocardial infarction, or stroke based on relative and absolute measures of association (23). No benefits at all!

Eating oily fish, however, reduces all-cause and coronary heart mortality (24), so here is a strong argument for throwing the capsules away and going back to eating wild salmon, herring and mackerel. But there may be a problem here too. Fish are not necessarily what they used to be, and it is possible that eating them may not be as cardio-protective as it used to be (25). Thanks to industrial pollution there are significant levels of contaminants in fish today including mercury, which can potentially harm the heart and other organs. Intake of fish is a major source of exposure to mercury, and some scientists believe this may overcome the beneficial effects of the Omega-3 fatty acids in the fish (26-27).

In this situation, the best way forwards may be to take purified fish oils that are free of contaminants, but fortified with the right antioxidants to provide a dual anti-inflamatory and antioxidative package. Vitamin E, the antioxidant most commonly used in fish oil capsules, is not the right candidate. It may protect the oils while they are in the capsule, but it does not protect them once they have been consumed. Supplementing the diet with purified Omega-3 fatty acids increases lipid peroxidation, as measured by plasma MDA release and lipid peroxide products, and this is *not* suppressed by vitamin E supplementation (30).

Anti-inflammatory Antioxidants

Some of the most potent antioxidants in the diet are polyphenols, important dietary compounds derived from various fruits and vegetables. Many of these not only protect cholesterol from oxidation in the body, but also target the linings of the blood vessels and other tissues, where they act as potent anti-inflammatory agents (31). Adding the right polyphenols back into overly refined fish oils would replace the anti-inflammatory compounds and effects lost during refining, and enable the fish oils to regain their original anti-inflammatory benefits.

One international group of scientists based in Norway and Italy focussed not on marine algae but on the olive, an important constituent of the Mediterranean diet. Olive fruits and leaves contain anti-inflammatory antioxidants that survive cooking, and are well absorbed when eaten. These compounds are called secoiridoids, and like the phlorotannins these polyphenols are oil-soluble. The best known secoiridoid is called oleuropein. Oleuropein is metabolised in the body to compounds which have exactly the right combination of anti-inflammatory and antioxidant properties that make the Mediteranean diet so cardio-protective (32-33).

Once the olive compounds enter the blood they become integrated into the lipoproteins which carry cholesterol round the body, and protect both the lipoproteins and the cholesterol from oxidation (34-35). (It is almost certain that the phlorotannins do exactly the same thing.)

Oxidized lipoproteins and oxidized LDL cholesterol play a fundamental role in the development of atherosclerosis leading to heart attack and stroke. Oxidized cholesterol compounds are highly toxic; they damage the linings of the arteries, creating foci of inflammation which are now thought to be the initial step in the process of cardiovascular disease.

The olive compounds protect the cholesterol from oxidation, and at the same time target the artery walls and quench any inflammation that may have already started there (36). This is a powerfully cardio-protective strategy, and if we add Omega-3 fatty acids then we achieve a very potent anti-inflammatory and cardio-protective environment (37-40). It is not the Eskimo diet or the Mediteranean diet, but a combination of the best of both.

New pharmaceutical research, which combines fish oils with aspirin, shows that this is a highly effective way to suppress chronic inflammation (41). This represents progress from the medical / pharmaceutical complex, but it is a sub-optimal strategy with adverse effects inclusing peptic ulceration and haemorrhagic stroke. The fish oil & oil-soluble polyphenol combination would protect against both, and provide many more benefits. Eating two portions of oily fish a week has already been shown to reduce the risk of premature death by a quarter (27); adding polyphenols would, in my estimate, reduce the risk of premature death by 75% or more.

More on polyphenols in the next chapter.

Chapter 13. Nutrition & Politics: The Armed Forces

The Omega-3 story has been building for many years, thanks to the work of such outstanding scientists as Professors Michael Crawford, John Stein, Joe Hibbeln, John Brenna, Stephen Cunane, Philip Calder, Helga Refsum, Andy Sinclair, Peter Willatts and others; but even though the science to support wide-spread supplementation of the Western diet with Omega-3's is overwhelming, the politicians who profess an interest in public health have ignored it. They don't care that our unbalanced diet is not only harming us physically but also imposing a huge burden – individually and socially – of depressive illness and suicide. One of the most common disorders of our times, depression is unequivocally related to a diet depleted in Omega-3 fatty acids, and it responds well to Omega-3 supplementation (1-6).

But now the military are involved. Suicide rates among US military personnel on active duty are at record numbers, doubling since the quaintly named Operations 'Enduring Freedom' (Afghanistan) and 'Iraq Freedom' (Iraq). The Pentagon, concerned that the recent escalation of US military suicide deaths to record numbers is not only bad PR but is also impairing the effectiveness of their disastrous foreign policy adventures, has accelerated the search for reversible risk factors. In a recent study they found, firstly, that their boys and girls had VERY low levels of Omega-3 fatty acids in their blood; in other words, the serving personnel were eating the usual junk served by the cheap-skates and profiteers who run the army catering corps. And secondly, they found that those with the lowest levels of Omega-3's in their blood were the most at risk of committing suicide (7).

Extrapolating from this military study, it seems very likely that the current pandemic of depressive illness and self-harm up to and including suicide is exacerbated by the huge quantities of soy, corn and other vegetable oils we consume, and the diminishing amount of fish oils. Such a diet produces a dangerously high Omega 6/ 3 ratio in the body and brain. And this, in turn, emphasises the potential importance of stearidonic acid, introduced in the previous chapter.

I first understood what stearidonic acid could do back in the early 90's, and made enquiries with the UK-based company that was starting to grow Bugloss and extract its SDA-rich oil. I wanted to use this oil in supplements and in functional foods because I knew a number of depressive patients who were vegetarian and would not eat fish or fish oil. The regulators would not allow it. Bugloss was not a food plant, they said, the oil was experimental and could not be fed to humans. I told them the oil was pure, had been fully characterised, that SDA was a natural part of human fatty acid metabolism. In vain. Idiot bureaucracy won the day and has contributed to too much depression, too many deaths, and too much anti-social behaviour since then.

Chapter 14. Nutrition and Politics: Sport and the 5-Ring Circus

Reliable figures are thin on the ground, but it is hard to escape the impression that both atrial fibrillation (AF) and sudden cardiac death (SCD) are becoming more common in athletes. There may be some common causative, nutritional factors.

If AF is indeed increasing among athletes and sportspersons, it is doing no more than keeping up with the increase in AF in the general population. Atrial fibrillation is the most common abnormality of heart beat. Its prevalence doubles with each decade of age, from 0.5% at age 50-59 years to almost 9% at age 80-89 years. It is also becoming very much more prevalent, increasing in men aged 65-84 years from 3.2% in 1968-1970 to 9.1% in 1987-1989 (1), and until very recently nobody really knew why.

AF sufferers describe their condition as like having a bag of snakes writhing around inside the chest; and although it is unlikely to kill you right away, it does increase the risk of stroke, heart attack and heat failure. The drugs currently used to treat AF are not always effective and are quite toxic, so it would be very useful to be able to prevent it from developing in the first place.

The Omega-3's in fish oil have long been known to reduce mortality after a heart attack (2-3). They do this by reducing myocardial electrical excitability, and hence the potentially fatal ventricular arrhythmias that so often follow the heart attack; and by up-regulating the heart's antioxidant enzyme systems (4). Now fish oils have been shown to be associated with reduced arrhythmias in the upper heart also. In a survey of 3,326 US men and women with an average age of 74, the incidence of AF was 30% lower in those with the highest levels of DHA and EPA in their blood, than those with the lowest levels of these Omega 3 fatty acids (5). The cardio-protective effects of fish oil were further demonstrated by trials which showed that in AF patients that had been electro-converted (ie shocked back into normal rhythm), the rate of AF recurrence was reduced by long-term supplementation with Omega-3's (6-7). There is also evidence that Omega-3's exert immediate anti-arrhythmic effects (8).

As the electrochemistry of the upper heart is fundamentally the same as the electrochemistry of the lower heart, these findings makes perfect sense, and they provide a plausible explanation as to why the rates of AF are rising; they are probably being driven up by our declining intakes of oily fish. But I doubt this is the whole story. There is evidence that lowered intakes of magnesium may also be involved, and for us elderly chaps and athletes who would like to reduce the risk of AF even further, there is a case for adding magnesium supplements to our daily fish or fish oil (9-11).

Sudden cardiac death is a more serious proposition, but here too there are almost certainly nutritional factors, which can be modified. Even today, many athletes are still eating terrible diets based on chicken, pasta and soy products; a diet depleted in antioxidants and the anti-inflammatory beta-glucans, Omega-3's and polyphenols.

In older athletes (ie above the age of 35), SCD is generally caused by atherosclerotic disease, which affects them in the same way as it affects the general population. In younger athletes, however, we must look for other causes. In this latter group the risk of SCD is low, at around 1 case in every 200,000 (12-13), but this is still three times higher than in sedentary people (14).

Autopsies reveal that about half of SCD athletes have congenital anatomical abnormalities of the heart or have developed left ventricular hypertrophy due to training (15-17). Another 25% have genetic channelopathies, which affect ion transfers into and out of heart muscle cells and render them more vulnerable to arrhythmias (18). The final 25% of SCD in this group is idiopathic, ie its origins are unknown. In all groups the final, fatal sequence involves ventricular arrhythmia, either tachycardia or fibrillation.

As the incidence of congenital myocardial defects is likely to be identical in athletes and non-athletes, the three-fold increase in the risk of SCD in athletes must be due to left ventricular hypertrophy and the last, unknown category. The unknown category cannot, by definition, be screened out, and the group with left ventricular hypertrophy (which is a physiological adaptation and not in itself normally dangerous), can be difficult to differentiate from the hearts of non-athletes with heart disease (15).

If we cannot screen out the vulnerable, we should at least consider prophylactic strategies. Due to the evidence that a diet depleted in Omega-3 fatty acids makes both upper and lower heart arrhythmias more likely, Omega-3 supplementation seems a logical approach. However, the fact that it is not consistently protective (19) indicates that there must be other factors involved.

Intensive physical exercise creates oxidative and inflammatory stress (20). Myocardial arhythmias are linked to both oxidative stress (21-23) and inflammatory stress (24-25); and it is therefore highly likely that these are exacerbating and contributory factors in SCD. A simple combination of Omega-3's and polyphenols and magnesium would address all these problems, and reduce the risk of AF and SCD, without any downside. A completist would add an antioxidant program designed to support the main Redox ladder[17].

When such a nutritional program was proposed by a colleague to one (nameless) national Olympic Committee, they responded with insults. Sponsorship and spectacle are more important to certain Olympic administrators than the health and safety of the athletes who are the beating and vulnerable heart of the Games.

There is another apect to the exercise / omega 3 story, which is perhaps more relevant to the occasional and amateur athlete. Anyone who takes up a sport – or just changes his /

---

17. 'Redox ladder' describes the sequence whereby lipid peroxides are made safe in the body, under conditions of nutrient repletion. It typically starts with lipid peroxidation and ends with the excretion of the relatively stable ascorbate radicals in the urine. An antioxidant program designed to support the ladder would include lipophiles such as the tocopherols, tocotrienols, carotenoids and xanthophyls; a swing lipophile such as lycopene, and an asscorbate base. Polyphenols duplicate many but not all of these actions.

her routine – will be familiar with the dreaded post-exercise muscle pains that put so many off exercise. These have little to do with lactic acid build-up, and relate more to muscular micro-damage and inflammation (26-29). 1Life, an omega-3 / polyphenol combination, is highly effective in preventing the inflammation and the pain (personal experience).

Chapter 15. Your Omega-6 / -3 ratio, and how it reflects your diet

The Omega 6/3 ratio is critical in determining overall health, but doctors do not have access to the kind of technology needed to determine this ratio either in the diet or, more importantly, in the body. There is only one test available at this time; the 1Life Test, which was developed at the University of Trondheim.

This test generates an entire fatty acid profile. It gives an overview of the 11 different fatty acids present in your blood, and explains exactly what this means. The fatty acid profile is a reflection of the fatty acids in the diet, and test results provide the basis for dietary recommendations.

The 1Life test has been used to generate the largest human data base of fatty acid profiles in the world, with very large samples taken in Europe, North America, India and elsewhere. It was used as the basis for supplementing with a proprietary omega 3 / polyphenol combination which has been used with remarakable effects in a series of informal studies in Northern Europe.

In one ongoing trial, by far the largest of its kind, a total of over 15,000 subjects have now been tested in 8 countries on 4 continents. The latest results are shown below. People who did not take any fish oils supplements had an unhealthy 6/3 ratio of over 12 to1. Those taking a standard fish oil scored somewhat better at roughly 7 to 1, but only those who took the omega 3 / polyphenol combination achieved the ideal 2.5 to 1 ratio.

Trial Group	Individuals tested	Omega-6/Omega-3 balance
Group A. Do not take Omega-3 supplements	8396	12,4:1
Group B. Take a daily Omega-3 supplement	4107	6,7:1
Group C. Take Omega 3 / polyphenols for 3-4 months	1172	2,5:1
Total	13675	

This omega 3 / polyphenol combination was trialled with the Norwegian fotball club Lillestrøm Sports Club. LSK (www.lsk.no) had been plagued by illness and injuries during preparation for the 2008/2009 season, so they started a Preventative Health programme in October 2009 which included the omega 3 / polyphenol combination. At the outset the players had an omega 6:3 ratio of 12, but after supplementing this fell to 3. The effects were remarkable. Absence due to illness in the 2009/10 season fell by 85%, and absence due to injury fell by 57%, giving the players an additional 42 days per month to train together. Their physical test results improved significantly and the club made substantial progress in the foortball league.

Fatty acids in Foods

The fatty acids in your blood come from your diet. Almost all foods contain fatty acids, and any one food product can contain many different fatty acids. For example, milk and milk products contain C16: 0 palmitic acid (saturated), C18: 0 stearic acid (saturated) and C18: 1 oleic acid (monounsaturated). Almonds contain C18: 0 stearic acid (saturated), C18: 1 oleic acid (monounsaturated) and C18: 2 linoleic acid (polyunsaturated), together with other fatty acids.

Tables 1a and 1b provide examples of the different fatty acids in different food sources. Table 1a.

Palmitic acid C16:0 Saturated	Stearic acid C18:0 Saturated	Oleic acid C18:1 Omega-9	Linolic acid C18:2 Omega-6	Alpha- Linolenic acid C18:3 Omega-3*
Milk and milk products such as butter, cream, ice cream, sour cream, yoghurt, cheese	Milk and milk products, such as butter, cream, ice cream, sour cream, yoghurt, cheese and more	Vegetable oils such as olive, palm, rapeseed, corn, sesame, sunflower, Soy	Vegetable oils such as rapeseed, corn, sesame, sunflower, soy, linseed, olive and palm oils	Vegetable oils such as rapeseed and linseed oil
Red meat and meat products	Red meat and meat products	Red meat and meat products. Bovine fat and tallow		Spinach, brussels sprouts
	Pork meat, fat and pork products	Pork meat, fat and pork products Bovine fat and tallow	Pork meat, fat and pork products Bovine fat and tallow	Berries ie blueberries, lingonberry
Palm oil and products that contain palm oil such as pastry, crackers, fried potatoes, potato chips etc		Palm oil and products that contain palm oil	Palm oil and products that contain palm oil	
Coconut and coconut oil	Lamb	Fish oil		

Products of cocoa and cocoa butter ie chocolate	Products of cocoa and cocoa butter	Products of cocoa and cocoa butter		
Avocado		Avocado	Avocado	
Poultry and poultry products	Poultry and poultry products	Poultry and poultry products	Poultry and poultry products	
Egg and egg products		Egg and egg products	Egg and egg products	
Nuts such as almonds, peanuts and brazil nuts		Almonds, peanuts, walnuts, hazelnuts, brazil nuts	Almonds, peanuts, walnuts, hazelnuts, brazil nuts	Walnuts
Wheat and wheat products		Wheat and wheat products	Wheat and wheat products	

Gamma-linoleic acid C18:3 Omega-6	dihomo-Gamma-Linoleic acid C20:3 Omega-6	Arachidonic acid (AA) C20:4 Omega-6	Eicosapent-aenoic acid (EPA) C20:5 Omega-3	Docosapent-aenoic acid (DPA) C22:5 Omega-3	Docosah-exsaenoic acis (DHA) C22:6 Omega-3
Minor amounts in plant oils and meat	Minor amounts in evening primrose oil and blackcurrant seeds	Red meat and meat products	Oily fish	Oily fish	Oily fish
		Pork meat, fat and pork products	Cod liver	Cod liver	Cod liver
		Lamb and lamb products	Seafood and algae	Seafood and algae	Seafood and algae
		Poultry and poultry products	1Life Active products	1Life Active products	1Life Active products
		Egg and egg products			

*Alpha-linolenic acid (ALA) is a plant-derived Omega-3 fatty acid, but it is not a good source of the Omega 3's we need. Only 1-5 % of ingested ALA is converted to EPA and even less to DHA in the body. Conversion is even lower if the diet contains large amounts of the plant-derived Omega-6 fatty acid linoleic acid (LA), since alpha-linolenic acid and linoleic acid compete for the same enzymes for conversion (1).

The 1Life Test

The 1Life test measures approximately 98% of the fatty acids in the blood and gives a profile of 11 different fatty acids including saturated, monounsaturated (omega 9) and polyunsaturated (omegas 6 and 3)

A comprehensive report is then produced which includes:

- An explanation of how evolution has affected diet and health
- Dietary indicators
  - Your omega 3 levels
  - the omega 6/3 balance,
  - arachidonic acid formation efficiency,
  - cell membrane fluidity index (this measures how efficiently your cells interact with their environment)
  - mental strength index (this reflects mood and cognitive status)

All these values are accompanied by easy to understand explanations.

- Dietary advice
  - long term (dietary suggestions)
  - fast track (how to rectify levels using supplementation)
  - maintenance recommendations
  - special arachidonic dietary advice (if required)
  - The report include a section for those who engage in regular sport

The test is carried out at St Olav's Hospital, Trondheim, Norway.

You perform the test in your own home. It requires a few drops of blood from a finger prick which are absorbed onto a special filter paper. The test kit holds all the equipment and information required. You then stamp the pre-addressed envelope and return the sample to St Olav's Hospital. The test is completely anonymous. It contains a unique user code which you then use to access your results and report by typing it in online at www.1life63.com. Results take around 10 days to be posted on the site.

Chapter 16. Key Anti-Inflammatory Nutrients #3: Polyphenols[18]

The polyphenols are a large family of compounds that occur in many plants and plant foods (1). From the plant's perspective they are primarily defence compounds used to ward off infections, predators and UV stress; when we consume them they become part of our defence systems. The polyphenols have many potentially therapeutic effects in the body but perhaps most importantly, they are potent anti-inflammatory agents. They damp down the important inflammatory enzymes COX-1 and COX-2 (the same enzymes blocked by analgesic drugs such as aspirin and ibuprofen); but unlike the analgesics they also block the pro-inflammatory enzymes LIPOX-5 and -8, and the crucial matrix metallo-proteases (MMP's). This wide spectrum of anti-inflammatory activity makes the polyphenols far more effective than drugs at protecting tissues such as cartilage from inflammatory breakdown, although here I cannot quote you chapter and verse as the requisite clinical trials have not been done. I am forced to rely on a plethora of clinical reports, and my own personal experience.

The polyphenols are currently fashionable in scientific circles, but they are not new to medicine. Many years ago they were known, collectively, as Vitamin P. You won't find Vitamin P in the modern textbooks but back in the 1930's and early 40's Vitamin P was all the rage; a wonderful and natural medicine that would cure, it was claimed, just about every ill. These ideas were based on the work of one of the leading biochemists and nutritional researchers of the day – the very great Hungarian scientist Albert Szent-Györgyi.

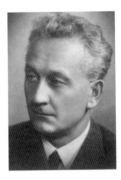

Born in 1893, Szent-Györgyi studied at the universities of Pecs, Leiden, Prague, Berlin, Groningen, Cambridge, where he obtained his second degree in biochemistry, and Woods Hole in Boston. In 1937 he won the Nobel Prize for his pioneering work on vitamin C.

---

18. The polyphenols are a family of plant compounds that share a phenolic molecular structure. Members of this family include the phenolic acids, tannins, stilbenes, lignans and flavonoids. The flavonoids themselves are divided into flavonols, flavones, isoflavones, flavanones, anthocyanins and flavanols (which include catechins and proanthocyanins). These groups have overlapping anti-inflammatory properties, but individual compounds have a wide range of different ancillary effects.

The political situation in Europe at that time was degenerating. Szent-Gyorgyi became one of the leaders of the anti-fascist movement, and worked as a diplomat at the Istanbul embassy to promote alliance with the Western powers. Hitler signed Szent-Gyorgyi's arrest papers personally; during 1944 and 1945, Albert was a fugitive from the Gestapo.

After the war Szent-Gyorgyi was talked about as the next President of Hungary, but he was not at ease with the Communist regime and left for America in 1947 where he actively campaigned against war and against nuclear weapons. He was much loved by his students, and perhaps you can tell why from this, one of my favourite quotes. In 1960, and at the age of 67, he said 'I learned from my parents that the only thing worth struggling for is the creation of new and beautiful things. This is why I run into my laboratory every morning."

Szent-Gyorgyi's work on Vitamin P (named either after Paprika, from which it was extracted, or vascular Permeability, which it reduced) fell into disrepute because its effects were so unpredictable. With hindsight we can see that the unpredictability was due to the fact that there was not one Vitamin P but a cloud of at least 4,000 related compounds which were present in different combinations and different levels in different plant extracts. The medical profession banished vitamin P from the textbooks, and it effectively disappeared.

But Vitamin P is making a comeback, with the P now also standing for Polyphenol. All the many compounds in this group share a polyphenolic molecular structure comprising multiple aromatic rings with multiple hydroxyl groups.

Impetus for polyphenol research partly comes from new findings which reveal their profound anti-inflammatory abilities. It was well known, for example, that polyphenols were good at inhibiting the important COX, LOX and MMP enzymes – but it was recently discovered that they go further, by inhibiting the cell's ability to produce these enzes in the first place [2]. At the same time they tone down some of the deepest and most pivotal inflammatory mechanisms including the caspases, nf-kappa B and related pathways [3-4], and inflammasome activation [5-6]. They also have some ability to up-regulate AMPK [7]. These findings indicate that the polyphenols should have very significant health-protecting effects, and increasing numbers of senior scientists are rallying to their standard.

Norman Hollenberg, for example, the eminent professor of medicine at Harvard Medical School, recently issued a call to arms. 'The health benefits of a flavonol found in cocoa called epicatechin are so striking that it should be (re-)classified as a vitamin' [8].

Hollenberg's statements were based on many years of research into the benefits of cocoa drinking in the Kuna people who inhabit the San Blas islands off the coast of Panama. The islanders, who drink 5 or 6 cups of coca per day, have rates of stroke, heart failure, cancer and diabetes around one tenth of the rates found elsewhere in the developed world [8]. Hollenburg used death certificates to compare the causes of death of island-dwelling Kuna with those who live on the mainland, where the only cocoa drinks consumed are the well-known mass-marketed, sanitised and flavonol-free[19] commercial products. These showed that the relative risk of death from heart disease on the Panama mainland was 1,280 per cent higher than on the islands, and death from cancer was 630 per cent higher.

According to these findings, epicatechin could greatly reduce the impact of some of the most common diseases in the Western world. Profesor Hollenberg even suggested that 'epicatechin could rival penicillin and anaesthesia in terms of its importance to public health". He made an important proviso: "Although the findings are comparable with effect of the flavanol-rich cocoa on health, clearly a large number of alternative possibilities exist involving diet, physical activity, stress and genetic factors. An observation study of this kind cannot prove causality. Indeed, only a randomised, controlled clinical trial in which all of these factors can be controlled will lead to a definitive conclusion."

The Harvard team is exactly right. These findings, although highly suggestive, do not constitute scientific proof. That's why the regulators maintain the usual party line, and do not allow health claims to be made for cocoa and cannot bring themselves to recommend cocoa to their patients. They say that even if cocoa flavonols have dramatic effects in the Kuna people, they might not affect health in any other population. They say that we must wait until the definitive trial is done. But that will take many years, if it is ever done. No drug company would sponsor such a study, and if it ever was to be carried out Big Pharma would try every trick in the book to discredit the results, the researchers and the research institutions where it was carried out.

Rather than wait for the definitive study, which will never be done, I prefer to look at all the data that already exists and draw my own conclusions. From what I have seen it would be foolish not to include polyphenols in one's diet and supplementary regime.

Many clinical studies show the benefits of these compounds. One recent and rather good paper showed that higher intakes of dietary polyphenols are associated with a reduced risk of cardiovascular disease in Americans and Norwegians (9). This prospective cohort study of 34,489 postmenopausal women reported that high dietary intake of polyphenols reduced the risk of mortality from cardiovascular disease (CVD), coronary heart disease (CHD) and stroke by between 10 and 22 per cent. These are hugely significant reductions; not as extraordinary as in the Kuna study, but that is because even at the upper end of the dietary range, today's Americans and Norwegians do not reach the Kuna islanders' levels of intake.

But there are at least two groups that do, or did. The mid-Victorians consumed copious amounts of cocoa and this, along with their high intakes of fruits and vegetables, undoubtedly contributed to their strikingly good health (see chapter 6). The other group is found on the Greek island of Ikaria. Middle-aged and elderly Ikarians have one of the highest longevity rates in the world, and – like the Kuna islanders – they tend to live out their long lives in excellent health. They do not drink cocoa but Greek coffee, a unique beverage which combines low levels of caffeine with very high levels of polyphenols, and which protects them from chronic inflammation (10).

---

19. Commercial cocoa products today have most of their flavonol content removed, as flavonols have a slightly bitter taste and many consumers prefer bland sweetness.

Different types of polyphenol appeared to have slightly different protective properties, but their overall benefits were broadly similar (9). In terms of foodstuffs, intake of apples, pears, and red wine was associated with lower rates of CHD and CVD deaths, while grapefruit intake was linked to lowered CHD mortality. Interestingly, in this study no significant benefits for cardio-vascular health were observed for the consumption of tea, a polyphenol-rich beverage previously seen to have benefits. This may be because many people drink tea with milk, which binds polyphenols and may prevent them from being absorbed (11).

More data come from the University of Warsaw, where a team of clinicians gave a polyphenol-rich extract of chokeberry to patients who had survived a heart attack, and had been receiving statins for a period of 6 months (12). The chokeberry extract significantly reduced inflammation in the blood vessels of these patients, in whom the statins had had little effect. As the inflammation in the artery walls subsided, allowing them to relax, the patients' blood pressure fell by a very healthy amount: systolic pressure by 11 mm Hg, and diastolic pressure by 7.2 mm Hg.

At the University of Tehran another research group gave concentrated pomegranate juice, an equally rich source of polyphenols, to Type 2 diabetics with elevated cholesterol levels (13). Their 22 diabetic patients drank 40 g of the concentrated juice every day for 8 weeks, and at the end of this period significant reductions were seen in low-density lipoprotein-cholesterol, and total cholesterol. These two studies show that polyphenols from various food sources do everything that statins can do, and a good deal more besides.

Polyphenols seem to be good for mice also – especially the diabetic, obese mice often used as models for diabetic, obese humans. A Japanese team (14) fed their diabetic mice a diet laced with cocoa polyphenols for a mere three weeks. They found that in the cocoa-fed mice, blood glucose levels fell significantly, and concluded in their paper that "The dietary intake of food or drinks produced from cacao beans might be beneficial in preventing the onset of type-2 diabetes."

The mice were fed a concentrated cocoa extract, the equivalent of about 5 grams of polyphenols per day in human terms or 2.5 kilos of milk chocolate. This is an unfeasibly high dose but chocolate contributes significant amounts of antioxidants to the average diet; in fact, it is in the top three most important dietary sources of antioxidants, along with coffee (15). This and a related paper (16) suggested that the 'therapeutic dose' of dark chocolate could be as low as 50 g per day.

The flavonols in cocoa and chocolate reduce inflammation in the linings of arteries (112, 113) and lower blood pressure (114). There is evidence that as a result of these effects, chocolate may reduce the risk of coronary artery disease (115); and recently, a Californian research group with a sense of humour found 'dark chocolate receptors[20]' in the heart and blood vessels (116). Old-fashioned un-sweetened cocoa powder, the kind regularly consumed by the mid-Victorians, contains up to 50 mg flavonols per gram. 10 grams of cocoa powder (about

20. The 'dark chocolate receptors' were actually delta-opioid receptors

one heaped table spoon, which makes one cup of cocoa) will therefore deliver 500 mg of polyphenols. This has a huge antioxidant and anti-inflammatory payload (117).

At the William Harvey Research Institute at Barts Hospital in London, a team lead by Professor Roger Corder (17-19) has been investigating the cardio-protective properties of red wine. Regular, moderate consumption of red wine is linked to a reduced risk of coronary heart disease and to lower overall mortality, but the relative contribution of wine's alcohol and polyphenol components to these effects has long been unclear.

Corder's work identified a group of polyphenols called procyanidins as the principal vasoactive compounds in red wine. It also found that these valuable compounds were present in higher concentrations in wines from areas of south-western France and Sardinia, where traditional production methods ensure that these compounds are efficiently extracted during the wine-making process. It could be coincidence but these regions also happen to be associated with longevity...

Polyphenols, it would appear, are good for you from birth to old age, and everywhere in between. Pycnogenol, a mixture of polyphenols derived from the bark of the Maritime pine, is helpful in reducing the pain and discomfort of dysmennorhoea (20) and pregnancy (21). This was no instant effect – the intensity of the pain experienced by the women in the trial gradually fell over a course of four weeks – but unlike the pharmaceutical pain-killers, there were no adverse effects. At the other end of the scale, polyphenols have been strongly linked to a reduced risk of Alzheimer's disease (22), with high consumption of fruit juice, a potentially rich source of polyphenols, (23) conferring a reduction of risk of about three quarters.

The spices are particularly good sources of polyphenols. One of the best documented of these is haldi or turmeric, which has a long history of use in Ayurvedic medicine in the treatment of painful conditions from sore throats to arthritis (24). The polyphenols in turmeric, known as curcuminoids, are effective and safe anti-inflammatory agents (25-26).

The safety of turmeric is proven. In the US, the National Toxicology Program of the National Institute of Environmental and Health Sciences evaluated the safety of turmeric oleoresin containing concentrated and standardized levels of curcuminoids at the request of the National Cancer Institute and the FDA. Working with a variety of animal and human data, they concluded that turmeric extracts were non-toxic, and exhibited a variety of potentially therapeutic properties (27-28). The U.S. FDA includes turmeric powder and oleoresin on its list of substances generally recognized as safe (GRAS).

I will briefly review the curcuminoids here as they serve as a good example for the whole class of polyphenols.

Curcuminoids reduce pain and inflammation by inhibiting the inflammatory enzymes COX-1 and COX-2 (29-35), and the enxymes lipoxygenase or LIPOX-5 and -8 (36-38). These mechanisms have been thoroughly investigated and duplicated by researchers all over the world.

Unsurprisingly, given their mode of action, the anti-inflammatory and analgesic effects of the curcuminoids are considerable. Sadly there are only a limited number of clinical trials (39-41), as these are expensive and the drug companies have shown little interest in sponsoring them. I am personally aware, however, of a large and increasing number of case histories showing that the curcuminoids are useful and powerful tools in the management of pain. But they have many other clinical applications ....

Cardiovascular Protection

There is substantial and convincing evidence that the curcuminoids protect the cardiovascular system, in a number of complementary ways. They are powerful antioxidants (42-44). They lower LDL (the 'bad') cholesterol, and protect it against oxidisation (45-46). They reduce blood pressure by damping inflammation in the blood vessel walls (47-48, 107) and preventing the over-growth of smooth muscle cells in the artery walls (49-50). They make the blood less likely to form clots (51-54). They inhibit the glycation reactions that cause protein denaturation (55-56), and the loss of arterial compliance that is strongly linked to an increased risk of heart attack and stroke (106). They protect against reperfusion injury (57-58) and improve the so-called apo a/b ratio (59), a cardio-protective mechanism which the drug companies have not yet been able to access. All in all, this is a powerfully cardio-protective and anti-ageing combination of effects (60).

Gastro- and chemo-protection

The curcuminoids protect against ulcers and are used to treat dyspepsia (61) and as anti-ulcer treatments (62-63). This is partly because the curcuminoids block a group of enzymes called matrix metallo-proteases or MMP's, (64) which are centrally involved in the process of ulceration. Inhibiting the MMP's is considered not only to protect against ulceration, but also against some of the key steps in tumour growth and metastasis. For example, the curcuminoids have been shown to suppress angiogenesis (65), prevent the growth of a variety of cancers (25, 66-67) and actively kill cancer cells (68-69). This has lead to at least five Phase-1 clinical trials in colo-rectal cancer (70), with larger Phase 2 studies now enrolling (71).

Beyond Curcumin

Unsurprisngly, given the curcuminoids' many therapeutic effects, there have been attempts to produce semi-synthetic (and hence patentable) analagues (72-73). These may eventually appear on the market, once safety testing has been completed. In the meantime, another very exciting group of polyphenols are the secoiridoid polyphenols which occur in olives and olive oil, two central items in the Mediterranean diet. These have been discussed previously but are worth looking at in more detail.

Research into the health benefits of olive polyphenols was given impetus by a large multi-centre clinical tial by the EUROLIVE group, which showed that they improved multiple cardio risk factors (74). This stimulated a huge interest in olive polyphenols, and a rapidly growing number of studies looking at their impact on health. In the following chapter I have sampled a few of the research papers published in the last 18 months.

To begin with, these polyphenols are highly bioavailable. In one critically important study, test animals were given a single dose of olive extract (75). The secoiroids were readily absorbed, metabolized and distributed through the blood stream to practically all parts of the body, and even across the blood-brain barrier into the brain. This latter finding is very interesting, as it highlights a potential role for these olive phenolics in the prevention and the treatment of various neurodegenerative disorders, including Alzheimer's. That concept is supported by a group of three papers which document the anti-inflammatory and neuro-protective effects of oleuropein (76-78); reducing or preventing chronic inflammation in the brain is considered to be critical to slowing or stabilising Alzheimer's. But there is more.

Over and above this generally protective anti-inflammatory effect, oleuropein also does something much more specific; it modifies the way in which amyloid precursor protein is cleaved (79), and this is a central element in the pathoaetiology of the disease. These dual protetive effects of the olive polyphenols would be expected to be highly protective against dementia, and even more so when you factor in the olive compounds' ability to protect blood flow.

Skeptics will have noted that I quoted an animal bioavailability study, but let me reassure you that olive polyphenols are very well absorned in humans too (80-82).

Many polyphenols are cardi- and vaso-protective, and the secoiridoids are no exception. Two papers show that they protect arteries and the tissues they supply against anoxia and reperfusion injury (83-84), a brace of effects which protect against the development of atheroma and hypertension. The anti-inflammatory properties of olive polyphenols also protected the liver (85), joints (86) and gastrointestinal tract from painful and dangerous inflammatory conditions; they prevented gastric ulcers (87) and alleviated colitis (88).

The anti-cancer effects linked to many polyphenols are most certainly shared by the olive compounds, which have a range of properties that variously kill cancer cells (89), stop them from proliferating (90), and inhibit both tumour growth and metastasis (91-93). Somewhat unexpectedly, the secoiridoids also have some ability to inhibit the formation of adipose tissue (94-95), and so could find a place in weight control regimes.

Finally, by combining all the above benefits with hormetic activity (ie acting rather like adaptogens), the secoiridoids have powerful anti-ageing effects (96-97). They trigger the up-regulation of genes which increase anti-oxidant activity (98-99). It is likely that they also activate AMP kinase, a very important energy switch which improves muscular fitness, lowers both blood glucose and cholesterol levels, and reduces body fat.

Like the Omega-3 fatty acids, the polyphenols confer a powerful range of health and longevity promoting benefits. The combination of Omega-3's and the right polyphenols will do more for you than the entire contents of any high street pharmacy. For example ....

Inflammation and the brain

Inflammation in the brain not only drives dementia (118) but is also a central part of the entire ageing process. Inflammation in a specific part of the brain called the hypothalamus seems to be particularly critical, as the hypothalamus secretes hormones which affect almost every system in the body. Inflammatory damage to the hypothalamus affects levels of these hormones including growth hormone, which controls rates of tissue growth and repair, and gonadotropin-releasing hormone (GnRH) (100). Unsurprisingly, a fall in these hormones accelerates the ageing process; in experimental mice, hypothalamic inflammation lead to a rapid loss of muscle strength and size, skin thickness, ability to learn – and life expectancy. Conversely, blocking inflammation in the hypothalamus slowed ageing and increased longevity by about 20%; and adding extra GnRH increased the ability of the mice to grow new brain cells (101-104).

Preventing inflammation and nerve cell damage and death in the hypothalamus is a very important anti-ageing strategy – but you don't need to treat yourself with GnRH. A number of the anti-inflammatory polyphenols have already been shown to slow or prevent brain ageing (108); as have the omega 3 fatty acids (109-111). It is a sure bet that the combination of omega 3 fatty acids and polyphenols will be far more effective than either nutrient on its own.

Dietary enhancement and excercise are particularly important because there is good evidence that obesity (which is pro-inflammatory) accelerates inflammation in the hypothalamus, which in turn causes and exacerbates diabetes (105). Diabetes causes further chronic inflammation, creating a further twist in a vicious circle which drives the ageing process even faster and further increases the risk of dementia (119). This is yet another example of how our defective diets and lifestyles create a perfect metabolic storm which drives so many of us to premature and unnecessary disability and death.

But our overwhelmingly unhealthy lifestyle is damaging our brains in other ways too. As well as the rapidly rising tide of dementia, the incidence of mental illness is also accelerating. Between 1987 and 2007, the US mental disability rate more than doubled, rising from 1 in every 184 Americans to 1 in every 76. Among American children the figures are even more alarming. A recent CDC report found that 1 in 5 (ie over 10 million children) had a mental health disorder with the most common, ADHD, diagnosed in over 4 million (120).

Poor diet has undoubtedly contributed to this disaster – after all, our brains are built from and maintained by fatty acids and other constituents in our diets - and a diet that fails to provide the brain with what it needs inevitably leads to brain dysfunction of some sort. Tragically, our drug-centric model of mental healthcare ignores this. Even more tragically, although Prozac, Ritalin, Haloperidol, Valium and other psychiatric medications can suppress unwanted mental symptoms in the short term, follow-up studies show that they increase the likelihood that a person will become chronically and often more seriously ill over the longer term (121).

The recorded fall in average IQ since the 19th century (122) is a terrible indictment of today's shoddy lifestyles and drug-centred 'health care' systems. The evidence that we can reverse this decline with simple dietary enhancement, though circumstantial, is very persuasive (123). Even if you don't think enough of yourself to live more healthily, the prospective health and happiness of your children may provide a better motive.

Chapter 17. Key Anti-Inflammatory Nutrients #4: selenium, Vitamins D, E and K, and the Lipophillic (Fat-Soluble) Phytonutrients

Selenium

Once ingested, selenium is incorporated into a group of specific proteins (seleno-proteins) which have many different functions in the body. One seleno-protein, glutathione peroxidase (GPX), is an important antioxidant enzyme that protects lipids in the body from oxidative cascades; and as many lipid peroxidation products are pro-inflammatory, it was thought that GPX might be the main anti-inflammatory mechanism.

We now know, however, that selenium exerts anti-inflammatory effects via multiple mechanisms (1). Selenium depletion affects many genes involved in inflammation (2-3), and recent research suggests that the most important anti-inflammatory mechanism is not GPX but the enzyme Iodothyronine Deiodinase-2 or DIO2 (4). Formerly thought to be solely active in thyroid function, DIO2 is now, like many other enzymes, thought to play different roles in different tissues.

'Vitamin' D and the Lipophiles

D's anti-inflammatory effects are subtle and modified by dietary and genetic factors, so the literature on this vitamin is not always consistent. On balance, however, the evidence suggests that D depletion and deficiency is linked to an increased risk of a number of chronic inflammatory conditions including the autoimmune diseases (5).This is probably due to D's ability to modify the activity of cells in the adaptive immune system called T-regulator cells (6-7); and, possibly, to D's ability to enhance anti-bacterial defences and thus reduce the risk of infections. D deficiency may also be linked to an increased risk of allergy (8) but the evidence here is conflicting (9).

As D and the other lipohillic micronutrients (vitamins A, E, K and the carotenoids) are fat-soluble, they concentrate in adipose tissue. This is important, because adipose tissue is a not only a site for storing spare calories but also a highly active endocrine organ. In normal weight individuals adipose tissue is involved in metabolic homeostasis. In obesity, however, it becomes a pathological organ, inflamed and causing chronic inflammation elsewhere in the body (10-11). This inflammatory process is modified and subdued by a diet containing adequate amounts of the lipophiles, all of which have now been shown to exert damping, anti-inflammatory effects inside adipose tissue (12). Fat-soluble polyphenols such as the secoiridoids in olives appear to do exactly the same thing (13).

As well as their anti-inflammatory effects, this interesting and important group of micro- and phyto-nutrients exert multiple effects on gene expression, and in this way exert multiple beneficial effects on their target tissues. Most if not all of these lipophiles are capable of switching off cancer cells, and many of them seem to be able to inhibit the growth of adipose tissue (12, 13).

Now we come back to the terrible, depleted modern diet, stuffed with empty calories and depleted or deficient in the lipophillic micronutrients (and all the other micronutrients). This dangerous combination is creating too many people with too much adipose tissue; and not enough of the damping lipophiles (14-15). Their fat is in the fire, and it is inflaming the rest of their bodies.

You can actually see this during surgery. When vegetarians are cut open their fatty tissues are coloured from yellow to orange, which is the hallmark of healthy fat. The fat inside junk food enthusiasts, which is typically pearl to pale yellow, is toxic and pro-inflammatory[21].

It looks very much as if a diet rich in the lipophiles will help to minimise weight gain, and it will certainly reduce the inflammatory effects of existing adipose tissue.

21. Surgeons who specialise in bone work are familiar with this colour code. Yellowish bone is generally healthier, better structured and stronger than white bone.

Chapter 18. Key Anti-Inflammatory Factors #5: Exercise, Carbs, Blood Sugar Control

These three factors are closely inter-related. Blood sugar levels are determined by the amount of digestible carbohdrates consumed (sugars and starches in foods are largely broken down to glucose); and how much glucose can be removed from the blood – which is largely into muscle, and determined by how much that muscle is exercised.

Physical exercise

The "baby boomers", the generation currently in their 60's, 70's and 80's, are fatter, weaker and sicker than their parents (1). Those currently in this age group are more susceptible to degenerative diseases than were previous generations of elders, with problems stemming primarily from poor diet and lack of proper exercise. The combination of disease and unfitness is creating enormous socio-economic problems, by dramatically increasing the numbers unable to perform normal daily activities. Ten years ago, 12% of over-60's required assistance to carry out routine daily activities such as walking a quarter mile, climbing a small flight of stairs, or even getting out of a chair. Today, that figure has risen to an alarming 20% (2).

Technological advancements have played a significant role. As urbanised folk have increasingly been weaned off of physical labour and instead placed in front of computer screens, the level of physical activity among the population has dropped significantly. People's calorific needs have declined, and this, too often combined with poor food choices, means that their nutritional standards have declined. Type B malnutrition is now rife.

Ironically, the technological advancements that benefited the Baby Boomers when they were younger are proving to be their downfall in later life. And if anything, things are getting worse. Due to increasing use of the internet and games consoles, and increasing obesity, children's fitness levels are falling – and nowhere more rapidly than in Britain. Levels have been falling by around four per cent per decade on average worldwide, but in the UK they have plummeted by eight per cent (3).

'Children don't climb trees or use their bikes any more', said the researchers. 'They are inactive.' Guidelines recommend children undertake at least 60 minutes of moderate to vigorous exercise a day, including taking part in sports, brisk walking and running – but children today are managing less than a quarter of that.

'Lack of activity destroys the good condition of every human being, while movement and methodical physical exercise save it and preserve it.' ~Plato

It has long been known that physical inactivity is unhealthy, and increases all-cause mortality. Governments and health agencies get all hot and bothered about this sort of thing, and run around issuing recommendations. For example, the updated physical activity and health recommendations from the American College of Sports Medicine and the American Heart

Association emphasize participation in at least 30 minutes of moderate-intensity physical activity, which should be accumulated in bouts of at least 10 minutes, on 5 days per week; or relatively more intense exercise for less time ie 20 minutes on 3 days per week [4].

These recommendations map out a strict and strenuous route to better health, but are ignored by most folk who find it impossible to integrate this level of activity into their urban and time-poor lives. But now there is an easier way forwards ....

It turns out that there is far more to the exercise / health connection than we originally thought, and that maybe all we need to do is simply to spend less time sitting down. And if even standing up seems too onerous, there is a pill for that too ...

A sedentary lifestyle is hazardous to your health. Sitting (or more specifically prolonged soitting) has been identified as a serious health hazard, and an independent risk factor for vardiovascular diseae and early death by researchers at the Baker Heart and Diabetes Unit in Melbourne [5-8]. This is true even in adults who take regular exercise and maintain a healthy weight; too much sitting is distinct and separate from from taking too little exercise [5,9-10], but if you do both you are even more at risk. The critical factor seems to be putting tension on the main muscles of the legs and back. It is difficult to undertake aerobic exercise without working these muscles, but you can work these muscles without getting out of breath.

The loss of local contractile stimulation induced through sitting leads to both the suppression of skeletal muscle lipoprotein lipase (LPL) activity (which is necessary for triglyceride uptake and HDL-cholesterol production) and reduced glucose uptake. Conversely standing, which involves isometric contraction of the anti-gravity (postural) muscles and only low levels of energy expenditure, improves skeletal muscle LPL and glucose uptake. This is why the more time you spend siting down, the higher your LDL cholesterol and glucose tend to be, as well as your blood pressure and waist size [11].

Today's excessively sedentary lifestyles are undoubtedly harmful, but regular and moderate exercise reduces the risk of all cause mortality. It reduces or normalises the symptoms related to the metabolic syndrome, and is an effective treatment in patients with chronic heart diseases, type 2 diabetes and many cancers. The level of physical activity needed to generate these benefits is surprisingly low; brisk walking for an hour or so, three or more times a week, seems to be adequate.

In one study, men who walk briskly for 3 hours per week or more had a 57% lower rate of progression of prostatic cancer compared to those who walked at an easy pace for less than 3 hours per week [12]. Disease progression was slowed or halted to a similar extent in breast cancer patients who walked briskly to a similar schedule [13], in colorectal cancer patients [14-17] and also in patients with Alzheimer's disease [18], cardiovascular disease [19] and Metabolic Syndrome / diabetes [20]. Increased levels of physical activity are benefical in cardiovascular disease also, and free of risk [21].

Moderate exercise is really a wonder treatment. There are multiple protective mechanisms involved here but one is undoubtedly the ability of regular exercise to reduce or suppress chronic inflammation.

When muscle fibers contract they produce a master anti-inflammatory cytokine called IL-6. IL-6 has a dual effect; it stimulates the synthesis and release of other anti-inflammatory compounds such as IL-1ra and IL-10, and simultaneously inhibits the production of the proinflammatory cytokine TNF-alpha (22-23).

Moderate exercise exerts other key anti-inflammatory benefits. Increased metabolic activity in exercised muscle causes a localised increase in free radicals, falls in local oxygen and glucose levels, and increased local cAMP (24). The combination of low oxygen and high cAMP levels in muscle switches on the central energy switch, a very important enzyme called AMP-Kinase (25).

When AMP-Kinase is activated it triggers a cascade of downstream effects. It switches on muscle LPL and inhibits the synthesis of cholesterol – so cholesterol levels naturally fall. It stimulates the dissolution of fat *and* its subsequent oxidation (25-26). Excessive adiposity is pro-inflammatory, so this is a longer-term anti-inflammatory effect of exercise (27). More immediately, AMP-K activation inhibits inflammatory activity in fat depots (28) – a genuinely exciting finding, but there is more.

Activated AMP-kinase restores insulin sensitivity, thus reducing or removing the pro-inflammatory effects of hyperglycemia. It achieves this via two other inter-related mechanisms, both of which enhance the ability of muscle to soak up glucose from the blood stream. AMP-kinase increases the numbers of GLUT4 glucose uptake pumps on muscle cell membranes that 'pull' glucose into the muscle; and it triggers autophagy, a process of tissue renewal in the muscle that increases numbers of the mitochondria where that glucose will be 'burned' (27-30). Mitochondria are highly dynamic organelles that fuse and divide in response to environmental stimuli, developmental status, and energy requirements. The increase in mitochondria triggered by activated AMP-K explains why, when you take exercise you get fitter and achieve better blood glucose control. As blood glucose levels come under control, insulin levels fall also; and this is another anti-cancer mechanism (31-32).

The classical way to activate AMP-Kinase is by taking aerobic exercise; as noted above, the fall in muscle oxygen levels and the increase in cAMP iduced by aerobic exercise have long been known to activate AMP-K. AICAR, a synthetic form of cAMP, is widely thought to have played a critical role in the Tour de France in 2009 (and was banned in 2011). It is an interesting drug, but its cost, at around a half million euros per course, rules it out for most people.

But AMP-Kinase is a complicated enzyme, and it can be switched on, more effectively, via a different route. Tensions in skeletal muscle, and probably torque on bone, trigger the release of very special proteins known as sestrins. These are members of the family of stress-responsive proteins charmingly called 'alarmins' which include the better known Heat Shock Proteins and Anti-Microbial Proteins. Sestrin is unique in that it activates the 'central energy switch' AMP-kinase (33), and in this way produces all the health benefits of exercise.

Now we can see why too much sitting is harmful. It deactivates AMPK, and that in turn leads to reduced muscle LPL activity (so LDL cholesterol goes up), and fewer mitochondria and glucose uptake pumps in the muscle (so blood glucose and insulin go up). Cholesterol synthesis is dis-inhibited (which also increases blood cholesterol levels); fat burning is suppressed and fat synthesis is accelerated – so you get fatter. And all of these things are pro-inflammatory.

So now you know how to switch on your own AMPK without breaking a sweat. Spend less time siting; get up and down more, go to the kitchen, walk round the room, walk to the newsagent or off-license; don't sit still for more than a half hour at a time (34-36). You can speed up the process by standing on a vibrating plate, which send waves of tension and relaxation through the main muscle groups. This is as good as orthodox exercise in older people in terms of increasing musle strength, power and balance control (37).

If you don't want to go to the trouble of standing on a vibrating plate, there are even easier alternatives. A number of plant derivates have been shown to activate AMP Kinase by mimicking or triggering the production of sestrin. These compounds therefore generate all the physiological and health benefits of exercise – although perhaps not all of its psychological benefits. The most effective of these appears to be Damulin B, a sapogenin derived from Gynostemma pentaphyllum (38).

This herb (Chinese – 'Jiaogulan') has been used for thousands of years in the Far East as a health tonic for the elderly and infirm, and is known colloquially as the Immortality Herb. Recent research shows that it does indeed reverse many aspects of metabolic and physiological senescence. Actiponin, the standardised extract of this herb, can best be described as 'exercise in a capsule'. It increases muscle fitness, lowers blood glucose and cholesterol levels, and promoted the loss of body fat in pre-clinical and clinical studies (38, 74, 75). Reproducing the effects of exercise, Actiponin is particularly effective at reducing visceral (abdominal) fat (75). This is a combination of effects that powerfully reduces the burden of chronic inflammation.

Fucoxanthin, a compound found in the edible brown seaweed Petalonia Binghamiae (39-40) has a similar if lesser effect; as do extracts of cumin (41), the peel of young citrus fruits (42), the edible bamboo grass Sasa quelpaertensis (43), and even apples and onions if eaten in large quantities (44), via the polyphenol quercitin.

NB Intensive and excessive exercise is pro-inflammatory (45), and should always be combined with anti-inflammatory supplementation. Moderation in all things!

Blood Sugar

Levels of sugar (more accurately glucose) in the blood must be maintained within a relatively narrow range; too low and we become comatose, too high and the glucose molecules initiate damaging glycation reactions. These cause chronic inflammation and damage to multiple tissues including blood vessels, nerves, the retina, the kidneys and the liver; in a complex and interlinking set of pathologies that cause oxidative damage, telomeric shortening and accelerated ageing (46-49)[22]. To make matters more complicated, rates of glucose entry into the blood fluctuate wildly, depending on the amount and nature of the carbohydrates and other macronutrients we eat. Rates of glucose removal from the blood can be just as erratic as they largely depend on how much glucose is needed a fuel by the muscles – and that depends on levels of physical activity. Glucose requirements by other tissues are more or less stable.

Under almost all conditions, blood glucose levels are satisfactorily controlled by a network of sensors and feedback loops. Eat more carbs than you need and insulin kicks in, lowering blood sugar by increasing glucose uptake into liver and muscle; consume fewer carbs and glucagon takes over, releasing glucose from the liver into the blood. So why is Type 2 diabetes so common today? The answer lies, as so often, in the past …

Diabetes is not a new disease. Up until the 11th century (and as late as the 19th century in some remote areas), the condition was diagnosed by 'water tasters' who made their diagnosis by tasting the sweetness of the sugars excreted in diabetic urine. In the 16th century the remarkable physician and alchemist Philippus Aureolus Theophrastus Bombastus von Hohenheim (who took the name Paracelsus, and is regarded by many as the father of toxicology and metabolic medicine) described diabetes as a serious general disorder. During the 19th century the towering French scientist Claude Bernard developed an understanding of pancreatic and liver metabolism; the German medical student Paul Langerhans first identified the pancreatic structures that still bear his name; and Oskar Minkowski and Joseph von Mering at the University of Strasbourg carried out the first experimental pancreatectomy.

The French physician Apollinaire Bouchardat saw his diabetic patients improve as a result of food rationing during the siege of Paris in 1870, and by 1875 was advocating patient education, exercise and weight reduction for all diabetics. His results were effectively duplicated 135 years later by Professor Roy Taylor's team at Newcastle University (50). Bouchardat developed the first self-test for glucose in the urine, and fully deserves his title as the founder of diabetology.

But the disease itself was rare. Towards the end of the 19th century, the great William Osler records 10 cases of diabetes among the 35,000 patients treated at Johns Hopkins (51)[23]. The

22. While a minor degree of glycative and other types of stress triggers and enhance repair mechanisms, today's pathogenic diet overloads the body with glycative and inflammatory stress and drives us towards the grave.
23. Osler famously said, 'The philosophies of one age have become the absurdities of the next, and the foolishness of yesterday has become the wisdom of tomorrow.' Pharmaceutical medicine may be the philosophy of our age, but nutrition will undoubtedly be the wisdom of tomorrow.

contemporary records of the Massachusetts General Hospital show 47,899 admissions, of whom 151 (a mere 0.3%!) were diagnosed with adult onset diabetes (52).

In the 19th century diabetes was an esoteric disorder. In 2001 the American Diabetes Association estimated that there were 20 million cases of diabetes world-wide; in 2011 a more extensive survey came up with a figure of 350 million (53). On current trends we will all become diabetic, and the implications kill the current medical philosophy (thank you William!) stone dead.

In 2003 – a lifetime ago in tems of diabetes figures - the estimated lifetime risk of developing diabetes for individuals born in the USA in 2000 was 32.8% for males and 38.5% for females (54); rising among Hispanics to 45.4% in males and an astonishing 52.5% in females. These figures show that the statements made by idiot politicians and polyanna physicians about rising life expectancy are largely baloney; diabetics suffer from accelerated ageing, and have large reductions in life expectancy. For diabetics diagnosed at age 40, men lose 11.6 life-years and 18.6 quality-adjusted life-yers and women lose 14.3 life-years and 22.0 quality-adjusted life-years (54).

Why has diabetes become such a universal disease? The answer is simple; it is a combination of eating too many carbohydrates, and taking too little exercise. Under these conditions more glucose enters the blood than can be removed, overwhelming all the checks and balances that formerly kept us healthy. We need to address both sides of this equation; we have already discussed exercise, so now let us review carbs.

Some interesting research papers show that contrary to the diabetes associations, which are mainly funded by drug companies and therefore have deeply conflicting loyalties, an effective way of reducing the risk of pre-diabetes (Metabolic Syndrome) and type 2 diabetes is to reduce the intake of sugars and refined carbohydrates (55-56). A low-glycemic diet has also been shown to reduce the risk of complications of diabetes such as macular degeneration, the loss of sight that affects so many diabetics (57). A low-glycemic diet lowers the body's production of insulin, and insulin is, among other things, an ageing hormone. A low-carb, low-insulin lifestyle should therefore have other anti-ageing benefits, and another excellent review has indeed revealed that the low-glycemic diet protects against a range of ageing diseases including heart disease, gallbladder disease and breast cancer (58). Improved diet and increased exercise levels confer similar benefits (59-60)

Needless to say, these findings have been down-played by the diabetes industry because they do not constitute a profit opportunity. Hopefully they won't be able to down-play it for much longer, because in the latest Chapter of this intriguing story Cynthia Kenyon, an eminent ageing specialist at the University of California, has published a series of papers which show just how carbs speed up the ageing process. This is in addition to the telomeric ageing caused by glycative and oxidative stress.

Inhibiting insulin/IGF-1 signalling extends lifespan and delays age-related disease in species throughout the animal kingdom. Professor Kenyon's recent work reveals how this works. She found that turning down the gene that controls insulin switches on another gene which acts like an elixir of life, by enhancing cellular repair processes. A high-carb, high-glycemic diet forces the body to switch on insulin production; and prevents the 'elixir' gene from being switched on. Cellular repair then slows down, and the ageing process speeds up ..... (61-62). Conversely, a low-glycemic diet reduces insulin, and thus switches on the elixir gene and boosts the cellular repair mechanisms.

Professor Kenyon's initial work was done in roundworms, where she found that specific genetic manipulation at this insulin / 'elixir' gene locus increased life span a staggering 6 times. The genes that control aging in worms do the same thing in rats and mice, probably monkeys, and there is evidence that they are active in humans too.

The technical name of the 'elixir' gene which brings all the anti-ageing benefits is DAF 16, but it was quickly nicknamed 'Sweet Sixteen' because it turned the worms into teenagers. ‹It sends out instructions to a whole range of repair and renovation genes,› says Professor Kenyon. 'The Sweet Sixteen gene also boosts compounds that make sure the skin and muscle-building proteins are working properly, the immune system becomes more active to fight infection and genes that are active in cancer get turned off.'

Professor Kenyon has changed her diet as a result of her work with the Sweet Sixteen gene, as have many others. Colleagues of mine who have followed this regime for years generally look and are in almost every sense decades younger than their chronological ages.

You won't hear much about this from your GP or nutritionist. After all, this flies in the face of 30 years of health advice to 'have a lower fat intake and eat plenty of long-lasting complex carbohydrates to keep the body supplied with energy'. Received wisdom was hopelessly wrong on this, and it has become clear that official advice has harmed and killed many. It is another black chapter in medico-pharmaceutical history.

The drug companies will inevitably introduce an exciting new range of products designed to target the 'elixir' gene, and these exciting new products will equally inevitably introduce an exciting new range of unexpected adverse effects. Or, you could switch to a low-carb diet. If you have a sweet tooth, switch from sugar and honey to intensive sweeteners such as saccharin, newly declared safe by the EPA; aspartame, recently given the all-clear (63-64); or stevia, monksfruit extract and others.

If you crave starchy foods switch from digestible to fermentable carbs. This means switching from grains and potatoes to pulses and legumes, but there are other techniques you can use. For example, by cooking, cooling and re-heating starchy foods such as potatoes, you convert the starch from digestible to fermentable. In this state it no longer convers to blood glucose, and instead develops healthy prebiotic properties. Prebiotics help to normalise the gut microbiota, in a way which will exert primary anti-inflammatory effects in the gastro-intestinal tract and secondary anti-inflammatory effects elsewhere in the body (65-68). This is covered in more detail in the next chapter[24].

The basic causes of Metabolic Syndrome and diabetes are quite well understood. The typical Western diet pours excessive amounts of glucose into the bloodstream which, when combined with under-exercised muscle, pretty much guarantees insulin resistance. As this diet / low exercise combination generally leads to an accumulation of adipose tissue which has an excessive omega 6:3 ratio and is unprotected by lipophile nutrients, that adipose tissue becomes an important source of inflammation. Growing inflammation makes the insulin resistance worse (69), and this – together with glycation reactions – leads to accelerated ageing and a spectrum of diabetic complications including liver, kidney and brain damage, blindness, cardiovascular disease and cancer. There is a vicious cycle here because the process of chronic inflammation and increased insulin resistance causes muscle wasting (73); and this makes insulin resistance worse.

Given our pathological lifestyles it is not surprising that diabetes figures are soaring – in fact, it is suprising that the disease is not more prevalent. But diabetics have a choice. They can reverse this mess of metabolic imbalances with simple lifestlyle changes, with a good chance of curing themselves. Or they can opt for a pharma approach, and suppress some of the symptoms of their disease with variously toxic drugs. The pharma approach is generally promoted, but it is an irresponsible and feeble-minded strategy.

Diabetes is a public health problem due to the sheer numbers of cases, and the huge drain on health resources. But it is a problem that is starting to affect non-diabetics directly, because diabetes reduces resistance to infection. Increasing numbers of people with impaired resistance to infection in any given population puts the entire population at increased risk of infection. Diabetics are significantly more vulnerable to tuberculosis than non-diabetics (70-71), and as the numbers of diabetics among us increase the likelihood of a TB epidemic also increases (71-72). Tuberculosis is becoming more and more difficult to treat, culminating in the recent emergence of totally drug-resistant strains (see chapter 10). If we continue to rely on pharmaceutical crutches and do not mend our ways, a wave of untreatable TB will arrive in due course.

---

24. The Biagi and Bengmark papers (65, 66, 68) are superb, and essential reading for anyone interested in the mechanisms of ageing and how they can be modified.

Chapter 19. Foods and Cooking Techniques

When foods containing proteins are cooked at high temperatures, the protein binds with glucose or other sugars in the food to produce compounds called Advanced Glycation End Products, or AGEs. Many foods brown at high temperatures, and this discolouration is a sign of AGE production. AGE compounds are very pro-inflammatory, and very ageing.
The best known AGE compound is acrylamide. This forms when starchy foods are cooked at high temperatures, and sugar molecules in the starch react with an amino acid called asparagine. It has been found in crisps, french fries, toast, Pringles and other foods. Acrylamide is classified as carcinogenic in humans.

AGEs can also be formed within the body. Some glucose molecules are bound by enzymes to proteins in the body, forming glycoproteins which are essential to normal body functioning. But when glucose binds to proteins (or fats) in the body through non-enzyme action, it creates AGE products. Non-enzymatic binding occurs when levels of glucose are too high for too long, as happens in diabetes. This drives the formation of AGE's and leads to inflammation – which helps to explain why diabetics suffers from excessive inflammation and accelerated ageing.

AGEs are aging because they stimulate inflammation, but this is not the only way they accelerate the ageing process. The binding of glucose to proteins in the body also causes cross-linking between proteins, binding them together in a random and dysfunctional manner. Externally, this shows up as skin ageing, wrinkling and reduced elasticity. Internally, this drives diseases such as cataracts, hypertension, blood clotting and kidney damage.
Dr Levi of the American Journal of Kidney Diseases says: "AGE reactions … gradually accumulate over the lifetime of the protein. The goal must be to prevent AGEs forming in the first place".

AGEs in the diet can be reduced by adopting different cooking techniques, and the AGE's formed internally in diabetes can be reduced by controlling blood sugar levels. So here are two more ways to shift from an inflammatory to an anti-inflammatory and healthier way of living.

It is not just AGEs we have to be careful of - high temperature cooking also creates ALEs, which might sound friendlier but are just as harmful. Advanced Lipoxidation End products are created when fats and oils are heated, and are highly pro-inflammatory.

Foods containing high levels of both AGEs and ALEs include powdered milk as used in enteral nutrition, numerous industrially produced foods and baby formulae (!), high temperature fried and grilled meat and poultry, deep fried and shallow fried fish, coffee and colas[25], soy sauces, balsamic products and smoked and cured foods – in short, fast food staples (1).

Daily consumption of fast foods for as little as a month causes liver damage equivalent to hepatititis (2). In one area where fast foods are a staple (San Antonio, Texas), the incidence

---

25. Coffee may contain AGE's but it also contains also a range of anti-inflammatory polyphenols, and is on balance a Good Thing (author's bias). Colas have few redeeming qualities.

of diet-related liver damage in a largely middle-aged population was found to be over 50%; with non-alcoholic fatty liver disease (NAFLD) at 46% and the more serious non-alcoholic steatohepatitis (NASH) at 12% (3). Fast foods generally combine high levels of AGE and ALE compounds with large amounts of salt and fat, and it is not eay to separate out the exact causes and effects. What is certain, however, is that high intakes of AGE and ALE's cause tissue damage in the short and in the long term.

Higher levels of these pro-inflammatory compounds in the blood are linked to higher rates of **many** degenerative diseases, including neurodegenerative diseases (4-5), cardiovascular diseases and diabetes (6-7), liver disease (8), lung disease (9) and a wide range of cancers (10-14).

How to Reduce Intakes of AGE's and ALE's

AGE and ALE levels in the diet can be greatly reduced by using lower temperature cooking methods.

Meat and fish: Cooking procedures that create a crust, such as the crispy borders of meats prepared at very high temperatures, produce AGE's. Grilling, deep-frying, barbequing and roasting all do this, and ground meats such as hamburger are particularly bad in this respect; as is the use of sugar or honey in glazes. Stewing, boiling or microwaving, cooking methods which do not exceed 100 degrees C, are far less prone to AGE and ALE formation. Minimise or avoid ground (minced) meat.

Eggs. Fried eggs contain relatively high levels of AGE's and ALE's; poaching, scrambling or boiling are better in this respect.

Deep-frying: avoid

Shallow frying: minimise; do not allow oils to over-heat to the point where they smoke, use cooker hood or other ventilation.

Stir frying: there is indirect but persuasive evidence that stir frying is the safest of all forms of frying, due to the short cooking time (15).

More of: fruits, vegetables, prebiotics found in foods such as oats, Jerusalem artichokes, pulses and legumes

Chapter 20. Internal affairs: inflammation and the microbiota

You are never alone. In fact, you are a minority element in a crowded ecosystem because, like everyone else, you are only 10% human. 90% of the cells in your body are alien, in that they are microbes, and most of these live in the large bowel. They have evolved to live inside us, and we have evolved to be dependent on them. Some scientists believe that the human body has evolved as "an elaborate vessel optimized for the growth and spread of our microbial inhabitants" (1), collectively known as the microbiota.

From a genetic perspective the odds are stacked even further against us. More than 99% of the genetic information inside us is microbial, and this 'second genome' or microbiome, may exert as much of an effect on our health as the genes we inherit from our parents. One key research group stated that human health should now "be thought of as a collective property of the human-associated microbiota," and a function of the community, not the individual (2). And here is another point where diet, and certain other aspects of lifestyle (such as stress levels) can cause, or reduce, chronic inflammation.

Some bacteria are strongly linked to better health. The probiotic species bifidobacteria and lactobacilli produce short chain fatty acids such as butyrate, which provides fuel for the epithelial cells that line the intestines and is essential for gut health. However, the probiotics can only produce butyrate when they are fed the right fuel, an extensive range of non-digestible carbohydrates or fibers found in fruits, vegetables, legumes and whole grains. These fibers are called prebiotics. When prebiotics are consumed the probiotic bacteria multiply, levels of butyrate increase and gut health is enhanced. If there are insufficient plant fibers in the diet probiotic bacteria decline, butyrate production drops and the epithelial cells become dysfunctional. The gut wall becomes more permeable and harmful agents enter the bloodstream including harmful microbes, bacterial toxins and other substances which trigger chronic inflammation.

This is worsened by the fact that as probiotic numbers fall, less friendly bacteria rush in to take their place. Bacteria are divided into Gram positive and Gram negative species, depending on the nature of their cell walls. Most probiotic species are Gram positive, but as their numbers fall they are replaced by Gram negative bacteria. Gram negative bacteria produce compounds called lipopolysaccharides (LPS), powerfully pro-inflammatory compounds which cause damage locally in the gut and throughout the body and are linked to *all* the important degenerative diseases (3), and to increased mortality (4).

A diet low in plant foods adds another insult, as it is almost inevitably low in polyphenols. Polyphenols have powerful and direct anti-inflammatory effects in the body, referred to elsewhere in this book, but new research has found that they have another important protective effect. Not all polyphenols are absorbed in the small bowel, and so they arrive in the large bowel. Here they are metabolised by the gut bacteria, forming dihydroxylated metabolites which strongly inhibit the inflammatory effects of LPS (5-6). On a junk diet, therefore, more LPS is produced and its inflammatory and disease-causing effects are enhanced.

This is a further reason why the Mediterranean and mid-Victorian diets are so healthy, and how they protect us by preventing chronic inflammation. And it is another reason why the high fat, high sugar, low-prebiotic junk and fast food diet promotes inflammation, disease and premature death. Perhaps the clearest link is with insulin resistance, metabolic syndrome and Type 2 diabetes, a family of progressively worsening conditions driven by chronic inflammation, and which accelerate the ageing process.

In animal models, a high fat junk food diet has been shown to lead to increased levels of increased gut permeability, LPS, inflammation and insulin resistance (7-8). There is good evidence that exactly the same mechanism operates in humans (9-12).

Woryingly, similar results were found when the gut microbial ecosystem was damaged by a course of antibiotics (8). Antibiotics can be life-saving, but a very high proportion of antibiotic prescriptions are grotesquely unnecessary; 50 million useless and unnecessary courses of antibiotics a year in the USA alone (13). These drugs are too often given uncritically by doctors unaware of the microbial havoc and potential long-term harm they are inflicting on their patients.

So how does all of this fit into an already over-crowded anti-inflammatory diet? The simple answer is that it is already baked into the cake. A diet rich in fruits, vegetables, legumes and whole grains already contains a range of the non-digestible cardbohydrates that fuel the probiotic species that help keep LPS low, together with the polyphenols that damp down the inflammatory effects LPS still further. But there is another aspect to this story, relating to food storage.

Fresh fruits, vegetables, legumes etc are obviously a good thing. However, it is important that these are fresh or at least frozen or canned. Foods left on the shelf quickly acquire significant microbial populations, and rising levels of LPS. Supermarkets love MPV's (minimally processed vegetables), which give them a higher profit margin – but these foods are rich sources of LPS, with particularly high levels in bean sprouts, diced onion and chopped root vegetables such as carrots (14). LPS levels increase in fresh meats too, even in the fridge, and especially in ground (minced) meat products (15).[26]

If all of this is making you feel stressed, I apologise. Stress is another way in which the host / microbe interface can go wrong, via what is known as the microbiome / gut / brain axis. This acts as a complex feedback loop whereby the gut and the brain 'talk' to one another. For example, stress can adversely impact on microbial populations in the gut, thereby increasing both levels and activity of LPS (6, 16); and cumulatively creating an unhealthy environment which affects our brain and our behaviour (17). Conversely, certain strains of probiotic bacteria have positive effects on the brain (18), and reduce signs of anxiety and depression (19-20). The scientists involved coined the term 'psychobiotics', which will doubtless be appearing on a yoghurt pot near you soon. Much of this work is done at the excellent University of Cork, a supremely relaxing city which is also – perhaps coincidentally – a global centre of culinary excellence.

---

26. Game meats which are typically hung for days contain extremely high levels of LPS. Caveat consumptor!

Probiotics are undoubtedly coming of age. There are so many different strains of probiotic bacteria that it is hard to pick a favourite, but I am impressed by the body of data supporting Lactobacillus reuteri. This has anti-inflammatory effects in the gut (21-22) and other tissues (23-24), and, like many other lactobacilli (25) it also provides its host with vitamin D (26). I am even more impressed by the catchily named Bifidobacterium bifidum CECT 7366, a microbe which is able to keep Helicobacter pylori under control (27).

H pylori is a bacterium which inhabits the stomach, where it is implicated in gastric and duodenal ulcers, and stomach cancer. This is not the whole picture, however. When H pylori becomes too dominant the risk of gastric cancer increases, but if it is eradicated we become more prone to asthma (28) and TB (29). Some scientists believe that the absence of H pylori may also increase the risk of esophageal cancer (30), although this is currently under review (31).

The emerging paradigm amongst microbiologists is that it is generally preferable to maintain a healthy balance of microbial species whenever possible, rather than opting for the nuclear option of antibiotics. Medical doctors, however, are obsessed with H pylori eradication and routinely use complex antibiotic regimes to achieve this. These regimes are unpleasant and have a rising failure rate, due to antibiotic resistance; and in any case, now there is evidence that this whole approach may carry significant risks. Taking Bb CECT 7366 in a daily yoghurt, wafer or capsule would almost certainly be a better and more pleasant way to maintain a healthy microbiome[27].

A note to IBS sufferers. You will probably not react well to prebiotics, and may have to avoid them in the short term (32). This is the basis of the so-called FODMAP diet (33). Your symptoms could be due to probiotic species which have inappropriately colonised the small bowel, so a preliminary clear-out with polyphenols is advised before re-admitting prebiotics to the diet.

A note to people with poor oral hygiene. If your gums bleed after brushing you have periodontal disease, a chronic infection of the gums. The bacteria involved produce LPS, which has long been suspected to be the link between periodontal disease and an increased risk of heart disease (34-35). More recently, it has been identified as a possible risk factor for another inflammatory condition, Alzheimer's Disease (36).

A note to students of history. While chronic exposure to LPS appears to be a risk factor for almost all diseases, acute exposure to high levels of LPS might conceivably have some uses. In the late 19th century the US surgeon William Coley developed the use of dead bacterial cultures to trigger fever and – occasionally – cure in his cancer patients. These cultures, known as Coley's Toxins, utilise gram negative bacteria and contain high levels of LPS (37). High levels of LPS affect the immune system in ways which would be expected to enhance cancer cell killing (38). The dangers of this approach, however, are significant, and it should not be tried at home.

---

27. To enable probiotic species to work effectively it is always best to combine them with the appropriate prebiotic, which is the probiotic's substrate (or food). As prebiotics are all derived from plant foods, this is another argument for a plant-based diet. The combination of a probiotic and its prebiotic is termed a symbiotic.

Chapter 21. Genetic factors: inflammation, mutrients & telomeres

Chronic inflammation causes tissue damage, but it also harms our health prospects in another, even more insidious way; it reduces the ability of the body to heal that damage, and shortens our life-span, by reducing our cells' ability to renew themselves.

The lifespan of normal cells is controlled by telomeres, sections of DNA at the end of each chromosome; and by the telomere shortening mechanism, which limits cells to a fixed number of divisions. With each dell division the telomeres shorten. When the telomeres are totally consumed cells can no longer replicate, and commit suicide (apoptosis). The telomeres' main function is to ensure, during cell division, that the cell's chromosomes are properly paired and allocated to each daughter cell, and do not fuse with each other or rearrange, creating genetic errors which could lead to cancer.

Telomere length is usually measured in leucocytes, white blood cells which are easily accessible via blood samples. Reduced telomere length is invariably linked to worse health outcomes and higher death rates, and is increasingly regarded as a deep biomarker of biological ageing. Chronic inflammation, a very major cause of disease and death [1], causes telomere shortening – and telomere shortening may in turn cause inflammation [2-4]. Oxidative stress, which overlaps with inflammatory stress, also causes telomere shortening [5]. All these factors are inter-connected and probably mutually reinforcing [6].

Individuals who experience chronic oxidative and inflammatory stress such as diabetics, the obese, smokers and those exposed to chronic air pollution [7-10] have shorter telomeres than people of the same age who are lean, non-smokers and not exposed to chronic air pollution. It is very reasonable to assue, therefore, that those nutrients which reduce oxidative and inflammatory stress should slow telomere loss, and biological ageing.

There is extensive evidence, coming from multiple labs and research centres, that the Omega-3 fatty acids and the polyphenols do just this.

In 2010, a research team at San Francisco Hospital were studying patients with coronary artery disease. They found a clear inverse relationship between baseline blood levels of marine omega-3 fatty acids and the rate of telomere shortening over 5 years [11]. This suggested that eating enough Omega-3's could slow biological ageing, but there was more. In a subsequent study at Ohio State University College of Medicine, just 4 months of supplementation with Omega-3's in healthy but sedentary and overweight middle-aged and elderly subjects, sufficient to improve the Omega-6 / -3 ratio, was linked to reduced inflammation and a *lengthening* of telomeres in immune cells [12]. This indicated that Omega-3's might actually reverse biological ageing, or at the very least set it back to where it was before chronic inflammation started to erode the telomeres.

Support for this comes from UCLA, where a pilot study lead by the redoubtable Dean Ornish showed that a 3-month life style intervention program, which included Omega-3's and selenium with a healthy diet and moderate exercise, increased levels of the enzyme telomerase (13). As telomerase regenerates telomeres, this and the Ohio data suggest that a healthier diet and lifestyle can achieve telomeric repair. In contrast, increasing intakes of the pro-inflammatory Omega-6 fatty acids have been linked to shorter telomeres (14-15).

Polyphenols appear to be as protective as the Omega-3's. Green tea is a rich source of polyphenols, and in one study, researchers from the Chinese University of Hong Kong found that the telomeres of people who drank an average of three cups of green tea per day were significantly longer than people who drank an average of a quarter of a cup a day (16). The difference in telomere length corresponded to approximately a difference of 5 years of life. The concept that an increased intake of polyphenols slows telomere loss is supported by larger studies (14).

Based on their complementary modes of action, one would expect the combination of Omega-3's and polyphenols to be more protective than either one alone.

Chapter 22. Canaries in the Coalmine: inflammation, nutrients and infertility

Sometimes it is necessary for the old order to fail utterly before a new order can be considered, particularly when there are powerful groups (health insurance companies, the pharmaceutical industry, the medical profession) with vested interests in the status quo. Most of us can only hear warnings that the old system is at the point of failure when we are ready to hear them, and it helps if those warnings are couched in language that touches us. Here is one such warning.

It comes from France, where a recent nation-wide survey has shown that male sperm counts are falling precipitously (1). Researchers found that during the 16 years between 1989 and 2005, sperm counts in French men progressively dropped by an average of 32.3%. Numbers of normally formed sperm also fell by a third.

The French results confirm research over the past 20 years that has shown sperm counts declining in many countries across the world (2-3), and indicate that masculinity itself is under threat. Further evidence for this comes from the rise in rates of testicular cancer which have doubled in the last 30 years, prostate cancer (the second leading cause of cancer death in males in the West) and other male sexual disorders such as undescended testes (4).

Dr. Joelle Le Moal, an environmental health epidemiologist and one of the study's authors, described the French findings as "… a serious public health warning." Richard Sharpe, the internationally renowned professor of reproductive health at the University of Edinburgh, agreed. "There can be little doubt that the decline in sperm counts is real,' he said. 'Something in our modern lifestyle, diet or environment is causing this and it is getting progressively worse.'

Nature has engineered a good deal of redundancy into us, and healthy men produce far more sperm than necessary for conception, but we are reaching the point where fertility is being substantially compromised. Historical data show that in the 1940's, semen samples from young men averaged over 100 million sperm per ml. However, sperm counts in the majority of 20 year old European men are now so low that we have reached the crucial tipping point of 40 mill/mL spermatozoa, which is where sub-fertility kicks in. In Denmark, 40% of young males are now below that figure (5), and the French are in the same bateu. Significant and increasing numbers of males are presenting with sperm counts below 15 million /ml, which is well into the infertile range.

It is always dangerous to project current trends uncritically into the future – and it is important to note that fertility rates have not yet shown any untoward variations (6). However, if sperm counts continue to fall at the current rate, our children and grandchildren will experience ever-increasing rates of infertility and human populations will start an exponentially accelerating collapse as early as 2030.

If this is not, finally, a call to action to the scientifically illiterate and predominantly male politicians who currently lord it over over us, I don't know what is. And it is almost certainly another symptom of the more general and more wide-spread problem of chronic inflammation. The causes of falling sperm counts are not fully understood, and there is always some well-intentioned buffoon ready to tell us that the real problem is tight underwear; but the evidence indicates that our lousy, pro-inflammatory diets and lifestyles are doing most of the damage[28].

As men instinctively know, the testes are very privileged organs. 'Immune privilege' means that they are able to tolerate foreign tissues without triggering an inflammatory immune response. This is entirely logical, as otherwise sperm would be attacked and destroyed by our own immune systems, and we would be unable to reploroduce. Other sites with immune privilege include the fetus and placenta, for the same reason.

The testes still have to be able to defend themselves against infection, and so must maintain a very complex and delicate balance of pro- and anti-inflammatory forces inside a very small volume of highly complex tissue which has the dual role of producing both sperm and the sex hormone testosterone. The situation is complicated further by the fact that the process of formation of sperm cells involves many of the elements of a controlled chronic inflammatory reaction (7).

In health, a broadly immunosuppressive and anti-inflammatory microenvironment in the testicles protects the germ and sperm cells from immune attack. In inflammatory conditions, tolerance is disrupted and local immune cells start to damage and destroy the germ and sperm cells (8). Maintaining the right balance of pro- and anti-inflammatory factors is therefore critical to sperm formation and healthy sperm counts.

In the testis, as in many tissues throughout the body, the number of germ and sperm cells is determined by a dynamic balance between cell proliferation and programmed (apoptotic) cell death. (9). Seventy-five percent of all germ cells produced in the testis are discarded through the process of apoptosis (10). This means that sperm counts are rapidly affected by changes in sperm formation or death rates.

Excessive chronic inflammation increases sperm death rates; and external sources of inflammation (infection, chronic inflammatory conditions, LPS) all cause a fall in sperm counts (11-16). Conversely, excessive chronic inflammation in the testes and reduced sperm counts can be reversed by those sterling anti-inflammatory agents, the polyphenols (17-19). These will likely work even better when combined with Omega 3 fatty acids, which have also been shown to be positively related to sperm quality and numbers (20-23).

From a historical and dietary perspective, the wide-spread problem of falling sperm counts is closely linked to the decline in our intake of the key dietary anti-inflammatory nutrients. It is just another manifestation, along with the huge increases in the chronic degenerative diseases, of our pro-inflammatory lifestyle. This manifestation won't kill us individually but could, if left unchecked, kill us off as a species.

---

28. Environmental pollutants know as xenoestrogens are also implicated.

Chapter 23. RDA's and RNI's: How much Nutrition Do We Really Need?

One of the serious problems with the anti-inflammatory nutrients is that the officially recommended doses are, in some cases, very wrong. The Recommended Daily Allowance (RDA) of foods and supplements has traditionally been set by government health bodies in the UK, Europe and USA. In the UK the Department of Health first gave the RDA for vitamins A, C, and D, three of the B vitamins, and three minerals in 1979. In 1991, the UK government issued a report suggesting new guidelines for daily requirements of vitamins and minerals, which would replace the RDAs. These are called, collectively, Dietary Reference Values (DRVs), and include the terms Estimated Average Requirement (EAR), which should meet the requirements of half of the population; and Reference Nutrient Intake (RNI), which replaces the former RDA, and supposedly represents the nutrient requirements of 97% of the population.

The RDA's and latterly the RNI's of macro- and micronutrients are constantly being re-evaluated, in an on-going process that started in the late 1930's and continues to this day. Currently published tables of RNI values should be regarded as a work in progress; they are known to contain at least five major classes of inaccuracies, all of which are under some level of review.

One substantial deficiency in the current tables is that some of the current RNI's have not yet assimilated recent expert findings and are clearly too low to promote good health at the population level. This is addressed in Section 2.

A second problem is that a number of phyto-nutrients and miscellaneous molecules which have the characteristics of vitamins (ie organic compounds that must be obtained in small amounts in the diet to maintain good health), do not yet have RNI's. As our understanding of human metabolic chemistry develops it has become increasingly hard to justify the fact that methyl groups, for example, the equivalent of what was once termed vitamin U, and which feed one carbon metabolism, have no RNI. Cyanogenic groups, essential for the activity of the vitally important antimicrobial enzyme lactoperoxidase, have no RNI. Key carotenoids including lycopene, lutein and possibly zeaxanthin have no RNI; neither do the omega 3 PUFA's, the polyphenols or the (1-3), (1-6) beta-glucans, even although these compounds fulfil all the vitamin criteria. One could also include the fermentable carbohydrates in this category, although health-promoting intakes of these compounds exceed those of the classical vitamins. These multiple and substantial omissions are partly due to the conservatism of the bodies which designate RDA / RNI values, and partly due to the lack of sufficient data.

A third, more structural problem with the concept of the RDA's / RNI's is that they have been calculated in human populations within the 20th and 21st centuries, and do not take previous epidemiological information into account. This in turn means that they are predicated on prevailing models of senescence which focus primarily on degenerative diseases, which are widely and uncritically accepted as being generally entropic in nature. Recent research, however, has established that current patterns of ageing and dying are not intrinsic, and should be more accurately regarded as socio-cultural artefacts. It is known that in at least one previous historical period (1850-1890), and in a population in which adults had a similar life expectancy to that which exists today, degenerative disease was relatively rare (1). This absence of degenerative disease has been linked to higher levels of physical activity, and to significantly higher intakes of micro- and phyto-nutrients than are consumed, and considered normal, in the 21st century. Intakes of phyto-nutrients, in particular, were approximately ten times higher than exist in today's low-calorie and depleted diets. Conversely, the pattern of multiple micro- and phyto-nutrient depletion caused by the contemporary diet is emerging as the most important cause of degenerative disease today. This is very much in line with Bruce Ames' triage theory (2, 3).

A fourth problem with RDA's refers to their mathematical derivation. The RDA is calculated as the EAR (Estimated Average Requirement) + 2xSD (EAR); where EAR is the amount of a micronutrient needed to ensure the health of 50% of a specific population, based on a review of the scientific literature. According to this calculation, the RDA is anticipated to be sufficient to cover the needs of up to 98% of the population in question. However, the calculation can only be meaningfully performed when the Standard Deviation of the EAR is known, which is not always the case; and when the requirement for the nutrient is symmetrically distributed, which is also not always the case. For example smokers, athletes, pregnant women, the elderly, obese and/ or diabetic subjects and dark-skinned ethnic groups may have distinct requirements for certain micronutrients.

An inter-related additional problem is one of time-frame; the EAR filter only looks at the short- to medium-term impact of 'sub-optimal' levels of any nutrient (such as the relationship between severe hypo-vitaminosis C and scorbutism, which emerges within weeks), and is generally unable to take into account longer-term patho-aetiological sequences such as the link between multiple micronutrient depletion, including moderate hypo-vitaminosis C, and an array of degenerative diseases, which typically develop over decades.

A fifth major problem with micronutrient RDA's is that they have been estimated on the basis of single entities, as if they all had separate, non-overlapping metabolic roles. There are many examples where this is manifestly not the case; one such is the ability of polyphenols to reduce the requirement for vitamin C (4), thus effectively modulating vitamin C's RDA. Calcium provides another example. The RDA for calcium has been set at a level of intake that supposedly supports bone health, but this was calculated in populations which are commonly depleted in many or all the other bone trophic micronutrients (including vitamins D and K); and for this reason is so ludicrously high that it increases the risk of heart disease (5, 28). In a nutritionally replete population the RDA for calcium would be substantially lower.

These multiple problems were partially recognised at a recent Institute of Medicine workshop entitled "The Development of DRIs 1994–2004: Lessons Learned and New Challenges." (6). At this meeting the current Dietary Recommended Intakes (DRI's) were criticised as being largely based upon the very lowest rank in the quality of evidence pyramid, that is, opinion, rather than the highest level – randomized controlled clinical trials. There was a call for a higher standard of evidence to be utilized when making dietary recommendations. It is unclear whether this will be enacted in the near future.

RDA's for the trace elements other than calcium are relatively well characterised and will not be addressed here. There is insufficient evidence to make recommendations regarding the phytonutrients, other than the historical data which indicates RDA's approximately 10 times current dietary average values [1]. This short review accordingly focuses on a number of vitamins where the current RDA's are under sustained attack, and where substantial changes in RDA values are likely. The term SODA is used; this neologism refers to Suggested Optimal Daily Allowances.

1. Specific Cases

Vitamin E: Current RDA 30 IU (30 mg of dl-alpha-tocopherol or equivalents)

Vitamin E is a family of eight tocochromanols consisting of four tocopherols and four tocotrienols, but is generally calculated in terms of d-alpha tocopherol equivalents for RDA purposes. This is because the d-alpha form is the most potent anti-oxidant in most measurement systems, and this in turn dates back to a time when vitamin E was thought of as being nothing more a lipophile antioxidant. It is now known, however, that the various tocopherols and tocotrienols have a range of different functions, many of which are not antioxidant, and partition differently in the body. Among the tocopherols, for example, the gamma form plays a preferential role in maintaining cell membrane viability [7], while the alpha form has a distinct ability to prevent certain types of apoptosis [8]. Other substantive differences are known [9]; and are equally prominent among the tocotrienols [10, 11], which have inter alia specific anti-cancer effects [12, 13].

It would perhaps be more relevant to calculate multiple RDA's based on the functionalities of all 8 tocochromanols, but this has not been attempted. In the meantime, we have derived a SODA for total tocochromanols based on a retrospective analysis of the dietary intake in the period 1850-1890 [1]. This is approximately 50-60 mg, roughly double the current RDA.

It is not possible at this time to make specific recommendations regarding optimal tocopherol / tocotrienol ratios, but a roughly equal distribution seems reasonable, based on the individual functionalities of the eight compounds in the group and the differential composition of dietary sources of these compounds. This would not fall outside the known range of dietary intakes.

Vitamin D: Current RDA for 50-70 yrs, 400 IU (1 mcg).

Typical diets provide about 100 IU/day, ie one quarter of the current RDA, which is itself generally considered to be grossly inadequate (see below). Unsurprisingly, hypo-vitaminosis D is prevalent in the temperate nations, particularly among dark-skinned groups. New research estimates that inadequate levels of vitamin D cause / contribute to about 37,000 premature deaths in Canada every year, and cost the country 14 to 15 billion dollars annually (14). These results, if extrapolated to the UK, indicate that low vitamin D levels contribute to 75,000 premature British deaths per year; and conversely, that properly designed supplements could save over £200 billion of EU healthcare costs per year. It is therefore critically important that we move rapidly towards an effective RDA for vitamin D.

According to Osteoporosis Canada's most recent recommendations (15), adults under the age of 50 should be taking up to 1,000 International Units of vitamin D and people over 50 should be taking supplements up to 2,000 IU. The NIH has a "Tolerable Upper Intake Level (UL)" of 2,000 IU/day, but newer studies indicate a UL as high as 10,000 IU/day (16).

The Institute of Medicine (IOM) is conducting a review of vitamin D science and is due to deliver its findings. Many expect them to recommend RDA's as high as 2000 IU, in line with Osteoporosis Canada's position. The IOM are also examining UL's. Their decision to do so was influenced by papers by Dr Reinhold Vieth on vitamin D's safety and therapeutic index (17, 18), and by the simple fact that for most skin types, a full body minimal erythemal dose of UVB results in the production of about 20,000 IU of cholecalciferol (19). This is about 100 times more vitamin D than the current RDA: indeed, normal rates of endogenous D synthesis constitute a convincing argument that current RDA values are conceptually unsound, and gravely inadequate. It is noteworthy that Ian Monroe, the chair of the relevant Institute of Medicine (IOM) committee which sets vitamin levels, wrote a letter to the Journal in which he complimented Vieth's paper and promised that his findings would be considered in the IoM review (20).

Additional data regarding the true safe upper limit of D can be derived from clinical studies in which high doses of vitamin D were used therapeutically, and without signs of toxicity. For example, hyperparathyroidism has been successfully managed with 50,000 to 200,000 IU of vitamin D daily (21), while rickets generally requires a dose of 1,600 IU/day, and may require a daily dosage of 50,000 to as much as 300,000 IU in resistant cases (22). Based on the sun exposure and existing safety data, I rate the SODA at around 5000 IU / day. Given regulatory concerns, a compromise of 2500 IU seems reasonable.

The current epidemic of vitamin D depletion and deficiency is due in no small measure to ill-advised recommendations to avoid exposure to what is deemed excessive sunlight; recommendations which were issued in an attempt to stem the rising tide of skin cancers. There are many things wrong with the current guidelines, not least the fact that melanoma, the most serious of the skin cancers, has little to do with sun exposure (See following chapter on vitamin D and UV)

There are very few good food sources of 'vitamin' D. Oily fish are a good source but not many people eat these today. Mushrooms the next best but vary wildly depending on the degree of exposure to UV – in this sense fungi are very like us (23, 24).

Vitamin K: Current RDA: 80 mcg or 1 mcg / kg body weight

Vitamin K is a group name for K1 (phylloquinone, dietary source green leaves) and K2 (menaquinones, dietary source bacterial fermented foods such as natto and cheeses). Both forms contribute to tissue vitamin K status. The current RDA is derived from doses require to maintain normal (hepatic) clotting functions, and is based on K1. This fails to take account more recently discovered functions of the vitamin K group, which include the calcification of osteoid and the prevention of calcification of soft tissues such as muscle and blood vessesls. The doses of K needed to maintain healthy bones and to inhibit or reverse the calcification of soft tissues are significantly higher than doses needed to maintain clotting functions (25); in any case, due to pharmacokinetic considerations, the K2 form is specifically indicated for these latter two functions (26, 27).

Given the current pandemic of osteoporosis, vitamin K2 supplements would be recommended more widely were it not for the fact that there is still widespread misunderstanding about K requirements and safety. Current recommended K intakes (1 microgram / kg body weight) were originally set for liver function, and as stated above are far too low to maintain healthy bones (26). Vitamin K has been shown to be safe at doses several hundred times greater than the RDA values; it does not, for example, induce hyper-coagulation at doses up to 20 mg (28).

A common concern relates to the interaction between vitamin K and warfarin, which operates by acting as a K antagonist. Counter-intuitively, there are positive advantages to supplementing with K. Warfarin responses tend to fluctuate, making it a leading cause of ADR's; a recent study showed that in subjects with higher intakes of K, the long-term anticoagulation effects of warfarin were actually more stable (28).

Based on the work on K2 and bone metabolism, and levels of K2 intake in prefectures in Japan where natto is consumed and where osteoporotic fracture is relatively uncommon (29), the SODA is considered to be around 1mg. A compromise of 500 mcg seems reasonable.

This brings us back to the thorny issue of calcium where the RDA, originally set in an attempt to preventing osteoporosis, is manifestly far too high. The EU RDA for calcium is a flat 800 mg/ day, while the USA RDA values are age-related. Below the age of 50, men are and women are recommended to take 1000 mg/day. After the age of 50 the RDA rises to 1,200 mg / day for both sexes. Even at these ridiculous doses calcium is ineffective in protecting against osteoporosis, either on its own or when combined with vitamin D; and in any case, the correlation between calcium status and osteoporosis risk is notoriously poor. Bone is a very dynamic tissue, and its quality and quantity are determined by the balance between bone growth and bone resorption (breakdown). As the rate of resorption is accelerated by a pro-inflammatory environment in the body, it is hardly surprising that age-related osteopenia and osteoporosis are so prevalent.

Consider a tiled roof which has not been maintained, so that the nails holding the slates on the roof are corroded or missing. The slates start to fall off; the medical answer is to throw slates (calcium) back onto the roof in the hope that some of them might stick. But if there are insufficient nails, and if the wind is blowing hard (inflammation), then the calcium supplement will be useless and bone will continue to be lost. Simply adding vitamin D (which basically enhances calcium absorption) is equally misguided. Adding vitamin K (which, in the roof metaphor, acts rather like a nail) to calcium + D will greatly help matters; and if you were to add an anti-inflammatory program containing Omega-3 fatty acids and polyphenols, rates of bone resorption would fall and the net loss of bone should slow, stop and even go into partial reverse.

The absurdly high doses of calcium currently being recommended are not only ineffective; they appear to be counter-productive in that they raise the risk of myocardial infarctions (30-32).

2. SUMMARY

It is notable that the largest discrepancies between RDA and SODA occur with lipophiles, which are more likely to accumulate in the body than are the water-soluble vitamins. This has undoubtedly contributed to the conservatism around RDA's and UL's described above; the inadequacy of which has been high-lit by the issues of multiple vitamin forms and emerging functionalities.

A second level of bias has been introduced via the use of inappropriate and incomplete risk analysis models, which are based on pharmaceutical approaches. Regulators have measured the risks of additional intakes of single nutrients and applied mathematical screening systems based on the application of xeno-molecules. They have failed to incorporate into their models the vastly greater risks of not adding these nutrients to the diet. This failure was due, in turn, to an inadequate uederstanding of the multiple depletion of the Western, low-calorific throughput diet, and its subsequently pathogenic properties. On-going research into superior diets such as the Mediterranean and mid-Victorian diets shows that the risks of not supplementing the diet are substantial, and if rigorously defined must include the bulk of the pandemics of degenerative disease that we currently think of as inevitable and 'normal'. The IoM's current debate about the RDA for vitamin D will, hopefully, start to move this issue forwards.

Further complications regarding vitamin D are addressed in the next chapter.

Chapter 24. Sunshine, shadows and showers: the dangers of living in glasshouses

'Vitamin' D is not a vitamin but a hormone. A very few foods contain this compound, but most of us produce most of our own vitamin D ourselves in our skin, when it is exposed to sunlight. In Nothern Europe, however, we don't expose much skin to sunlight after the end of September, and we don't take our shirts off again until May at the earliest. This is why most Europeans are depleted in D for most of the year, a pattern that has been worsened by the blizzard of anti-sunshine PR from various Departments of Health that seem hell-bent on convincing us that sunlight is dangerous and unnatural.

This campaign was started partly as a result of input from an eminent cancer specialist, whose Scottish patients were showing an increasing incidence of melanoma. The UK Department of Health jumped on board and soon, in the public's mind, the link between sunlight and melanoma was established. We all had to wear hats, UV-blocking clothing, tons of sunscreen, and not even venture into the midday sun.

Seen from an historical perspective, this makes little sense. We were 'designed' to be outdoors animals, and the very idea that sunlight is somehow dangerous for us shows just how ignorant of history many scientists (and of course politicians) are. In the mid-Victorian period, when life expectancy equalled or exceeded our own, rural workers laboured in the fields from dawn to dusk throughout the spring, summer and autumn. Yet despite the shocking absence of sunscreen, cancer was very rare indeed; it occurred at about 10% of today's levels (1).

Today, however, when more and more of us work indoors, and are less exposed to sunlight than ever before, the incidence of melanoma continues to climb – and appearing, not infrequently, on parts of the body not exposed to sunlight such as the sole of the foot. It has trebled since 1960 and is continuing to increase (2-3); to the point where in the UK this once rare condition is now the most common cancer in the 15 – 34 age group (4). Part of the increase in melanoma is probably due to increased sun bed use, but this cannot be the only factor...

The mid-Victorians provide us with one valuable clue. They ate huge amounts of fruits and vegetables containing a range of compounds that migrate into the skin, give it a golden colour, and protect it against solar damage (5-7). These protective compounds have antioxidant, anti-inflammatory and anti-cancer properties. Due to our less physical lifestyles and impoverished food intakes, our skins do not receive the same level of dietary protection. This is one major reason why we are more vulnerable to skin cancer. If, in addition, you eat a terrible diet – such as is routinely eaten Scotland – levels of these protective compounds in the skin will be even lower. I say this from personal experience, as I was raised in Scotland; the reason why so many Scots are so pale is not only because they have Celtic genes, but also because the only vegetable that many of them eat is the chip. The resulting lack of dietary protection in their skin exacerbates their Celtic pallor and leaves their skin very vulnerable.

The other reason for the increase in melanoma is that more and more of us work under glass. By that I mean that we mostly see sunlight through windows, rather than exposing ourselves to the sunlight directly. Sunlight through glass is very different from direct sunlight, and while glasshouses may be good for strawberries, evidence is accumulating that they are not good for us. This is because glass lets the UV-A component of sunlight through, but blocks UV-B. This is a doubly dangerous combination because UV-A is potentially dangerous, and we need UV-B.

UV-B is a higher frequency component of sunlight, and it is UV-B that triggers vitamin D synthesis in the skin. Vitamin D has a range of anti-cancer properties, and we would therefore expect the overall effect of moderate exposure to UV-B to be cancer-protective, especially if the skin is also protected with dietary compounds. Three major papers have recently been published making a very strong case for vitamin D being cancer-protective (8-11); in one of these, Professor Cedric Garland of the University of California predicted that a 50 mcg dose of vitamin D daily would prevent an estimated 200,000 cases of breast cancer and 250,000 of bowel cancer worldwide.

The rural mid-Victorians were exposed to long periods of direct sunlight, with plenty of UV-B, and as a result had far higher levels of vitamin D than we do today. In addition, their high intakes of fruit and vegetables meant that they had outstanding dietary skin protection. As a result of these two factors, they had very little cancer of any kind.

We are in exactly the opposite situation. We eat far less fruit and vegetables, and have more vulnerable and more easily inflamed skin as a result. To make matters worse, our glazed offices and conservatories mean that we are bathed in UV-A. UVA can cause cancerous mutations, and it breaks down any vitamin D that had been formed in skin after outdoor UVB exposure. This is an imbalance of effects that would be expected to raise the incidence of cancer in indoor workers –and this is exactly what we see today (12).

The opposing effects of UV-A and UV-B on vitamin D levels creates a protective mechanism, which prevents prolonged sun exposure from causing Vitamin D overdose.

The way to better health is to eat more fruit and vegetables, and get the midday sun on your back – just enough to cause slight reddening. This will produce up to 200 mcg of D in your skin (13), the right amount to keep your bones healthy and reduce your risk of cancers such as breast and colon cancer. It all makes a mockery of the government's decision to keep the RNI of vitamin D at 10 mcg/day.

This sad story is yet another example of the dangers of medical specialism, and doctors who know everything about drugs but little about anything else. The cancer specialist who initiated the anti-sun campaign was (rightly) concerned about skin cancer. Unfortunately the medical profession's lack of awareness of history and nutrition lead to ill-advised and counter-productive advice about staying out of the sun which lowered vitamin D levels across the nation, did nothing to reduce skin cancer, and contributed to many unnecessary cancer deaths. The fact that more recent evidence has shown that the typically Celtic colour scheme (pale skin and red hair) is intrinsically prone to skin cancer even without UV exposure (14), has weakened the official sun = danger story further.

One last note. I mentioned showers, and now it turns out that excessive cleanliness may also be contributing to the increase in melanoma and other cancers. You might think this is crazy, but bear with me…

Vitamin D is a steroid hormone, and like all steroids it is lipid soluble. When it is formed in the upper layers of the skin after exposure to UV-B, it doesn't get into the blood stream right away. It remains in the lipid layers of the skin (such as the sebum) for some time before it can be absorbed into the deeper layers of the skin and passed into the bloodstream. This is a slow process of diffusion, and is not completed for up to 8 hours (15) or even longer (16). If you de-grease your skin by washing with soap before that time, you will wash away a considerable part of the freshly formed vitamin D. Better leave the protective sebum on the skin until the next morning, and wash before (or after) breakfast. But if you are still scared of the sun, here are the best food sources of this sunshine 'vitamin'.

	mcg D	% RNI
Cod liver oil, 1 tablespoon	36	360
Salmon, cooked, 3.5 ounces	90	090
Mackerel, cooked, 3.5 ounces	80	90
Tuna fish, canned in oil, 3 ounces	50	50
Sardines, canned in oil, drained, 1.75 ounces	60	70
Mushrooms, per 100g fresh weight*	30	35

* Mushrooms vary from 0.2 ncg to 30 mcg / 100 g fresh weight; depending on species and degree of UV expoure.

Chapter 25. Nutrition and Politics: The Cruelty of Business and the Persistence of Hope

During the 20th and 21st centuries, the degenerative diseases have steadily increased in frequency; so much so that today, most consider them to be an integral part of the ageing process. This is an obvious fallacy[29] but it suits the food industry which can continue to sell us foods that are intrinsically unsafe; and it suits the pharmaceutical industry because it enables them to sell us repeat prescriptions of the toxic and ineffective drugs we use to suppress the symptoms of our degenerative diseases. These drugs are not curative, nor have they prevented the increasing burden of these diseases – which, it is increasingly acknowledged, have become so prevalent largely because of our failure to maintain the anti-inflammatory standards of the diet our great-grandparents ate (1).

To greatly enhance the chances of health and healthy ageing, it is glaringly obvious that we should increase our intakes of dietary anti-inflammatory compounds. Speaking as a pharmacologist, it is irrelevant to me whether you do this via foods, supplements or both. If we want to empty the hospitals, more of the anti-inflammatory phytonutrients must be put back into the diet in one form or another.

Under the thumb of the food and pharma lobbies[30], however, regulators will continue to drag their heels until their hand is finally forced by a body of evidence large enough to outweigh the protests of the vested interests, a consumerist demand for better nutrition and the bankruptcy of the healthcare services.

I cannot talk for the consumers, or for the medeconomists, but I can try to talk for the science, which has now reached critical mass. On the top of a mountain of data showing that anti-inflammatory nutrients are health-protective, and the overwhelming historical evidence, we now have what is hopefully just the first solid, prospective, randomised clinical trial that proves the benefits of anti-iflammatory nutrition.

A team at the prestigious Karolinska Institute has just found that in women who eat higher levels of dietary anti-inflammatory compounds, the risk of heart attack is reduced by a very significant 20% (2). So here is another link in the dose-response curve, with a total of four data sets showing improved health prospects as we move from the degraded Western diet to the Karolinska diet, to the Mediterranean diet and finally to the mid-Victorian diet. We now have enough data to show, UNEQUIVOCALLY, that as we become less prone to inflammation, we become progressively more immune to the so called diseases of ageing.

We have the science to create far better public health, but science is meaningless unless it can be put into practice. What is needed is a politician of a rare kind; one with a brain and a

29. Coronary heart disease was a rarity in 1900, but had become the No. 1 killer by 1960. This is not natural, but the result of our dangerously unhealthy diets.
30. Regulatory capture describes a situation where regulatory agencies become owned by the industries they were set up to regulate. Given the vast number of personnel who shuttle between the food and phrama industries, and given that the food/pharma complex spends more than twice as much on lobbying government as the defence industries, it is not surprising that the regulatory bodies no longer serve their original purpose.

backbone to match, who can take up these ideas and buld them into a political platform for change and a new form of healthcare to be delivered not in the surgery or pharmacy but at the supermarket checkout. A political hero could make a name for him or herself by changing the regulations, and encouraging food companies to produce foods with higher, mid-Victorian nutrient density. This kind of pharmaco-nutritional approach would make us less prone to chronic inflammation, and lead to dramatic falls in the incidence of degenerative disease. It would also save a great deal of money.

Healthcare spending currently swallows 19% of GDP (3). The mid-Victorian data show that if national nutritional programs involving the food manufacturers and retailers could be fully implemented, pharmaconutrition could reduce the burden of the chronic degenerative diseases by up to 90%. Most folks would live healthier and longer, but finally die of short term illnesses such as overwhelming infections which consume far less healthcare resources. Preliminary calculations indicate that health care spending requirements could be cut by as much as 95%, equating in the UK to savings of over 17% of GDP or £119 Billion[31].

Let us be less ambitious and assume that a less extensive roll-out of nutritional programs, hampered by Big Pharma and their lackeys on the regulatory committes, only reached 30% of the population. This would cut degenerative disease by approximately 27%, and health care costs by roughly 30%, resulting in savings of a little over £40 Billion in the UK alone.

Mid-Victorian nutrition would save lives, years, suffering and vast amounts of money – and the only obstacles to achiving these goals are political.

Our lifestyles have changed more drastically in the last half century than in the whole of our previous history, and they have changed in ways that have made the formerly rare degenerative diseases, universal. The sedentary lives we now lead and the foods we eat today constitute a lifestyle far from the one we evolved within, and are 'designed' for. We are paying a high price for the great and unplanned lifestyle experiment that we have all, however unwittingly, agreed to participate in. And the food and drug industries, far from supporting our desires for health, conspire to undermine them.

I spend a good deal of time travelling around the world, and nowhere is this more evident than in North America. In many urban areas there is little food choice, especially if you cannot afford a car. Most convenience foods are low in nutrients, high in calories, salt and sugar; vegetable dishes in most restaurant chains are inevitably breaded and deep-fried, as is much of the rest of their food, and many children never eat fresh fruit. Most cities are not designed for walking, so most folks travel everywhere by car. With all these factors working against them, it is no wonder that so many Americans are overweight and obese. The restaurants and shopping malls are full of these unhappy, bloated, self-harming folk; imprisoned not only in their cultural wasteland but also within their own diseased bodies.

---

31. This is being developed formally in a series of papers currently being written by Dr Judith Rowbotham, myself and a group of medeconomists. We hope to publish in 2014.

They are unaware that the diet they eat is loaded with pro-inflammatory compounds and simultaneously deficient in anti-inflammatory nutrients; or that their sedentary lifestyles interact with this diet to create deposits of pro-inflammatory adipose tissue. They are unaware that this combination of factors is driving them down to road to degenerative disease, accelerating the ageing process and degrading their health and life expectancy. They are largely unaware that the drugs they will inevitably come to depend on will not cure their ills – and will very likely harm them. But it is not just the North Americans. The urbanised populations of Central and South America, South East Asia, Europe and Africa are all following in their footsteps.

How on earth did we allow ourselves to forget the nutritional wisdom of our great grand-parents? How did we allow the food industry to sell us foods that are so intrinsically unsafe? And why, when we inevitably developed heart disease, dementia or cancer, did we throw ourselves so uncritically on the cruel alter of an inept and fundamentally obsolescent pharmaceutical industry?

I have attempted to answer these questions in the next chapter.

Chapter 26. Food fights, drug wars and the way ahead

The food industry has been captured by a cadre of agro-business companies (Google them!) who grow a very limited number of staple foods such as corn, soy, wheat, potatoes, pork, beef and chicken; and by a slightly larger number of multinational but predominantly American food manufacturers. These corporate players form an oligopoly large and wealthy enough to rent all the regulators and politicians they need, and get them to do more or less what they like. They use this kind of leverage to kill off competitors and force through government subsidies for themselves, enabling them to produce cheap foods and spend billions advertising their shoddy products[32]. Cooked and processed burgers, fries and shakes are significantly cheaper than fresh fruits and vegetables, because these are not subsidised.

The food manufacturers are also very good at persuading us to eat their processed foods. They know exactly how to hit what they call the 'bliss point', combining salt, sugars, fats and texturisers with clever marketing strategies to make foods which, scientists increasingly believe, are psychologically addictive (1-6).

In short, given the ways in which foods are grown, designed and marketed today, our ill health is baked into the pie.

Our political masters are aware of this and could, if they wished, implement the kinds of policy changes that would allow more of us to live healthier and happier lives. For example, relatively minor changes in the way we tax and subsidise different agricultural sectors would change food prices in a way that would lead to significant health gains; yet would be revenue neutral (7). An excellent Danish paper demonstrated that reducing taxes on vegetables, fruits and wholegrains from 25% to 22%; increasing the taxes on butter, cheese, beef, pork and fatty meats from 25% to 31%; and introducing a sugar tax, would lead to significant dietary improvements without costing the government a cent (8). There are, however, many obstacles to overcome.

In 1965, Ralph Nader's book 'Unsafe at Any Speed: The Designed-in Dangers of the American Automobile', created a climate of opinion which forced the dinosaurs of Detroit to start to develop the safety features which dominate automobile design today (9). The problems with our food chain are rather different. There are no foods that are intrinsically dangerous, although many of them are harmful when they become an overly large part of the diet. And whereas the fatal car crashes Nader wrote about could be linked to specific design flaws, the slow-motion car crash that best describes our mass progress towards degenerative disease has many, albeit related causes. It will require coordinated changes across the food chain involving food producers and retailers, regulators and politicians.

That this is possible was shown by the brave Finnish North Karelia experiment in which sodium chloride (table salt) was removed from the food chain and replaced with PanSuola. PanSuola

---

32. More on food production can be found in the books 'Fast Food Nation', 'Pandora's Lunchbox', 'Salt, Sugar, Fat: How the Food Giants Hooked Us', and the films 'Food Inc' and 'King Corn'.

is a mix of magnesium and potassium chlorides with the amino acid l-lysine developed by the wonderful Heikki Karppanen, who was then at Helsinki University, together with Pekka Puska. This had amazing effects.

During the last 30 years the Finns, much like everyone else, have become less physically active and as a result have grown heavier. They are consuming more alcohol. Men are smoking slightly less than in 1972, women slightly more. The Finns differ from Brits and Americans, however, in that their average systolic blood pressure has fallen by 15 mm Hg, and diastolic blood pressure by 12 mm Hg (10). This is more than double the effect you would achieve if you were to put every man, woman and child on anti-hypertensive drugs. Average cholesterol levels fell by 1.1 mmol/l. This is roughly 100 times more effective than the effects of statins at the population level.

More importantly, because blood pressure and cholesterol levels are merely biomarkers, Finnish rates of cardio- and cerebrovascular disease have fallen dramatically. Since the dietary programmes started, death rates from heart attacks and strokes have both been reduced by around 80% (10-12). As the numbers of drugs prescribed have fallen, so has the incidence of adverse drug reactions. Life expectancy has increased by 5 to 6 years (12) - and all of this has been achieved by minor dietary modifications.

In Finland, Finnish food laws compel the well-known fast food chains to use burger buns made with PanSuuola; these fine American companies continue to sell sub-standard products everywhere else. Heikki's pioneering research was attacked by lesser scientists shilling for companies which relied on table salt as a cheap flavour enhancer, but it has been repeatedly substantiated (13).

Given the hostility of powerful vested interests, it would be unwise to rely on the good governance, good will and good sense of our governments. We elect scientifically illiterate men and women who are out for themselves, enslaved to the electoral cycle and dependant on guidance from advisors, many of whom are deeply compromised by their links to industry. And from a costs perspective, they don't like healthy people.

The obese and the smokers are sicker than lean non-smokers but they die young. Lean non-smokers, who are thought of as 'healthy' live longer but also incur healthcare costs for longer. Under current conditions, from the age of 20 on, thin non-smokers consume, on average $417,000 worth of healthcare; while the shorter-lived obese people and smokers consume $371,000 and $326,000 respectively (14).

These figues have lead many politicians to think that a healthier population is a more expensive one – which is why they don't much care for it. But what they don't realise is that today's 'healthy' individuals are, in reality, far from healthy. They may be lean and non-smokers, but if they have low-energy lifestyles and the inevitable Type B malnutrition, they are guaranteed to have a very high incidence of degenerative (expensive) disease (15-20).

The most cost-effective citizen is a lean non-smoker with enhanced nutrition and a low risk of degenerative disease; a truly healthy individual who will live and work (if necessary) for longer, and incur substantially lower healthcare costs. This is a win-win-win project, and all it requires is a brave and honest politician – if you can find one – willing to take on the vested interests, and make it happen[33].

Drug Wars

Speaking of vested interests, Big Pharma makes a very good living from chronic inflammation. In 2010, global sales of anti-inflammatory drugs amounted to over $35 Billion, with the major disease categories being (in descending order of financial significance) asthma and chronic obstructive pulmonary disease, rheumatoid arthritis, multiple sclerosis, inflammatory bowel disease and psoriasis.

Now consider the vast numbers of people (between a quarter and a third of the population!) who suffer from intermittent or chronic pain (21-25). If we add the NSAID painkillers, which are primarily anti-inflammatory agents, we are up above $100 billion. Most of the rest of the drugs on offer do little more than suppress the diseases caused by chronic inflammation; and now we are talking about a total global drug economy worth in excess of $800 Billion. Subtract sales of antibiotics, which have relatively little to do with inflammation, and this is still well in excess of $750 billion per annum.

The vast sums of money generated by pharmaceutical sales are closely matched by the global market in recreational drugs, which (at about 1% of global GDP) are reckoned at around $700 Billion (72). Illicit drug money corrupts customs, police, judiciary, politicians and indeed entire governments; the cocabuck has become a shadow currency to the shadowy petrodollar, and operates – as we have seen in Mexico and elsewhere – via bribery, intimidation, extortion and extreme violence.

Pharmadollars operate in a rather more civilised manner, but the end results are surprisingly similar – and on a much larger scale. Over 100,000 deaths are caused by adverse drug effects every year in the USA alone (26-27), and another 100,000 die as a result of medical errors and other causes due to the medical treatment of avoidable diseases (28-29). If we add the hundreds of millions of deaths caused by illnesses that we now know are avoidable, but which our doctors insist on treating with drugs (because they are trained to do so in institutions largely funded by Pharma money), it becomes obvious that pharmadollars have created an on-going, slow-motion holocaust.

Pharmadollars are also deeply implicated in the systemic corruption of regulatory and educational systems. For example, regulators such as EFSA and the FDA restrict

---

33. Anti-smoking groups successfully lobbied the political classes to try to phase out tobacco consumption, using concepts such as the dangers of passive smoking to justify smoke-free zones. It is not easy to see how this logic could easily be extended into the food chain.

manufactures of food and supplements from giving out information to the public that people could use to materially improve their health. Indeed, the constant re-cycling of key personnel between the regulatory agencies and the pharmaceutical companies has led to a general understanding that, as with food industry, the regulators have been captured by the companies they nominally regulate.

There was a time when governments cared about these matters, and developed agricultural and food policies specifically designed to enhance public health. During the second world war, the 'Dig for Victory' and related campaigns were considered essential to build healthier soldiers and workers. Those programs are gone, and those who promoted them were marginalised or assassinated (Google Sir Jack Cecil Drumond). Wars no longer require vast manpower, and our dear leaders now prefer to cure their political headaches with meta-data and drones. The historical rationale for the middle classes has long gone, which is why they are being crushed. We are witnessing the emergence of a neo-feudal world in which the richest 200 people in the world have about $2.7 trillion, which is more than the poorest 3.5 billion people who have only $2.2 trillion *combined* (30).

As the playing field is so sharply tilted to favour Big Pharma and Big Government, and as public health has suffered so much as a result, the obvious answer is to take matters into your own hands. Beating chronic inflammation via nutrition is cheap, easy, safe and considerably more effective than relying on the tender mercies of the current healthcare model. You could entrust your health to the wisdom and benevolence of our politicians, and die. Or you could adopt an anti-inflammatory lifestyle, and live.

It is worth stressing that I am not against doctors, many of whom provide a valuable service; and I am not against the pharmaceutical approach per se, as it has an invaluable role to play in acute medicine. I am against its uncritical use by doctors who do not understand how this system evolved, and who therefore do not understand its limitations. If you do not know where you come from you cannot know where or even who you are – so you have to look back, in this case to the origins of modern medicine.

Modern medicine starts with the antibiotics. Antibiotics were the first great triumph of pharmaceutical medicine. They heralded the start of an era of clinical science in which, for the first time, patients who went to their doctor seeking help had a better than even chance of benefiting from the encounter. The antibiotics were the first genuinely curative medicines, and they not only laid the foundations of the pharmaceutical model that still dominates healthcare today, but also created a legacy of expectations of pharmaceutical cures for all ills.

The vast sums of money to be made in selling drugs also lead to a great deal of pharmaceutical fraud, from the withholding of negative trial data to the outright falsification of data and the bribing of doctors. The blame for this mass deception of the public has little to do with the scientists and clinicians involved in developing new drugs. Instead, it lies closer to the marketing and financial sectors within the industry, whose only motivation is to boost the flagging rates of return in the pharmaceutical sector. Pharmaceutical breakthroughs, however, are getting fewer and further between. Products spun off from research into the human genome are unlikely to redress the balance books and neither will the fancy new model of pharma networking, whereby the drug companies out-source non-core elements of their business.

These 'breakthroughs' cannot accomplish the anticipated miracles because Big Pharma is knocking on the wrong door. A glance through any pharmacopeia reveals that we have many hundreds of specific and potent drugs - so potent, in fact, that iatrogenic illness (disease caused by the side effects of drugs) has become an important cause of death. Yet with the notable exception of the antibiotics, most of which are fast losing their efficacy, we have hardly any cures. Almost all the drugs we use are palliatives which sooth or suppress the symptoms of disease but are unable to cure the underlying condition, which consequently generally continues to deteriorate.

The degenerative diseases have such long latency periods. Coronary artery disease, Type 2 diabetes, cancer, Alzheimer's and osteoporosis do not occur overnight, although the first symptoms might do. These are slowly progressing conditions, which develop for decades before symptoms finally emerge.

In other words, the majority of apparently healthy adults are, in reality, pre-ill. They contain, in their bodies, the growing seeds of the illness(es) which will eventually become overt, and perhaps kill them. Fat is accumulating, arteries are beginning to silt up, bones and joints are thinning, brain cells are dying; leading inevitably, eventually, to obesity, a heart attack, osteoporotic fracture, or clinically confirmed dementia. By that very late stage, of course, once symptoms have emerged, the ability of the current medical system to put things right is very limited and generally restricted to suppressing the symptoms of the disease.

This is a truly bizarre situation. It is as if we taught car mechanics to carry out crash repairs, but nothing of maintenance. It is a lethal inheritance from the early successes of pharmaceutical medicine, the sulpha drugs and penicillins which so effectively cured infectious diseases, the dominant diseases of that time, and laid the foundations of the modern pharmaceutical industry. Unfortunately, they also created models of disease treatment that are no longer appropriate to the diseases which are important today. Even more unfortunately, these ideas still underpin the ruinously expensive system of crisis-management medicine currently on offer. They hugely influence the medical curriculum, dominate medical post-qualification training, and determine the bulk of clinical research.

Drugs developed from the concept of 'magic bullets', and the closely related idea of specificity, are appropriate when dealing with infectious illness. They are not the right tools, however, for dealing with a degenerative disease caused by adverse life-style factors, and consequently many metabolic imbalances, going subtly wrong over many years. The drugs do not and cannot work. The huge increases in obesity, diabetes, asthma, auto-immune disease, osteoporosis and cancer described elsewhere in this book, the recent declines in life expectancy reported in parts of the former Soviet Union, Italy, the UK and the USA (15), the relative fall in average height now occurring in the United States (16-18), the fact that numbers of children and adolescents with a chronic health condition has increased from 1.8% in the 1960s to more than 7% in 2004 (19), the related fact that 1 in 2 adults now has one or more chronic diseases (20), and the persistent failure of the pharmaceutical model to find cures for any of these problems, are all telling us that we need a new way of looking at health; one which takes life-style and nutritional factors into account.

The major diseases today are driven by chronic inflammation caused by multiple dietary imbalances. These cannot be rectified by throwing pharmaceutical spanners into the incredibly complex workings of a sick (or healthy) individual.

Sadly, despite the fact that the majority of risk factors and protective factors for degenerative disease are nutritional, nutrition as a subject is almost absent from medical schools. And because micronutrients are generic (ie they are not owned by any one company), there is little commercial incentive to do the studies that would provide the levels of proof that are required, for example, in the licensing of new drugs.

Fortunately, this situation is beginning to change. Thousands of small-scale studies carried out by scientists with an interest in nutrition now chart many of the detailed relationships between diet, micro-nutrition and health. Governments, alarmed by spiralling healthcare costs, have also started to study the potential of diet to lower the burden of disease. Between them, they have given birth to the new science of pharmaco-nutrition.

Pharmaco-nutrition starts by analysing the multiple metabolic errors that drive a disease such as coronary artery disease. It then cross-references these against the known pharmacology of food derivates; and finally assembles a comprehensive micronutritional support programme designed to rectify all the metabolic errors, or as many as can be identified. This is not a magic bullet, but a comprehensive support programme. Using this approach, for example, the chemistry of the blood and the physiology of the blood vessel walls can be re-programmed and re-configured in a way that effectively immunises the owner against cardio-vascular disease. If disease is present it can be forced to regress, as the catabolic processes that drive it are damped and the healing processes that clean and remodel the arterial beds are supported and strengthened.

In a more general sense, the pharmaco-nutritional approach teaches us that the pattern of decline that generally runs in parallel with ageing is not inevitable. Diseases we thought of as inherently progressive are not; just as atheroma can be made to shrink, so can worn joints be re-built and dying brain cells in ARCD patients coaxed back to life. These diseases are called degenerative because, in a typical patient on a typically Western diet, they do worsen with age. But to assume that because this is what we always see, this is the way things must be, is a substantial and all-too common philosophical error.

Pharmaco-nutrition, then, is a hugely significant shift in the way we think about, and treat, illness and the symptoms of ageing. I believe that pharmaco-nutrition will prove to be as effective in treating and curing the degenerative diseases as the antibiotics were, for a while, in curing the bacterial illnesses. If that sounds too radical for the average doctor, they have probably forgotten (if they ever knew) that antibiotics were initially scorned by many practitioners who felt that the infectious diseases were 'natural' and therefore untreatable.

20th century medicine was largely based on the work of the very great French scientist Louis Pasteur, whose science laid the foundations of the pharmaceutical 'magic bullet'. The medicine of the 21st century belongs to Claude Bernard, Pasteur's friend and equal, who is described as the father of physiology but can equally be regarded as the father of pharmaco-nutrition.

Chapter 27. Finally, an apology ...

Nutrition and its offspring pharmaco-nutrition are rapidly developing and relatively new sciences. Like all new sciences they progress from observations to hypotheses to trials, and then – based on the results of those trials - to further hypotheses. Plenty of mistakes are made along the way, but these are important; it is only by finding out that an idea is wrong that we can re-gather our forces, re-assess our observations and form new hypotheses to be tested, to destruction if possible. Even if we can never arrive at an ultimate truth the scientific method allows us to move, in a crab-like and perhaps an asymptotic way, towards the truth. Or at least, towards an understanding of things that is less wrong.

Of course it is not as cut and dried as this. In the real world scientists have egos, and often identify with and cling to a particular hypothesis even when the data have moved on. And many of us work for commercial institutions, which have a need to invest in and profit from the latest project. This means that intemperate statements are all too often made and used to sell products before the scientific case can be settled. And when those statements are revealed to be wrong, and the promise of the latest white hope revealed to be false, the pharma and supplement industries simply move on without explanation or apology to sell the next unproven nostrum. As my grandmother used to say whenever a new patent medicine was announced, 'Let's take it while it's still effective!' (A doctor's daughter and married to a well-known physicist, she was an early skeptic).

When a science touches on people's lives as much as the health sciences do, this creates understandable confusion and anger. How can the experts tell us one year that beta carotene protects smokers against cancer, and the following year that it makes matters worse? That margarine was healhier than butter, but now butter is best? That the monoclonal antibodies would save us all from cancer, when they turned out to be so cost-ineffective that NICE was forced to pull them from them from the National Health Service?

On behalf of my science, I apologise. I've been wrong many times – and never more so (as far as I know) than in the late 90's when I believed, along with many of my colleagues, that free radicals were the cause of all disease and the ageing process itself; and that anti-oxidants were the cure-alls. There is a germ of truth here, in that excessive levels of oxidative stress are undoubtedly damaging. But at the same time there is evidence that many of the strategies that mediate longevity do so by inducing low-level oxidative and other forms of stress (1-3). (This takes us back to the beginning of Section 2 where I talked, briefly, about stress and hormetics; too much of anything is usually a bad thing, but a little is often a good thing).

In hindsight, the mistake was an easy one to make. The chemistries of inflammation and oxidative stress overlap. Some inflammatory processes generate free radicals, and excessive oxidative stress causes inflammation. Even more confusingly, some antioxidants are highly effective anti-inflammatory agents, and vice versa. We backed the wrong horses, focussing on the antioxidant vitamins when, as we now know, anti-inflammatory nutrients such as the Omega-3's and the anti-inflammatory phyto-nutrients play a far more important role in personal and public health.

Progress in science is rarely linear. It is more often a series of knight's moves across a checker-board of politics, finance and ambition, leavened with only a little logic. Things change. The mono-clonal antibodies which were so ineffective against cancer, for example, have been given an unexpected new lease of life by combining them with the yeast-derived 1-3, 1-6 beta glucans (4-6). The latest knight's move, however, which is the subject of this book, is the real breakthrough. Chronic inflammation has emerged as a common cause of most of the diseases which are important today, and natural ways of preventing chronic inflammation are the obvious and logical way to protect ourselves. Unless it is blocked by the usual vested interests, the next wave in anti-inflammatory nutrition will improve and extend our lives, and restore the majority of us to the kind of good health we have always wanted.

I have relied in this book on the work of many good and great scientists. Any errors of interpretation are mine.

Acknowledgements

I would like to express my gratitude to Professor Arne Reimers (St Olav's Hospital, University of Trondheim) for his critical input, Professors Stig Bengmark (University College, London) and Jan Raa (University of Tromsø) for their inspiration, Professors John Stein (Oxford), Michael Crawford (Imperial College, London) and Jonathan Brostoff (Kings College, London) for their brilliance and kind support over the years.

I also thank Drs Judith Rowbotham, Alex Richardson, Bernard Gesch, Szabolcs Ladi, Julian Kenyon and Steve Hodges, comrades in arms; Colin and Joanna Rose, for their generosity and forward radar; Jith Veeravalli and Ramasamy Venkatesh for their trust and strategic thinking; Frances Jackson for her belief in me; Jan Bakke and Kenneth Birn for their friendship and support; Örjan Saele and Hilde Rismyhr-Saele for encouraging me to finish this, the first edition of this book. My thanks also to Richard Stead, Bengt Hanson, Takis and Kyriakos Zervakakis, Samo Borko, Allen Porter, Don Cox, Rich Mueller, Svein-Erik Nilsen, Randy Larsen, Phil Hawes, Peter Wallace, Bruce and Carol Nadeau, Jarmo Hörkkö, Danilo Massari, Matti Kaarlas, Costas Papaikonomou, David Walker and many other good friends in the academic and business worlds.

This book is dedicated to the shades of two very great scientists, Louis Pasteur and Claude Bernard. Their work and friendship laid the foundations not only for the pharmaceutical model of medicine that dominated the 20th century, but also the pharmaco-nutritional model that will largely replace it. I have taken the liberty of selecting a quote from each of these remarkable men, two pillars of an arch through which we obtain a beautiful and complementary vision of how science develops.

Louis Pasteur: 'Science knows no country because knowledge belongs to humanity, and is the torch which illuminates the world.'

Claude Bernard: "Our feelings lead us at first to believe that absolute truth must lie within our realm; but study takes from us, little by little, these chimerical conceits."

Finally, this book is dedicated to Pearl Gray Clayton, who may one day walk through that arch; and to Stacy Harrison-Clayton, for her courage and honesty.

REFERENCES

SECTION 1: Putting out the Flames – Quick Start

SECTION 2: Putting out the Flames – An Intermediate Course

Chapters 1 - 3

1. Willcox DC, Willcox BJ, Wang NC, He Q, Rosenbaum M, Suzuki M. **Life at the extreme limit: phenotypic characteristics of supercentenarians in Okinawa.** J Gerontol A Biol Sci Med Sci. 2008 Nov;63(11):1201-8.
2. Krebs-Smith SM, Guenther PM, Subar AF, Kirkpatrick SI, Dodd KW. **Americans do not meet federal dietary recommendations.** J Nutr. 2010 Oct;140(10):1832-8
3. Fulgoni VL 3rd, Keast DR, Bailey RL, Dwyer J. **Foods, fortificants, and supplements: Where do Americans get their nutrients?** J Nutr. 2011 Oct;141(10):1847-54
4. Troesch B, Hoeft B, Mcburney M, Eggersdorfer M, Weber P. **Dietary surveys indicate vitamin intakes below recommendations are common in representative Western countries.** Br J Nutr. 2012 Aug;108(4):692-8
5. James WPT, Ralph A, FerroLuzzi A. (1988). **Energy needs of the elderly.** In *Nutrition and Ageing.* (Munro, H.N. & Danford, D.E., Ed.) , 129151. Plenum Publishing Corporation, New York.
6. Komlos J, Breitfelder A. **Are Americans shorter (partly) because they are fatter? A comparison of US and Dutch children's height and BMI values.** Ann Hum Biol. 2007 Nov-Dec;34(6):593-606
7. Komlos J, Breitfelder A. **Height of US-born non-Hispanic children and adolescents ages 2-19, born 1942-2002 in the NHANES samples.** Am J Hum Biol. 2008 Jan-Feb;20(1):66-71.
8. Akbaraly T, Sabia S, Hagger-Johnson G, Tabak AG, Shipley MJ, Jokela M, Brunner EJ, Hamer M, Batty GD, Singh-Manoux A, Kivimaki M. **Does Overall Diet in Midlife Predict Future Aging Phenotypes? A Cohort Study.** *The American Journal of Medicine,* Volume 126, Issue 5 (May 2013) DOI:10.1016/j.amjmed.2012.10.028
9. Clayton P, Rowbotham J. **How the mid-Victorians worked, ate and died.** Int J Environ Res Public Health. 2009 Mar;6(3):1235-53.
10. Mori T, Beilin LJ. **Omega 3 Fatty Acids and inflammation.** Curr Atheroscler Rep. 2004 Nov;6(6):461-7. Review.
11. Mas E, Croft KD, Zahra P, Barden A, Mori TA. **Resolvins D1, D2, and other mediators of self-limited resolution of inflammation in human blood following n-3 fatty acid supplementation.** Clin Chem. 2012 Oct;58(10):1476-84.
12. Simopoulos AP. **Evolutionary aspects of omega-3 fatty acids in the food supply.** Prostaglandins Leukot Essent Fatty Acids. 1999 May-Jun;60(5-6):421-9.
13. Simopoulos AP. **Evolutionary aspects of diet, the omega-6/omega-3 ratio and genetic variation: nutritional implications for chronic diseases.** Biomed Pharmacother. 2006 Nov;60(9):502-7.
14. Simopoulos AP. **The importance of the Omega-6/Omega-3 fatty acid ratio in cardiovascular disease and other chronic diseases.** Exp Biol Med (Maywood). 2008 Jun;233(6):674-88. Review.
15. Zhang F, Altorki NK, Mestre JR, Subbaramaiah K, Andrew J. **Curcumin inhibits cyclooxygenase-2 transcription in bile acid- and phorbol ester-treated human gastrointestinal epithelial cells.** Dannenberg Carcinogenesis 1999;20(3):445-51.
16. Plummer SM, Hill KA, Festing MFW, Steward WP, Gescher A, Sharma RA. **Curcumin inhibits prostaglandin biosynthesis via cyclooxygenase-2 in human blood.** Cancer Epidemiol Biomarkers Prev2001; 10:1295–9
17. Surh YJ, Chun KS, Cha HH, Han SS, Keum YS, Park KK, Lee SS.. **Molecular mechanisms underlying chemopreventive activities of anti-inflammatory phytochemicals: down-regulation of COX-2 and iNOS through suppression of NF-kappa B activation.** Mutat Res. 2001;480-481:243-268.
18. Bengmark S. **Curcumin, an atoxic antioxidant and natural NFkappaB, cyclooxygenase-2, lipooxygenase, and inducible nitric oxide synthase inhibitor: a shield against acute and chronic diseases.** JPEN J Parenter Enteral Nutr. 2006 Jan-Feb;30(1):45-51. Review.
19. Rao CV. **Regulation of COX and LOX by curcumin.** Adv Exp Med Biol. 2007;595:213-26. Review
20. Mohan R, Sivak J, Ashton P, Russo LA, Pham BQ, Kasahara N, Raizman MB, Fini ME. **Curcuminoids inhibit the angiogenic response stimulated by fibroblast growth factor-2, including expression of matrix metalloproteinase gelatinase B.** J Biol Chem. 2000 Apr 7;275(14):10405-12.
21. Kleinewietfeld M, Manzel A, Wu C, Titze J, Kuchroo V, Linker R, Muller D, Hafler D. **High salt induces pathogenic Th17 cells and exacerbates autoimmune diseases.** *The Journal of Immunology,* 2012, 188, 60.13
22. Stott-Miller M, Neuhouser ML, Stanford JL. **Consumption of deep-fried foods and risk of prostate cancer.** Prostate. 2013 Jan 17. doi: 10.1002/pros.22643.
23. Bengmark S. **Gut microbiota, immune development and function.** Pharmacol Res. 2012 Sep 16. doi:pii: S1043-6618(12)00166-1

24. Cutolo M, Seriolo B, Villaggio B, Pizzorni C, Craviotto C, Sulli A. **Androgens and estrogens modulate the immune and inflammatory responses in rheumatoid arthritis.** Ann N Y Acad Sci. 2002 Jun;966:131-42.

25. Rasouli N, Kern PA. **Adipocytokines and the Metabolic Complications of Obesity.** J Clin Endocrinol Metab. 2008 November; 93(11 Suppl 1): S64–S73.

26. Kenyon N, Liu FT. **Pulmonary effects of diesel exhaust: neutrophilic inflammation, oxidative injury, and asthma.** Am J Pathol. 2011 Dec;179(6):2678-82.

27. Riedl MA, Diaz-Sanchez D, Linn WS, Gong H Jr, Clark KW, Effros RM, Miller JW, Cocker DR, Berhane KT; HEI Health Review Committee. **Allergic inflammation in the human lower respiratory tract affected by exposure to diesel exhaust.** Res Rep Health Eff Inst. 2012 Feb;(165):5-43

28. Robinson AB, Johnson KD, Bennion BG, Reynolds PR. **RAGE signaling by alveolar macrophages influences tobacco smoke-inducedinflammation.** Am J Physiol Lung Cell Mol Physiol. 2012a Jun 1;302(11):L1192-9.

29. Robinson AB, Stogsdill JA, Lewis JB, Wood TT, Reynolds PR. **RAGE and tobacco smoke: insights into modeling chronic obstructive pulmonary disease.** Front Physiol. 2012b;3:301.

30. Guiñazú N, Rena V, Genti-Raimondi S, Rivero V, Magnarelli G. **Effects of the organophosphate insecticides phosmet and chlorpyrifos on trophoblast JEG-3 cell death, proliferation and inflammatory molecule production.** Toxicol In Vitro. 2012 Apr;26(3):406-13

31. Miller MR, Shaw CA, Langrish JP. **From particles to patients: oxidative stress and the cardiovascular effects of air pollution.** Future Cardiol. 2012 Jul;8(4):577-602.

32. García JJ, Bote E, Hinchado MD, Ortega E. **A single session of intense exercise improves the inflammatory response in healthy sedentary women.** J Physiol Biochem. 2011 Mar;67(1):87-94.

33. Teixeira de Lemos E, Oliveira J, Páscoa-Pinheiro J, Reis F. **Regular physical exercise as a strategy to improve antioxidant and anti-inflammatory status: benefits in type 2 diabetes mellitus.** Oxid Med Cell Longev. 2012;2012:741545.

34. Teixeira de Lemos E, Oliveira J, Páscoa-Pinheiro J, Reis F. **Regular physical exercise as a strategy to improve antioxidant and anti-inflammatory status: benefits in type 2 diabetes mellitus.** Oxid Med Cell Longev. 2012;2012:741545.

35. Kournikakis B, Mandeville R, Brousseau P, Ostroff G. **Anthrax-protective effects of yeast beta 1,3 glucans.** MedGenMed. 2003 Mar 21;5(1):1.

36. Vedin O et al. **Tooth loss associated with cardiovascular risk factors in patients with chronic heart disease.** Presented at the American College of Cardiology's 62nd Annual Scientific Session, San Francisco, March 2013

37. Pasqualini D, Bergandi L, Palumbo L, Borraccino A, Dambra V, Alovisi M, Migliaretti G, Ferraro G, Ghigo D, Bergerone S, Scotti N, Aimetti M, Berutti E. **Association among oral health, apical periodontitis, CD14 polymorphisms, and coronary heart disease** in middle-aged adults. J Endod. 2012 Dec;38(12):1570-7.

38. Bokhari SA, Khan AA, Butt AK, Azhar M, Hanif M, Izhar M, Tatakis DN. **Non-surgical periodontal therapy reduces coronary heart disease risk markers: a randomized controlled trial.** J Clin Periodontol. 2012 Nov;39(11):1065-74.

39. Lockhart PB, Bolger AF, Papapanou PN, Osinbowale O, Trevisan M, Levison ME, Taubert KA, Newburger JW, Gornik HL, Gewitz MH, Wilson WR, Smith SC Jr, Baddour LM; American Heart Association Rheumatic Fever, Endocarditis, and Kawasaki Disease Committee of the Council on Cardiovascular Disease in the Young, Council on Epidemiology and Prevention, Council on Peripheral Vascular Disease, and Council on Clinical Cardiology. **Periodontal disease and atherosclerotic vascular disease: does the evidence support an independent association?: a scientific statement from the American Heart Association.** Circulation. 2012 May 22;125(20):2520-44.

40. Wolfe F, Freundlich B, Straus WL. **Increase in cardiovascular and cerebrovascular disease prevalence in rheumatoid arthritis.** J Rheumatol 2003; 30: 36–40.

41. Watson D, Rhodes T, Guess H. **All-cause mortality and vascular events among patients with RA, OA, or no arthritis in the UK General Practice Research Database.** J Rheumatol 2003; 30: 1196–202.

42. Fischer LM, Schlienger RG, Matter C, Jick H, Meier CR. **Effect of rheumatoid arthritis or systemic lupus erythematosus on the risk of first-time acute myocardial infarction.** Am J Cardiol 2004; 93: 198–200.

43. Esposito K, Marfella R, Ciotola M, Di Palo C, Giugliano F, Giugliano G, D'Armiento M, D'Andrea F, Giugliano D. **Effect of a mediterranean-style diet on endothelial dysfunction and markers of vascular inflammation in the metabolic syndrome: a randomized trial.** JAMA. 2004 Sep 22;292(12):1440-6.

44. de Lorgeril M, Salen P, Martin JL, Monjaud I, Delaye J, Mamelle N. **Mediterranean diet, traditional risk factors, and the rate of cardiovascular complications after myocardial infarction: final report of the Lyon Diet Heart Study.** Circulation. 1999 Feb 16;99(6):779-85.

45. Rautiainen S, Levitan EB, Orsini N, Akesson A, Morgenstern R, Mittelman MA, Wolk A. **Total Antioxidant Capacity from Diet and Risk of Myocardial Infarction: A Prospective Cohort of Women.** Am J Med 2012, 125(10); 974-980.

46. Stavitsky K, Brickman AM, Scarmeas N, Torgan RL, Tang MX, Albert M, Brandt J, Blacker D, Stern Y. **The progression of cognition, psychiatric symptoms, and functional abilities in dementia with Lewy bodies and Alzheimer disease.** Arch Neurol. 2006 Oct;63(10):1450-6.

47. Scarmeas N, Luchsinger JA, Mayeux R, Stern Y. **Mediterranean diet and Alzheimer disease mortality.** Neurology. 2007 Sep 11;69(11):1084-93.

48. Laurin D, David Curb J, Masaki KH, White LR, Launer LJ. **Midlife C-reactive protein and risk of cognitive decline: a 31-year follow-up.** Neurobiol Ageing. 2009 Nov;30(11):1724-7

49. Cederholm T, Palmblad J. **Are omega-3 fatty acids options for prevention and treatment of cognitive decline and dementia?** Curr Opin Clin Nutr Metab Care. 2010 Mar;13(2):150-5.

50. Kariv-Inbal Z, Yacobson S, Berkecz R, Peter M, Janaky T, Lütjohann D, Broersen LM, Hartmann T, Michaelson DM. **The isoform-specific pathological effects of apoE4 in vivo are prevented by a fish oil (DHA) diet and are modified by cholesterol.** J Alzheimers Dis. 2012;28(3):667-83.

51. Hjorth E, Zhu M, Toro VC, Vedin I, Palmblad J, Cederholm T, Freund-Levi Y, Faxen-Irving G, Wahlund LO, Basun H, Eriksdotter M, Schultzberg M. **Omega-3 Fatty Acids Enhance Phagocytosis of Alzheimer's Disease-Related Amyloid-β42 by Human Microglia and Decrease Inflammatory Markers.** J Alzheimers Dis. 2013 Jan 1;35(4):697-713

52. Geleijnse JM, Giltay EJ, Kromhout D. **Effects of n-3 fatty acids on cognitive decline: a randomized, double-blind, placebo-controlled trial in stable myocardial infarction patients.** Alzheimers Dement. 2012 Jul;8(4):278-87.

53. Joseph JA, Shukitt-Hale B, Denisova NA, Prior RL, Cao G, Martin A, Taglialatela G, Bickford PC: **Long-term dietary strawberry, spinach, or vitamin E supplementation retards the onset of age-related neuronal signal-transduction and cognitive behavioral deficits.** J Neurosci. 1998 Oct 1;18(19):8047-55.

54. Masoumi A, Goldenson B, Ghirmai S, Avagyan H, Zaghi J, Abel K, Zheng X, Espinosa-Jeffrey A, Mahanian M, Liu PT, Hewison M, Mizwickie M, Cashman J, Fiala M. **1alpha,25-dihydroxyvitamin D3 interacts with curcuminoids to stimulate amyloid-beta clearance by macrophages of Alzheimer's disease** patients. J Alzheimers Dis. 2009;17(3):703-17

55. Kelavkar UP, Hutzley J, McHugh K, Allen KG, Parwani A. **Prostate tumor growth can be modulated by dietarily targeting the 15-lipoxygenase-1 and cyclooxygenase-2 enzymes.** Neoplasia. 2009 Jul;11(7):692-9.

56. Salomon JA, Wang H, Freeman MK, Vos T, Flaxman AD, Lopez AD, Murray CJ. **Healthy life expectancy for 187 countries, 1990-2010: a systematic analysis for the Global Burden Disease Study 2010.** Lancet. 2013 Dec 15;380(9859):2144-62.

57. Charlton J, Murphy M, editors. The Health of Adult Britain 1841–1994. 2 vols. London: National Statistics; 2004.

58. McNay K, Humphries J, Klasen S. Cambridge Working Papers in Economics. Cambridge: 1998. Death and Gender in Victorian England and Wales: Comparisons with Contemporary Developing Countries.

59. Office for National Statistics 2011. http://www.ons.gov.uk/ons/rel/health-ineq/health-inequalities/trends-in-life-expectancy--1982---2006/trends-in-life-expectancy-by-the-national-statistics-socio-economic-classification-1982-2006.pdf

60. Lim et al 2012. **A comparative risk assessment of burden of disease and injury attributable to 67 risk factors and risk factor clusters in 21 regions, 1990-2010: a systematic analysis for the Global Burden of Disease Study 2010.** Lancet. 2013 Dec 15;380(9859):2224-60.

61. Vos et al. **Years lived with disability (YLDs) for 1160 sequelae of 289 diseases and injuries 1990-2010: a systematic analysis for the Global Burden of Disease Study 2010.** Lancet. 2013 Dec 15;380(9859):2163-96

62. Murray et al. **Disability-adjusted life years (DALYs) for 291 diseases and injuries in 21 regions, 1990-2010: a systematic analysis for the Global Burden of Disease Study 2010.** Lancet. 2013 Dec 15;380(9859):2197-223.

63. Clayton P, Rowbotham. **Victorian HeathCare; a Cost-Benefit Analysis** . In progress, 2013

64. UK Public Spending; http://www.ukpublicspending.co.uk/uk_budget_pie_chart

65. Sikora K '11. http://www.telegraph.co.uk/health/healthnews/8791979/The-big-C-cancer-treatment-is-increasingly-unaffordable.html

66. Sullivan R, Peppercorn J, Sikora K, Zalcberg J, Meropol NJ, Amir E, Khayat D, Boyle P, Autier P et al. **Delivering affordable cancer care in high-income countries.** Lancet Oncol. 2011 Sep;12(10):933-80

67. DEFRA 2012. http://www.defra.gov.uk/statistics/files/defra-stats-foodfarm-food-familyfood-2011-121217.pdf

68. Harstall C, Ospina M (June 2003). **How Prevalent Is Chronic Pain?** Pain Clinical Updates, International Association for the Study of Pain XI (2): 1–4

69. Mayday 2009. **A Call to Revolutionize Chronic Pain Care in America: An Opportunity in Health Care Reform.** The Mayday Fund. 2009.

70. Johannes CB, Le TK, Zhou X, Johnston JA, Dworkin RH. **The prevalence of chronic pain in United States adults: results of an Internet-based survey.** J Pain. 2010 Nov;11(11):1230-9

71. IoM 2011. Institute of Medicine of the National Academies Report (2011). **Relieving Pain in America: A Blueprint for Transforming Prevention, Care, Education, and Research.** Washington DC: The National Academies Press.

72. Phillips DP, Christenfeld N, Glynn LM (February 1998). **Increase in US medication-error deaths between 1983 and 1993.** *Lancet* 351 (9103): 643–4.

73. Lazarou J, Pomeranz BH, Corey PN (April 1998). **Incidence of adverse drug reactions in hospitalized patients: a meta-analysis of prospective studies.** *JAMA* 279 (15): 1200-1205

74. Leape L (May 1992). **Unnecessary Surgery.** *Annual Review of Public Health* 13: 363–383.

75. Starfield B (July 2000). **Is US health really the best in the world?** *JAMA* 284 (4): 483–5.

76. Brzozowski T, Konturek SJ, Majka J, Dembinski A, Drozdowicz D. **Epidermal growth factor, polyamines, and prostaglandins in healing of stress-induced gastric lesions in rats.** Dig Dis Sci. 1993 Feb;38(2):276-83.

77. Rao JN, Rathor N, Zhuang R, Zou T, Liu L, Xiao L, Turner DJ, Wang JY. **Polyamines regulate intestinal epithelial restitution through TRPC1-mediated Ca²+ signaling by differentially modulating STIM1 and STIM2.** Am J Physiol Cell Physiol. 2012 Aug 1;303(3):C308-17

78. Soda K. **The mechanisms by which polyamines accelerate tumor spread.** Journal of Experimental & Clinical Cancer Research 2011, 30:95

79. Gillis L, Gillis A. **Nutrient inadequacy in obese and non-obese youth.** Can J Diet Pract Res. 2005 Winter;66(4):237-42.

80. Cordain L, Eaton SB, Sebastian A, Mann N, Lindeberg S, Watkins BA, O'Keefe JH, Brand-Miller J. **Origins and evolution of the Western diet: health implications for the 21st century.** Am J Clin Nutr. 2005 Feb;81(2):341-54.

81. Amo T, Eide O. Industry data, personal communication '12

82. Bhopal RS, Rafnsson SB. **Could mitochondrial efficiency explain the susceptibility to adiposity, metabolic syndrome, diabetes and cardiovascular diseases in South Asian populations?** Int J Epidemiol. 2009 Aug;38(4):1072-81.

83. Akramas L, Akramienė D, Sakalauskienė J, Kubilius R, Gleiznys A. **Effect of (1→3),(1→6)-β-glucan on in vitro production of cytokines by leukocytes of patients with periodontitis.** Medicina (Kaunas). 2012;48(4):186-91.

84. Brown GD, Taylor PR, Reid DM, Willment JA, Williams DL, Martinez-Pomares L, Wong SY, Gordon S. **Dectin-1 is a major beta-glucan receptor on macrophages.** J Exp Med. 2002 Aug 5;196(3):407-12.

85. Elcombe SE, Naqvi S, Van Den Bosch MW, MacKenzie KF, Cianfanelli F, Brown GD, Arthur JS. **Dectin-1 regulates IL-10 production via a MSK1/2 and CREB dependent pathway and promotes the induction of regulatory macrophage markers.** PLoS One. 2013;8(3):e60086.

86. Clayton P. **Novel Therapeutic Strategies in Infection and Cancer management.** 2012 Current Ageing Science 5(3):1-7

87. Knoops KT, de Groot LC, Kromhout D, Perrin AE, Moreiras-Varela O, Menotti A, van Staveren WA. **Mediterranean diet, lifestyle factors, and 10-year mortality in elderly European men and women: the HALE project.** JAMA 2004 Sep 22;292(12):1433-9

88. USA stats: http://www.infoplease.com/ipa/A0005140.html

89. Kindig DA, Cheng ER. **Even as mortality fell in most US counties, female mortality nonetheless rose in 42.8 percent of counties from 1992 to 2006.** Health Aff (Millwood). 2013 Mar;32(3):451-8

90. Shoelson SE, Goldfine AB. **Getting away from glucose: fanning the flames of obesity-induced inflammation.** Nature Medicine, vol. 15, no. 4, pp. 373–374, 2009.

91. Sampey BP, Vanhoose AM, Winfield HM, Freemerman AJ, Muehlbauer MJ, Fueger PT, Newgard CB, Makowski L. **Cafeteria diet is a robust model of human metabolic syndrome with liver and adipose inflammation: comparison to high-fat diet.** Obesity (Silver Spring). 2011 Jun;19(6):1109-17.

92. Naja F, Nasreddine L, Itani L, Adra N, Sibai AM, Hwalla N. **Association between dietary patterns and the risk of metabolic syndrome among Lebanese adults.** Eur J Nutr. 2013 Feb;52(1):97-105.

93. Erwin RB, Ogden CL. **Consumption of Added Sugars Among U.S. Adults, 2005–2010.** NCHS Data Brief Number 122, May 2013. http://www.cdc.gov/nchs/data/databriefs/db122.htm

94. Brenna T. Personal communication July 2013

95. Woodley MA, Nijenhuis J, Murphy R. **Were the Victorians cleverer than us? The decline in general intelligence estimated from a meta-analysis of the slowing of simple reaction time.** Intelligence (2013), http://dx.doi.org/10.1016/j.intell.2013.04.006

96. Khalatbary AR, Zarrinjoei GR. **Anti-inflammatory effect of oleuropein in experimental rat spinal cord trauma.** Iran Red Crescent Med J. 2012 Apr;14(4):229-34.

97. Khalatbary AR, Ahmadvand H. **Neuroprotective effect of oleuropein following spinal cord injury in rats.** Neurol Res. 2012 Jan;34(1):44-51

98. Impellizzeri D, Esposito E, Mazzon E, Paterniti I, Di Paola R, Bramanti P, Morittu VM, Procopio A, Perri E, Britti D, Cuzzocrea S. **The effects of a polyphenol present in olive oil, oleuropein aglycone, in an experimental model of spinal cord injury in mice.** Biochem Pharmacol. 2012 May 15;83(10):1413-26

99. Belviranlı M, Okudan N, Atalık KE, Oz M. **Curcumin improves spatial memory and decreases oxidative damage in aged female rats.** Biogerontology. 2013 Apr;14(2):187-96.

100. Latour A, Grintal B, Champeil-Potokar G, Hennebelle M, Lavialle M, Dutar P, Potier B, Billard JM, Vancassel S, Denis I. **Omega-3 fatty acids deficiency aggravates glutamatergic synapse and astroglial aging in the rat hippocampal CA1.** Aging Cell. 2013 Feb;12(1):76-84

101. Denis I, Potier B, Vancassel S, Heberden C, Lavialle M. **Omega-3 fatty acids and brain resistance to ageing and stress: Body of evidence and possible mechanisms.** Ageing Res Rev. 2013 Mar;12(2):579-94.

102. Kiecolt-Glaser JK, Epel ES, Belury MA, Andridge R, Lin J, Glaser R, Malarkey WB, Hwang BS, Blackburn E. **Omega-3 fatty acids, oxidative stress, and leukocyte telomere length: A randomized controlled trial.** Brain Behav Immun. 2013 Feb;28:16-24

103. Rees GA, Doyle W, Srivastava A, Brooke ZM, Crawford MA, Costeloe KL. **The nutrient intakes of mothers of low birth weight babies - a comparison of ethnic groups in East London, UK.** Matern Child Nutr. 2005 Apr;1(2):91-9.

SECTION 3: Putting out the Flames – An Advanced Course

Chapter 4. Why have we become so unhealthy?

1. Hulsegge G, Susan H, Picavet J, Blokstral A, Nooyens ACJ, Spijkerman AMW, van der Schouw YT, Smit HA, Verschuren WMM. **Today's adult generations are less healthy than their predecessors: generation shifts in metabolic risk factors: the Doetinchem Cohort Study.** European Journal of Preventive Cardiology April 10, 20132047487313485512

2. Wang YC, Mcpherson K, Marsh T, Gortmaker SL, Brown M. **Health and economic burden of the projected obesity trends in the USA and the UK.** Lancet 2011;378:815–25.

3. Boyle JP, Thompson TJ, Gregg EW, Barker LE, Williamson DF. **Projection of the year 2050 burden of diabetes in the US adult population: dynamic modeling of incidence, mortality, and prediabetes prevalence.** Population Health Metrics 2010;8:29.

4. Alzheimer's Association. **2012 Alzheimer's disease facts and figures.** Alzheimers Dement. 2012;8(2):131-68

5. Bray F, Møller B. **Predicting the future burden of cancer.** Nature Reviews Cancer 2006;6:63–74.

6. Gallup Survey 2013. http://www.gallup.com/poll/162344/poor-health-tied-big-losses-job-types.aspx

7. Joseph JA, Shukitt-Hale B, Denisova NA, Prior RL, Cao G, Martin A, Taglialatela G, Bickford PC. **Long-term dietary strawberry, spinach, or vitamin E supplementation retards the onset of age-related neuronal signal-transduction and cognitive behavioral deficits.** J Neurosci. 1998 Oct 1;18(19):8047-55.

8. Kelly L, Grehan B, Chiesa AD, O'Mara SM, Downer E, Sahyoun G, Massey KA, Nicolaou A, Lynch MA. **The polyunsaturated fatty acids, EPA and DPA exert a protective effect in the hippocampus of the aged rat.** Neurobiol Aging. 2011 Dec;32(12):2318.e1-15.

9. Kiso Y. **Pharmacology in health foods: effects of arachidonic acid and docosahexaenoic acid on the age-related decline in brain and cardiovascular system function.** J Pharmacol Sci. 2011;115(4):471-5.

10. Dyall SC, Michael GJ, Michael-Titus AT. **Omega-3 fatty acids reverse age-related decreases in nuclear receptors and increase neurogenesis in old rats.** J Neurosci Res. 2010 Aug 1;88(10):2091-102

11. Elks CM, Reed SD, Mariappan N, Shukitt-Hale B, Joseph JA, Ingram DK, Francis J. **A blueberry-enriched diet attenuates nephropathy in a rat model of hypertension via reduction in oxidative stress.** PLoS One. 2011;6(9):e24028.

12. Ahmet I, Spangler E, Shukitt-Hale B, Joseph JA, Ingram DK, Talan M. **Survival and cardioprotective benefits of long-term blueberry enriched diet in dilated cardiomyopathy following myocardial infarction in rats.** PLoS One. 2009 Nov 19;4(11):e7975. Doi 10.1371/journal.pone.0007975.

13. Martini C, Pallottini V, De Marinis E, Marino M, Cavallini G, Donati A, Straniero S, Trentalance A. **Omega-3 as well as caloric restriction prevent the age-related modifications of cholesterol metabolism.** Mech Ageing Dev. 2008 Dec;129(12):722-7.

14. Shukitt-Hale B, Lau FC, Carey AN, Galli RL, Spangler EL, Ingram DK, Joseph JA. **Blueberry polyphenols attenuate kainic acid-induced decrements in cognition and alter inflammatory gene expression in rat hippocampus.** Nutr Neurosci. 2008 Aug;11(4):172-8

15. Willis LM, Shukitt-Hale B, Joseph JA. **Recent advances in berry supplementation and age-related cognitive decline.** Curr Opin Clin Nutr Metab Care. 2009 Jan;12(1):91-4. Review.

16. Ji A, Diao H, Wang X, Yang R, Zhang J, Luo W, Cao R, Cao Z, Wang F, Cai T. **n-3 polyunsaturated fatty acids inhibit lipopolysaccharide-induced microglial activation and dopaminergic injury in rats.** Neurotoxicology. 2012 Aug;33(4):780-8.

17. Latour A, Grintal B, Champeil-Potokar G, Hennebelle M, Lavialle M, Dutar P, Potier B, Billard JM, Vancassel S, Denis I. **Omega-3 fatty acids deficiency aggravates glutamatergic synapse and astroglial aging in the rathippocampal CA1.** Aging Cell. 2013 Feb;12(1):76-84.

18. de Lorgeril M, Salen P, Martin JL, Monjaud I, Delaye J, Mamelle N. **Mediterranean diet, traditional risk factors, and the rate of cardiovascular complications after myocardial infarction: final report of the Lyon Diet Heart Study.** Circulation. 1999 Feb 16;99(6):779-85.

19. Esposito K, Marfella R, Ciotola M, Di Palo C, Giugliano F, Giugliano G, D'Armiento M, D'Andrea F, Giugliano D. **Effect of a mediterranean-style diet on endothelial dysfunction and markers of vascular inflammation in the metabolic syndrome: a randomized trial.** JAMA. 2004 Sep 22;292(12):1440-6.

20. Gu Y, Luchsinger JA, Stern Y, Scarmeas N. **Mediterranean diet, inflammatory and metabolic biomarkers, and**

risk of Alzheimer's disease. J Alzheimers Dis. 2010;22(2):483-92.

21. Knoops KT, de Groot LC, Kromhout D, Perrin AE, Moreiras-Varela O, Menotti A, van Staveren WA. **Mediterranean diet, lifestyle factors, and 10-year mortality in elderly European men and women: the HALE project.** JAMA. **2004** Sep 22;292(12):1433-9.

22. Varraso R, **Fung TT, Barr RG,** Hu FB, Willett W, Camargo CA Jr. **Prospective study of dietary patterns and chronic obstructive pulmonary disease among US women.** Am J Clin Nutr. 2007 Aug;86(2):488-95

23. **Varraso** R, **Fung TT, Hu** FB, Willett W, Camargo CA. **Prospective study of dietary patterns and chronic obstructive pulmonary disease among US men.** Thorax. 2007 Sep;62(9):786-91.

24. Calabrese V, Cornelius C, Trovato A, Cavallaro M, Mancuso C, Di Rienzo L, Condorelli D, De Lorenzo A, Calabrese EJ. **The hormetic role of dietary antioxidants in free radical-related diseases.** Curr Pharm Des. 2010;16(7):877-83. Review.

25. Calabrese V, Cornelius C, Dinkova-Kostova AT, Iavicoli I, Di Paola R, Koverech A, Cuzzocrea S, Rizzarelli E, Calabrese EJ. **Cellular stress responses, hormetic** phytochemicals and vitagenes in aging and longevity. Biochim Biophys Acta. 2012 May;1822(5):753-83

26. Clayton P, Rowbotham J. **How the mid-Victorians worked, ate and died.** Int J Environ Res Public Health. 2009 Mar;6(3):1235-53.

27. Griffith R. Institute of Fiscal Studies, 2013. Personal Communication.

28. Ahmed HM, Blaha MJ, Nasir K, Jones SR, Rivera JJ, Agatston A, Blankstein R, Wong ND, Lakoski S, Budoff MJ, Burke GL, Sibley CT, Ouyang P, Blumenthal RS. **Low-Risk Lifestyle, Coronary Calcium, Cardiovascular Events, and Mortality: Results From MESA.** Am. J. Epidemiol. First published online June 2, 2013 doi:10.1093/aje/kws453

29. Myint PK, Smith RD, Luben RN, Surtees PG, Wainwright NW, Wareham NJ,Khaw KT. **Lifestyle behaviours and quality-adjusted life years in middle and older age.** Age Ageing. 2011 Sep;40(5):589-95.

30. Loef M, Walach H. **The combined effects of healthy lifestyle behaviors on all cause mortality: a systematic review and meta-analysis.** Prev Med. 2012 Sep;55(3):163-70.

31. Akbaraly T, Sabia S, Hagger-Johnson G, Tabak AG, Shipley MJ, Jokela M, Brunner EJ, Hamer M, Batty GD, Singh-Manoux A, Kivimaki M. **Does overall diet in midlife predict future aging phenotypes? A cohort study.** Am J Med. 2013 May;126(5):411-419

32. Wijndaele K, Brage S, Besson H, Khaw KT, Sharp SJ, Luben R, Wareham NJ, Ekelund U. **Television viewing time independently predicts all-cause and cardiovascular mortality: the EPIC Norfolk** study. Int J Epidemiol. 2011 Feb;40(1):150-9.

33. Benhaddou-Andaloussi A, Martineau L, Vuong T, Meddah B, Madiraju P, Settaf A, Haddad PS. **The In Vivo Antidiabetic Activity of Nigella sativa Is Mediated through Activation of the AMPK** Pathway and Increased Muscle Glutᵗ Content. Evid Based Complement Alternat Med. 2011;2011:538671.

34. Nguyen PH, Gauhar R, Hwang SL, Dao TT, Park DC, Kim JE, Song H, Huh TL, Oh WK. **New dammarane-type glucosides as potential activators of AMP-activated protein kinase (AMPK) from Gynostemma pentaphyllum.** Bioorg Med Chem. 2011 Nov 1;19(21):6254-60.

35. Scarborough P, Burg MR, Foster C, Swinburn B, Sacks G, Rayner M, Webster P, Allender S. **Increased energy intake entirely accounts for increase in body weight in women but not in men in the UK between 1986 and 2000.** Br J Nutr. 2011 May;105(9):1399-404.

36. German AJ. **The Growing Problem of Obesity in Dogs and Cats.** *J. Nutr.* July 2006 vol. 136 no. 7 **1940S-1946S**

Chapters 5 - 6. What we can learn from the (Victorian) past, & The case for supplements

1. Clayton P, Rowbotham J. **An unsuitable and degraded diet? Part 1: Public health lessons from the mid-Victorian working class diet.** J. Roy. Soc. Med. 2008;101:282–289.

2. Clayton P, Rowbotham J. **An unsuitable and degraded diet? Part 2. Realities of the mid-Victorian diet.** J. Roy. Soc. Med. 2008;101:350–357.

3. Clayton P, Rowbotham J. **An unsuitable and degraded diet? Part 3. Victorian consumption patterns and their health benefits.** J. Roy. Soc. Med. 2008;101:454–462.

4. Hunt T. Building Jerusalem. The Rise and Fall of the Victorian City Weidenfeld and Nicholson; London, UK: 2004. Part 1.

5. Wohl AS. The Eternal Slum: Housing and Social Policy in Victorian London. Transaction Books; London, UK: 2001.

6. Hunt T. Building Jerusalem. The Rise and Fall of the Victorian City Weidenfeld and Nicholson; London, UK: 2004. Chapter 7.

7. Wohl AS. Endangered Lives Public Health in Victorian Britain. Dent and Sons; London, UK: 1983.

8. McKeown T. Reasons for the Decline in Mortality in England and Wales in the Nineteenth Century. Pop. Stud. 1962;16:94–122.

9. Inkster I, Hill J, Griffin C, Rowbotham J, editors. The Golden Age. Essays in British Social and Economic History

1850–1870. Ashgate; Aldershot, UK: 2000.

10. Overton M. Agricultural Revolution in England: The Transformation of the Agrarian Economy 1500–1850. Cambridge University Press; Cambridge, UK: 1996.

11. Overton M. Agricultural Revolution in England: The Transformation of the Agrarian Economy 1500–1850. Cambridge University Press; Cambridge, UK: 1996. pp. 2–10.

12. Daunton M. Wealth and Welfare: An Economic and Social History of Britain 1851–1951. Oxford University Press; Oxford, UK: 2007.

13. Bressey C. Down But Not Out; The Politics of the East End Poor and Those Who Investigated Their Lives. J. Urban Hist. 2008;34:688–694.

14. Burnett J. A Social History of Housing 1815–1985 Routledge; London, UK: 1986. Part II, Chapters 6 and 7.

15. Carlyle T. Chartism. James Fraser; London, UK: 1840.

16. Gaskell North and South. Smith, Elder and Co.; London, UK: 1855.

17. Daunton M. Wealth and Welfare: An Economic and Social History of Britain 1851–1951. Oxford University Press; Oxford, UK: 2007. pp. 5–9.

18. Pickering P, Tyrell A. The People's Bread The History of the Anti-Corn Law League. Leicester University Press; London, UK: 2000.

19. Crafts N, Harley C. Output growth and the British industrial revolution: a restatement of the Crafts-Harley view. Econ. Hist. Rev. 2008;45:704–730.

20. Auerbach J, Hoffenberg P. Britain, the Empire, and the World at the Great Exhibition of 1851. Ashgate; Aldershot, UK: 2008.

21. Kellett J. The Impact of Railways on Victorian Cities. Routledge and Kegan Paul; London, UK: 1969.

22. Burnett J. Plenty and Want A Social History of Food in England from 1815 to the Present Day Routledge; London, UK: 1989. Part II.

23. Mayhew H. London Labour and the London Poor 1861. 4 volumes; Penguin; Harmondsworth, UK: 1985. 1Chapters 1–7.

24. Charlton J, Murphy M, editors. The Health of Adult Britain 1841–1994. Vol. 2. National Statistics; London, UK: 2004.

25. Burnett J. Plenty and Want A Social History of Food in England from 1815 to the Present Day Routledge; London, UK: 1989. Chapter 10.

26. Leicester Burnett J, Oddy D, editors. The Origins and Development of Food Policies in Europe. University Press; London, UK: 1994.

27. Coleman T. The Railway Navvies. Pelican; London, UK: 1968.

28. Rowntree BS. Poverty. A Study of Town Life. Centennial Edition, Policy Press; London, UK: 2001.

29. Garrow J. Editorial. BMJ. 1994;308:934.

30. Floud R, Wachter K, Gregory A. Height, Health and History: Nutritional Status in the United Kingdom, 1750–1980. Cambridge University Press; Cambridge, UK: 1993.

31. Colquhoun A, Lyon P, Alexander E. Feeding minds and bodies: the Edwardian context of school meals. J. Nutrit. Health Sci. 2001;31:117–125.

32. McKeown T. The Modern Rise of Population. Edward Arnold; London, UK: 1976.

33. McNay K, Humphries J, Klasen S. Cambridge Working Papers in Economics. University of Cambridge; Cambridge, UK: 1998. Death and Gender in Victorian England and Wales: Comparisons with Contemporary Developing Countries.

34. Joyce M. The Right to Live: health, democracy and inequality Available at http://www.iwca.info/cgi-bin/iwcacte.pl?record=3 (accessed August 2006).

35. Harris B. Gender, health and welfare in England and Wales since industrialisation. Res. Econ. Hist. 2008;26:157–204.

36. Roberts E. A Woman's Place. Blackwell; Oxford, UK: 1984.

37. Ross E. Love and Toil Motherhood in Outcast London 1870–1918. Oxford University Press; London, UK: 2002.

38. Colgrove J. The McKeown Thesis: A Historical Controversy and Its Enduring Influence. Am. J. Public Health. 2002;92:725–729.

39. Steadman Jones G. Outcast London A study in the relationship between classes in Victorian Society. Penguin; London, UK: 1984.

40. 8thReport of the Medical Officer of the Privy Council, 1865, Parliamentary Papers, XXXIII, 1866.

41. Mayhew H. London Labour and the London Poor. Vol. 4. Penguin; Harmondsworth, UK: 1861. 1985. p. 1.

42. Kirton J. Buy Your Own Cherries. Jarrold and Sons; Norwich, UK: 1862.

43. Plain Cookery Recipes. Nelson; London, UK: 1875.

44. Halvorsen BL, Holte K, Myhrstad MC, Barikmo I, Hvattum E, Remberg SF, Wold AB, Haffner K, Baugerød H, Andersen LF, Moskaug Ø, Jacobs DR, Jr, Blomhoff RA. **Systematic screening of total antioxidants in dietary plants.** J. Nutr. 2002;132:461–471.

45. Walton JK. Fish and Chips and the British Working Class, 1870–1940. Leicester University Press; London, UK: 1992.

46. Wigglesworth E. The Brewers and Licensed Victuallers Guide. Green and Co.; Leeds, UK: 1849.

47. Newsholme A, Scott M. Domestic Economy. Swann Sonnenschein; London, UK: 1892.

48. Wood H. Danesbury House. Scottish Temperance League: Edinburgh, UK; 1860. pp. 112–156.

49. Harrison B. Drink and the Victorians: The Temperance Question in England, 1815–1872. 2nd Ed. Keele University Press; Edinburgh, UK: 1994.

50. Berridge V. Current and future alcohol policy: the relevance of history, CCBH. History and Policy; London, UK: Feb, 2006.

51. Hilton M. Smoking in British popular culture 1800–2000. Manchester University Press; Manchester, UK: 2000.

52. Brixius K, Willms S, Napp A, Tossios P, Ladage D, Bloch W, Mehlhorn U, Schwinger RH. **Crataegus special extract WS 1442 induces an endothelium-dependent, NO-mediated vasorelaxation via eNOS-phosphorylation at serine 1177.** Cardiovasc. Drug. Therapy. 2006;20:177–184.

53. Asgary S, Naderi GH, Sadeghi M, Kelishadi R, Amiri M. **Antihypertensive effect of Iranian Crataegus curvisepala Lind.: a randomized, double-blind study.** Drug. Exp. Clin. Res. 2004;30:221–225.

54. Kim SH, Kang KW, Kim KW, Kim ND. **Procyanidins in crataegus extract evoke endothelium-dependent vasorelaxation in rat aorta.** Life Sci. 2000;67:121–131.

55. Veveris M, Koch E, Chatterjee SS. **Crataegus special extract WS 1442 improves cardiac function and reduces infarct size in a rat model of prolonged coronary ischemia and reperfusion.** Life Sci. 2004;74:1945–1955.

56. Walker AF, Marakis G, Simpson E, Hope JL, Robinson PA, Hassanein M, Simpson HC. **Hypotensive effects of hawthorn for patients with diabetes taking prescription drugs: a randomised controlled trial.** Br. J. Gen. Pract. 2006;56:437–443.

57. Xie ML, Mao CP, Gu ZL, Chen KJ, Zhou WX, Guo CY. **Effects of xiaoyu tablet on endothelin-1, nitric oxide, and apoptotic cells of atherosclerotic vessel wall in rabbits.** Acta Pharmacol. Sin. 2002;23:597–600.

58. Eguale T, Tilahun G, Debella A, Feleke A, Makonnen E. **In vitro and in vivo anthelmintic activity of crude extracts of Coriandrum sativum against Haemonchus contortus.** J. Ethnopharmacol. 2007;110:428–433.

59. McCance RA, Widdowson EM. The Composition of Foods. 6th Ed. Food Standards Agency; London, UK: 2006.

60. O'Keefe JH, Jr, Cordain L. **Cardiovascular disease resulting from a diet and lifestyle at odds with our Paleolithic genome: how to become a 21st-century hunter-gatherer.** Mayo. Clin. Proc. 2004;79:101–108.

61. Harrison B. Drink and the Victorians: The Temperance Question in England, 1815–1872. 2nd Ed. Keele University Press; Edinburgh, UK: 1994.

62. Berridge V. Current and future alcohol policy: the relevance of history, CCBH. History and Policy; London, UK: Feb, 2006.

63. Swift R. 'Behaving Badly: Irish Migrants and Crime in the Victorian City' In: Rowbotham J, Stevenson K, editors. Criminal Conversations: Victorian Crimes, Social Panic and Moral Outrage. Ohio University Press; Edinburgh, UK: 2005.

64. Williams R. **The pervading influence of alcoholic liver disease in hepatology** Alcohol Alcoholism 2008. 43393–397.397Review.

65. Smith EB. The People's Health. Croom Helm; London, UK: 1979.

66. Woods R. The Demography of Victorian England and Wales. Cambridge University Press; Cambridge, UK: 2000.

67. Burns A. Observations on some of the most frequent and important diseases of the heart; on aneurism of the thoracic aorta; on preternatural pulsation in the epigastric region; and on the unusual origin and distribution of some of the large arteries of the human body. Bryce; Edinburgh, UK: 1809.

68. Heberden W. Some Account of a Disorder of the Breast. Presented to the Royal College of Physicians, London, 1768, and published in Medical Transactions. Royal College of Physicians; London, UK: 1772. pp. 59–67.

69. Morgagni GB. De sedibus et causis morborum per anatomen indagatis libri quinque. Remondini; Venice, Italy: 1761.

70. Virchow R. Die Cellularepathologie in ihrer begrundung auf physiologische und pathologische Gewebelehre. Hischwald; Berlin, Prussia, Germany: 1858.

71. Hyde Salter H. **On the treatment of asthma by belladonna.** The Lancet. 1869:152–153.

72. Paget J. **On the average duration of life in patients with scirrhous cancer of the breast.** Lancet. 1856;1:62–63.

73. USDA2 Food and Nutrient Intakes by Individuals in the United States, by Sex and Age, 1994–1996 Nationwide Food Surveys Report US Department of Agriculture, Agricultural Research Service; Washington DC, US: No. 96-2, 1998.

74. USDA1 The Continuing Survey of Food Intakes by Individuals and the Diet and Health Knowledge Survey US Department of Agriculture, Agricultural Research Service, Food Survey Research Group; Washington DC, US: 1994–1996.1996CD-Rom data.

75. Gregory J, Collins D, Davies P, Hughes J, Clarke P. National Diet and Nutrition Survey. HMSO; London, UK: 2000.

76. Elia M, Stratton R, Russell C, Green C, Pan F, editors. The cost of disease-related malnutrition in the UK: considerations for the use of oral nutritional supplements (ONS) in adults. British Association for Parenteral and Enteral Nutrition; Redditch, UK: 2005.

77. Bardia A, Tleyjeh IM, Cerhan JR, Sood AK, Limburg PJ, Erwin PJ, Montori VM. **Efficacy of antioxidant supplementation in reducing primary cancer incidence and mortality: systematic review and meta-analysis.** Mayo Clin. Proc. 2008;83:23–34.

78. Dennett DC. Sweet Dreams: Philosophical Obstacles to a Science of Consciousness. MIT Press; Cambridge, MA, USA: 2005. p. 178.

79. Clayton P. Pharmageddon: The Limits to Pharmacutical Medicine – and What Lies Beyond. In prepn.

80. Carbonaro M, Mattera M, Nicoli S, Bergamo P, Cappelloni M. **Modulation of antioxidant compounds in organic vs**

conventional fruit (peach, Prunus persica L., and pear, Pyrus communis L.) J. Agr. Food Chem. 2002;50:5458–5462.

81.   Dani C, Oliboni LS, Vanderlinde R, Bonatto D, Salvador M, Henriques JA. **Phenolic content and antioxidant activities of white and purple juices manufactured with organically- or conventionally-produced grapes.** Food Chem. Toxicol. 2007;45:2574–2580.

82.   Pérez-López AJ, López-Nicolas JM, Núñez-Delicado E, Del Amor FM, Carbonell-Barrachina AA. **Effects of agricultural practices on color, carotenoids composition, and minerals contents of sweet peppers, cv. Almuden.** J. Agric. Food Chem. 2007;55:8158–8164.

83.   Gill C.Personal communication, 2008.

84.   Lester GE, Manthey JA, Buslig BS. **Organic vs conventionally grown Rio Red whole grapefruit and juice: comparison of production inputs, market quality, consumer acceptance, and human health-bioactive compounds.** J. Agric. Food Chem. 2007;55:4474–4480.

85.   Halvorsen BL, Holte K, Myhrstad MC, Barikmo I, Hvattum E, Remberg SF, Wold AB, Haffner K, Baugerød H, Andersen LF, Moskaug Ø, Jacobs DR, Jr, Blomhoff R. **A systematic screening of total antioxidants in dietary plants.** J. Nutr. 2002;132:461–471.

86.   Ornish D, Magbanua MJ, Weidner G, Weinberg V, Kemp C, Green C, Mattie MD, Marlin R, Simko J, Shinohara K, Haqq CM, Carroll PR. **Changes in prostate gene expression in men undergoing an intensive nutrition and lifestyle intervention.** Proc. Natl. Acad. Sci. USA. 2008;105:8369–8374.

87.   Traka M, Gaspar AV, Melchini A, Bacon JR, Needs PW, Frost V, Chantry A, Jones AME, Ortori CA, Barrett DA, Ball RY, Mills RD, Mithen RF. PLoS ONE 2008. 3e2568doi: 10.1371/journal.pone.0002568.

88.   Ames BN, Elson-Schwab I, Silver EA. **High-dose vitamin therapy stimulates variant enzymes with decreased coenzyme binding affinity (increased K(m)): relevance to genetic disease and polymorphisms.** Am. J. Clin. Nutr. 2002;75:616–658.

89.   C.H. Denyer, 1983 'The Consumption of Tea and Other Staple Drinks', Economic Journal, vol 3, 33-51

90.   HO45/788, Admiralty, 5 Feb 1844, Request to Victualling Yard Deptford.

91.   Woodley MA, Nijenhuis J, Murphy R. **Were the Victorians cleverer than us? The decline in general intelligence estimated from a meta-analysis of the slowing of simple reaction time.** Intelligence 2013. tp://dx.doi.org/10.1016/j.intell.2013.04.006

92.   Huebner J. (2005). **A possible declining trend for worldwide innovation.** Technological Forecasting and Social Change, 72, 980–986.

93.   Murray, C. (2003). **Human accomplishment: The pursuit of excellence in the arts and sciences, 800 BC to 1950.** New York, NY: Harper Collins

94.   Woodley MA. (2012). **The social and scientific temporal correlates of genotypic intelligence and the Flynn effect.** Intelligence, 40, 189–204.

95.   Woodley MA, Figueredo A J. (2013). **Historical variability in heritable general intelligence: Its evolutionary origins and socio-cultural consequences.** Buckingham, UK: The University of Buckingham Press

Chapter 7. Why you cannot get everything you need from a 'Well-Balanced Diet'.   This chapter has no references.

Chapter 8. How we lost the nutritional wisdom of our ancestors

1.   Haahtela T, Klaukka T, Koskela K, Erhola M, Laitinen LA; Working Group of the Asthma Programme in Finland 1994-2004. **Asthma programme in Finland: a community problem needs community solutions.** Thorax. 2001 Oct;56(10):806-14.

2.   Mannino DM, Homa DM, Akinbami LJ, Moorman JE, Gwynn C, Redd SC. **Surveillance for asthma--United States, 1980-1999.** MMWR Surveill Summ. 2002 Mar 29;51(1):1-13.

3.   Kirmaz C, Bayrak P, Yilmaz O, Yuksel H. **Effects of glucan treatment on the Th1/Th2 balance in patients with allergic rhinitis: a double-blind placebo-controlled study.** Eur Cytokine Netw. 2005 Jun;16(2):128-34

4.   Clayton P, Rowbotham J. **How the mid-Victorians worked, ate and died.** Int J Environ Res Public Health. 2009 Mar;6(3):1235-53

5.   Owens, I. **Reports of the Collective Investigation Committee of the British Medical Association. Geographical distribution of rickets, acute and subacute rheumatism, chorea and urinary calculus in the British Islands.** Br. Med. J. 1889, 1, 113-116

6.   Kumar J, Muntner P, Kaskel FJ, Hailpern SM, Melamed ML. **Prevalence and associations of 25-hydroxyvitamin D deficiency in US children: NHANES 2001-2004.** Pediatrics. 2009 Sep;124(3):e362-70

7.   SACN 2997. **Scientific Advisory Committee on Nutrition ACN Update on vitamin D: position statement by the Scientific Advisory Committee on Nutrition.** http://www.sacn.gov.uk/pdfs/sacn_position_vitamin_d_2007_05_07.pdf 5

8. Lanham-New SA, Buttriss JL, Miles LM, Ashwell M, Berry JL, Boucher BJ, Cashman KD, Cooper C, Darling AL, Francis RM, Fraser WD, de Groot PGM, Hyppönen E, Kiely M, Lamberg-Allardt C, Macdonald HM, Martineau AR, Masud T, Mavroeidi A, Nowson C, Prentice A, Stone EM, Reddy S, Vieth R, Williams CM. **Proceedings of the Rank Forum on Vitamin D.** Br J Nutr. 2011 January; 105(1): 144–156.
9. Fulgoni VL 3rd, Keast DR, Bailey RL, Dwyer J. **Foods, fortificants, and supplements: Where do Americans get their nutrients?** J Nutr. 2011 Oct;141(10):1847-54. doi: 10.3945/jn.111.142257.
10. Krebs-Smith SM, Guenther PM, Subar AF, Kirkpatrick SI, Dodd KW. **Americans do not meet federal dietary recommendations.** J Nutr. 2010 Oct;140(10):1832-8.
11. Troesch B, Hoeft B, McBurney M, Eggersdorfer M, Weber P **Dietary surveys indicate vitamin intakes below recommendations are common in representative Western countries.** Br J Nutr. 2012 Aug;108(4):692-8
12. Landrier J-F, Marcotorchino J, Tourniaire F. **Lipophilic Micronutrients and Adipose Tissue Biology.** Nutrients. 2012 November; 4(11): 1622–1649.
13. Duntas LH. **Selenium and Inflammation – underlying anti-inflammatory mechanisms.** Horm Metab Res. 2009 Jun;41(6):443-7.
14. Rayman MP, Rayman MP. **The argument for increasing selenium intake.** Proc Nutr Soc. 2002 May;61(2):203-15. Review.
15. Singh U, Devaraj S, Jialal I. **Vitamin E, oxidative stress, and inflammation.** Annu Rev Nutr. 2005;25:151-74. Review.
16. Devaraj S, Yun JM, Duncan-Staley CR, Jialal I. **Low vitamin D levels correlate with the proinflammatory state in type 1 diabetic subjects with and without microvascular complications.** American Journal of Clinical Pathology 2011;135:429–33.
17. Khoo AL, Chai LY, Koenen HJ, Sweep FC, Joosten I, Netea MG, et al. **Regulation of cytokine responses by seasonality of vitamin D status in healthy individuals.** Clinical and Experimental Immunology 2011;164:72–9.

Chapter 9. Putting out the flames: an advanced course

1. Rayman MP. **The importance of selenium to human health.** Lancet. 2000 Jul 15;356(9225):233-41.
2. Rayman MP, Rayman MP. **The argument for increasing selenium intake.** Proc Nutr Soc. 2002 May;61(2):203-15. Review.
3. Reilly, C. 1996. **Selenium in food and health.** London, Blackie Academic and Professional. pp 215-217
4. Landrier J-F, Marcotorchino J, Tourniaire F. **Lipophilic Micronutrients and Adipose Tissue Biology.** Nutrients. 2012 November; 4(11): 1622–1649.
5. Goldberg T, Cai W, Peppa M, Dardaine V, Baliga BS, Uribarri J, Vlassara H. **Advanced glycoxidation end products in commonly consumed foods.** J Am Diet Assoc. 2004 Aug;104(8):1287-91.
6. Uribarri J, Woodruff S, Goodman S, Cai W, Chen X, Pyzik R, Yong A, Striker GE, Vlassara H. **Advanced glycation end products in foods and a practical guide to their reduction in the diet.** J Am Diet Assoc. 2010 Jun;110(6):911-16
7. Rohrman S and 45 others. **Meat consumption and mortality - results from the European Prospective Investigation into Cancer and Nutrition.** BMC Medicine 2013, Mar 7;11:63.

Chapter 10. Key Anti-Inflammatory Nutrients #1: Yeast-Derived (1-3), (1-6) Beta-Glucans

1. Kournikakis B, Mandeville R, Brousseau P, Ostroff G. **Anthrax-protective effects of yeast beta 1,3 glucans.** MedGenMed. 2003 Mar 21;5(1):1.
2. Berdal M, Appelbom HI, Eikrem JH, Lund A, Zykova S, Busund LT, Seljelid R, Jenssen T. **Aminated beta-1,3-D-glucan improves wound healing in diabetic db/db mice.** Wound Repair Regen. 2007 Nov-Dec;15(6):825-32
3. Lehtovaara BC, Gu FX. **Pharmacological, structural, and drug delivery properties and applications of 1,3-β-glucans.** J Agric Food Chem. 2011 Jul 13;59(13):6813-28
4. CDC '13: **Emergence and Spread of Extensively and Totally Drug-Resistant Tuberculosis, South Africa.** Emerging Infectious Diseases Volume 19, Number 3—March 2013
5. Rayman, M. (1997) **Dietary selenium: time to act.** British Medical Journal, **314**, 387- 8.
6. Rayman MP. **The importance of selenium to human health.** Lancet. 2000 Jul 15;356(9225):233-41. Review
7. MacFarlane GD, Sackrison JL Jr, Body JJ, Ersfeld DL, Fenske JS, Miller AB. **Hypovitaminosis D in a normal, apparently healthy urban European population.** J Steroid Biochem Mol Biol. 2004 May;89-90(1-5):621-2.
8. Gallagher-Allred CR, Voss AC, Finn SC, McCamish MA. **Malnutrition and clinical outcomes: the case for medical nutrition therapy.** J Am Diet Assoc 1996 Apr;96(4):361-6, 369.
9. Bistrian BR, Blackburn GL, Vitale J, Cochran D, Naylor J. **Prevalence of malnutrition in general medical patients.** JAMA 1976 Apr 12;235(15):1567-70.
10. Naber TH, Schermer T, de Bree A, Nusteling K, Eggink L, Kruimel JW, Bakkeren J, van Hereveld H, Katan MB.

REFERENCES

Prevalence of malnutrition in nonsurgical hospitalized patients and its association with disease complications. Am J Clin Nutr 1997 Nov;66(5):1232-9.

11. Daly JM, Hearne B, Dunaj J, et al. **Nutritional rehabilitation--patients with advanced head and neck cancer receiving radiation therapy**. *Am J Surg*. 1984;148:514-520.

12. Andrassy RJ, DuBois T, Page CP, et al. **Early postoperative nutritional enhancement utilizing enteral branched-chain amino acids by way of a needle catheter jejunostomy.** *Am J Surg*. 1985;150:730-734.

13. Fietkau R. **Principles of feeding cancer patients via enteral or parenteral nutrition during radiotherapy.** *Strahlentherapie und Onkologie*. 1998;174(Suppl 3):47-51

14. Edington J, Winter PD, Coles SJ, Gale CR, Martyn CN **Outcomes of undernutrition in patients in the community with cancer or cardiovascular disease.** Proc Nutr Soc 1999 Aug;58(3):655-61.

15. Bogden J. **Daily micronutrient supplements enhance delayed-hypersensitivity skin test responses in older people**. Am J Clin Nutr 1994; 60:437-447

16. Meydani SN, Meydani M, Blumberg JB, Leka LS, Siber G, Loszewski R, Thompson C, Pedrosa MC, Diamond RD, Stollar BD. **Vitamin E supplementation and in vivo immune response in healthy elderly subjects: a randomized controlled trial**. J Am Med Assn 1997; 277:1380-1386.

17. Jain AL. **Influence of vitamins and trace-elements on the incidence of respiratory infection in the elderly.** Nutrition Research 2002; 22:85-87.

18. DEFRA 2012. http://www.defra.gov.uk/statistics/files/defra-stats-foodfarm-food-familyfood-2011-121217.pdf

19. Nyquist AC, Gonzales R, Steiner JF, Sande MA. **Antibiotic prescribing for children with colds, upper respiratory tract infections, and bronchitis.** JAMA. 1998 Mar 18;279(11):875-7.

20. CDC '98: **Prescribing Guidelines.** *Pediatrics* 1998; 101:163—184

21. Yong D, Toleman MA, Giske CG, Cho HS, Sundman K, Lee K, Walsh TR. **Characterization of a new metallo-beta-lactamase gene, bla(NDM-1), and a novel erythromycin esterase gene carried on a unique genetic structure in Klebsiella pneumoniae sequence type 14 from India.** Antimicrob Agents Chemother. 2009 Dec;53(12):5046-54

22. Bushnell G, Mitrani-Gold F, Mundy LM. **Emergence of New Delhi metallo-β-lactamase type 1-producing Enterobacteriaceae and non-Enterobacteriaceae: global case detection and bacterial surveillance.** Int J Infect Dis. 2013 Jan 15. pii: S1201-9712(12)01318-5. doi: 10.1016/j.ijid.2012.11.025.

23. Hsu J, Santesso N, Mustafa R, Brozek J, Chen YL, Hopkins JP, Cheung A, Hovhannisyan G, Ivanova L, Flottorp SA, Saeterdal I, Wong AD, Tian J, Uyeki TM, Akl EA, Alonso-Coello P, Smaill F, Schünemann HJ. **Antivirals for treatment of influenza: a systematic review and meta-analysis of observational studies.** Ann Intern Med. 2012 Apr 3;156(7):512-24.

24. Whitley RJ, Boucher CA, Lina B, Nguyen-Van-Tam JS, Osterhaus A, Schutten M, Monto AS. **Global Assessment of Resistance to Neuraminidase Inhibitors: 2008-2011. The Influenza Resistance Information Study (IRIS).** Clin Infect Dis. 2013 May;56(9):1197-205.

25. Daszak P, Cunningham AA, Hyatt AD. **Anthropogenic environmental change and the emergence of infectious diseases in wildlife.** Acta Trop. 2001 Feb 23;78(2):103-16. Review.

26. Kernodle DS, Gates H, Kaiser AB: **Prophylactic Anti-Infective Activity of Poly-(1-6)-beta-D—Glucapyranosyl-(1-3)-beta-D-Glucapyranose Glucan in a Guinea Pig Model of Staphylococcal Wound Infection.** Antimicrob Agents & Chemother 42:545-549, '98

27. Wakshull E, Brunke-Reese D, Lindermuth J, Fisette L, Nathans RS, Crowley JJ, Tufts JC, Zimmerman J, Mackin W, Adams DS. **PGG-glucan, a soluble beta-(1,3)-glucan, enhances the oxidative burst response, microbicidal activity, and activates an NF-kappa B-like factor in human PMN: evidence for a glycosphingolipid beta-(1,3)-glucan receptor.** Immunopharmacology. 1999 Feb;41(2):89-107.

28. Mansell PWA, Ichinose I-I, Reed RJ, Krements ET, McNamee RB, Di Luzio NR: **Macrophage-mediated destruction of human malignant cells in vivo.** J Nat Cancer Inst 1975; 54: 571-580.

29. Hahn MG, Albersheim P: **Host-pathogen interactions. XIV. Isolation and partial characterization of an elicitor from yeast extract.** Plant Physiol 1978; 62: 107.

30. Robertsen B, Engstad RE, Jorgensen JB. **Beta- glucans as Immunostimulants in fish**. Immune Responses I994, V. 1 Fair Haven, NJ, USA.

31. Song Y-L, Hsieh Y-T. **Immunostimulation of tiger shrimp hemocytes for generation of microbicidal substances: analysis of reactive oxygen species.** Developmental and Comparative Immunology, Vol.I, No.3, pp.201-209, 1994.Elsevier Science.

32. Czop JK, Austen KF '85: **A b-glucan inhibitable receptor on human monocytes: its identity with the phagocytic receptor for particulate activators of the alternative complement pathway**. J Immunol 1985; 134: 2588-2593

33. Onderdonk AB, Cisneros RL, Hinkson P, Ostroff G: **Anti-infective effect of poly-beta-1,6-glucotriosyl-beta 1,3glucapyranose glucan in vivo.** Infection & Immunity 60:1642-1647, '92

34. Vetvicka V, Terayama K, Mandeville R, Brousseau P, Kournikakis B, Ostroff G: **Pilot Study:Orally-Administered Yeast Beta1,3-glucan Prophylactically Protects Against Anthrax Infection and Cancer in Mice**; J Am Nutraceutical Assocn 5:1-5, 2002

35. Rasmussen, LT, Konopski Z, Oian P, Seljelid R; **Killing of Escherichia coli by mononuclear phagocytes and neutrophils stimulated in vitro with beta-1, 3-D-polyglucose derivatives**, Microbiol Immunol 36(11):1173-1188. 1992.

36. Rasmussen, LT and Seljelid, R.: **Novel Immunomodulators With Pronounced In Vitro Effects Caused by Stimulation of Cytokine Release**, J Cell Biochem; 46:60-68. 1991. Quote: "Beta-1, 3-D-polyglucose derivatives protect mice against otherwise lethal bacterial infections."

37. Rasmussen LT, Seljelid R, **Dynamics of blood components and peritoneal fluid during treatment of murine E. coli sepsis with beta-1, 3-D-polyglucose derivatives. I: Cells.** Scand J Immunol 32(4): 321-331. Oct 1990.

38. Rasmussen LT, Seljelid R, **Dynamics of blood components and peritoneal fluid during treatment of murine E. coli sepsis with beta-1, 3-D-polyglucose derivatives. II. Interleukin 1, tumor necrosis factor, prostaglandin E2 and leukotriene B4,** Scand J Immunol 32(4): 333-340. Oct 1990.

39. Rasmussen LT, Seljelid R: **The modulatory effect of lipoproteins on the release of interleukin 1 by human peritoneal macrophages stimulated with beta 1 -3D-polyglucose derivatives.** Scand J Immunol 1989; 29: 477-484.

40. Rasmussen LT, Seljelid R, **Production of prostaglandin E2 and interleukin 1 by mouse peritoneal macrophages stimulated with beta-1, 3-D-glucan derivatized plastic beads** Scand J Immunol 26(6): 731-736. Dec 1987.

41. Rasmussen, LT, Fandrem. Jr., and Seljelid R., **Dynamics of Blood Components and Peritoneal Fluid During Treatment of Murine E. Coli Sepsis with beta-1, 3-D-polyglucose Derivatives;** Scand. J Immunol 63:73-80 1985.

42. Williams D.L. and Diluzio N.R.; **Modification of Experimental Viral Hepatitis by Glucan Induced Macrophage Activation.** In the Reticuloendothelial System and Pathogenesis of Liver Disease, Liehr and Grun, eds. Elsevier/North Holland Biomedical Press; pp. 363-368. 1983.

43. Williams D.L. and Diluzio N.R.; **Glucan-Induced Modification of murine Viral Hepatitis.** Science (1980), 208: 67-69. 1980.

44. Williams D.L., et al; **Protective Effect of Glucan in Experimentally Induced Candidiasis.** J. Reticuloendothel; Soc 23: 479-490. 1978.

45. Williams D.L, Diluzio NR, **Glucan induced modification of experimental Staphylococcus aureus infection in normal, leukemic and immunosuppressed mice.** Adv Exp Med Biol 121(A): 291-306. 1979

46. Leibovich SJ, Danon D: **Promotion of wound repair in mice by application of glucan.** J Reticuloendothelial Soc 1980; 27: 1-11.

47. Lahnborg G, Hedstrom KG, Nord CE: **The effect of glucan - a host resistance activator - and ampicillin on experimental intra-abdominal sepsis.** J Reticuloendothelial Soc 1982; 32: 347-353.

48. Di Luzio NR, Williams DL: **The role of glucan in the prevention and modification of microparasitic diseases.** In: Assessments of chemical regulation of immunity in veterinary medicine. Gainer JH, ed. NY: Scientific, Medical and Scholarly Pub., 1983

49. de Felippe J J, da Rocha-Silva F M, Maciel FM, Soares A de M, Mendes NF: **Infection prevention in patients with severe multiple trauma with the immunomodulator beta 1-3 polyglucose (glucan).** Surgery, Gynecology and Obstetrics 1993; 177(4): 383-388.

50. Babineau TJ, Hackford A, Kenler A, Bistrian B, Forse RA, Fairchild PG, Heard S, Keroack M, Caushaj P, Benotti P. **A phase II multicenter, double-blind, randomized, placebo-controlled study of three dosages of an immunomodulator (PGG-glucan) in high-risk surgical patients.** Arch Surg. 1994 Nov;129(11):1204-10.

51. Babineau TJ, Marcello P, Swails W, Kenler A, Bistrian B, Forse RA. **Randomized phase I/II trial of a macrophage-specific immunomodulator (PGG-glucan) in high-risk surgical patients.** Ann Surg. 1994 Nov;220(5):601-9.

52. Dellinger EP, Babineau TJ, Bleicher P, Kaiser AB, Seibert GB, Postier RG, Vogel SB, Norman J, Kaufman D, Galandiuk S, Condon RE. **Effect of PGG-glucan on the rate of serious postoperative infection or death observed after high-risk gastrointestinal operations. Betafectin Gastrointestinal Study Group.** Arch Surg. 1999 Sep;134(9):977-83.

53. Tzianabos AO, Cisneros RL; **Prophylaxis with the immunomodulator PGG glucan enhances antibiotic efficacy in rats infected with antibiotic-resistant bacteria,** Ann NY Acad Sci 797: 285-287; Oct 1996.

54. Kaiser AB, Kernodle DS. **Synergism between poly-(1-6)-beta-D-glucopyranosyl-(1-3)-beta-D-glucopyranose glucan and cefazolin in prophylaxis of staphylococcal wound infection in a guinea pig model.** Antimicrob Agents Chemother. 1998 Sep;42(9):2449-51

55. Mandeville R: Biophage Pharma Inc, personal communication

56. Jung K, Ha Y, Ha SK, Han DU, Kim DW, Moon WK, Chae C: **Antiviral effect of Saccharomyces cerevisiae beta-glucan to swine influenza virus by increased production of interferon-gamma and nitric oxide.** J Vet Med B Infect Dis Vet Public Health. 2004 Mar;51(2):72-6.

57. Patchen ML, D'Alesandro MM, Brook I, Blakely WF, McVittie TJ: **Glucan: mechanisms involved in its "radioprotective" effect..** J Leuc Biol 1987; 42: 95-105.

58. Patchen ML, McVittie TJ: **Stimulated hemopoesis and enhanced survival following glucan treatment in sublethally and lethally irradiated mice.** Int J Immunopharmac 1985; 7: 923-932.

59. Qi C, Cai Y, Gunn L, Ding C, Li B, Kloecker G, Qian K, Vasilakos J, Saijo S, Iwakura Y, Yannelli JR, Yan J. **Differential pathways regulating innate and adaptive antitumor immune responses by particulate and soluble yeast-derived β-glucans.** Blood. 2011 Jun 23;117(25):6825-36.

60. Williams DL, Sherwood ER, Browder IW, McNamee RB, Jones EL, Di Luzio NR: **Preclinical safety evaluation of soluble glucan.** Int J Immunopharmacol 1988; 10: 405-41 1.

61. Acute Oral Toxicity Study of NSC-24 in Rats. Essex Testing Clinic. 1990, NJ, USA.
62. Kirmaz C, Bayrak P, Yilmaz O, Yuksel H. **Effects of glucan treatment on the Th1/Th2 balance in patients with allergic rhinitis: a double-blind placebo-controlled study.** Eur Cytokine Netw. 2005 Jun;16(2):128-34.
63. Sugiyama A, Hata S, Suzuki K, Yoshida E, Nakano R, Mitra S, Arashida R, Asayama Y, Yabuta Y, Takeuchi T. **Oral administration of paramylon, a beta-1,3-D-glucan isolated from Euglena gracilis Z inhibits development of atopic dermatitis-like skin lesions in NC/Nga mice.** J Vet Med Sci. 2010 Jun;72(6):755-63.
64. Kawashima S, Hirose K, Iwata A, Takahashi K, Ohkubo A, Tamachi T, Ikeda K, Kagami S, Nakajima H. β-glucan curdlan induces IL-¹·-producing CD+⁺ T cells and inhibits allergic airway inflammation. J Immunol. 2012 Dec 15;189(12):5713-21
65. Washburn WK, Otsu I, Gottschalk R, Monaco AP: **PGG-glucan, a leukocyte-specific immunostimulant, does not potentiate GVHD or allograft rejection.** J Surg Res 62, 179-83, '96
66. Goldman R: **Characteristics of the b-glucan receptor of murine macrophages.** Exp Cel Res 1988; 174: 481-490.
67. Bjelakovic G, Gluud LL, Nikolova D, Whitfield K, Wetterslev J, Simonetti RG, Bjelakovic M, Gluud C. **Vitamin D supplementation for prevention of mortality in adults.** Cochrane Database Syst Rev. 2011 Jul 6;(7):CD007470.
68. Adams JS, Clemens TL, Parrish JA, Holick MF. **Vitamin-D synthesis and metabolism after ultraviolet irradiation of normal and vitamin-D-deficient subjects.** N Engl J Med.1982 Mar 25;306(12):722-5
69. Vieth R. **Vitamin D supplementation, 25-hydroxyvitamin D concentrations, and safety.** Am J Clin Nutr. 1999; 69(5):842-56.
70. Vieth R, Chan P-C, MacFarlane GD: **Efficacy and safety of vitamin D3 intake exceeding the lowest observed adverse effect level.** Am J Clin Nutr 2001;73:288–94.
71. Beck, M. A., Shi, Q., Morris, V. G., Levander, O. A. (1995) **Rapid genomic evolution of a non-virulent coxsackievirus B3 in selenium-deficient mice results in selection of identical virulent isolates.** Nat. Med. 1,433-436
72. Beck MA, Levander OA, Handy J (2003) **Selenium Deficiency and Viral Infection** J Nutr 133(5):1463S-1467S
73. Pinto JP, Dias V, Zoller H, Porto G, Carmo H, Carvalho F, de Sousa M. **Hepcidin messenger RNA expression in human lymphocytes.** Immunology. 2010 Jun;130(2):217-30.
74. Li M, Eastman CJ, Waite KV, Ma G, Zacharin MR, Topliss DJ, Harding PE, Walsh JP, Ward LC, Mortimer RH, Mackenzie EJ, Byth K, Doyle Z. **Are Australian children iodine deficient? Results of the Australian National Iodine Nutrition Study.** Med J Aust. 2006 Feb 20;184(4):165-9
75. Nawoor Z, Burns R, Smith DF, Sheehan S, O'Herlihy C, Smyth PP. **Iodine intake in pregnancy in Ireland—a cause for concern?** Ir J Med Sci. 2006 Apr-Jun;175(2):21-4.
76. Andersen SL, Sørensen LK, Krejbjerg A, Møller M, Laurberg P. **Iodine deficiency in Danish pregnant women.** Dan Med J. 2013 Jul;60(7):A4657.

Chapter 11. Key Anti-Inflammatory Nutrients #2: Omega-3 Fatty Acids

1. Simopoulos AP. **The importance of the omega-6/omega-3 fatty acid ratio in cardiovascular disease and other chronic diseases.** Exp Biol Med (Maywood). 2008 Jun;233(6):674-88. Review.
2. Colin A, Reggers J, Castronovo V, Ansseau M. **Lipids, depression and suicide.** Encephale. 2003 Jan-Feb;29(1):49-58 (French)
3. Schaeffer L, Gohlke H, Müller M, Heid IM, Palmer LJ, Kompauer I, Demmelmair H, Illig T, Koletzko B, Heinrich J. **Common genetic variants of the FADS1 FADS2 gene cluster and their reconstructed haplotypes are associated with the fatty acid composition in phospholipids.** Hum Mol Genet. 2006 Jun 1;15(11):1745-56.
4. Clayton P, Rowbotham J. **How the mid-Victorians worked, ate and died.** Int J Environ Res Public Health. 2009 Mar;6(3):1235-53.
5. Blasbalg TL, Hibbeln JR, Ramsden CE, Majchrzak SF, Rawlings RR. **Changes in consumption of omega-3 and omega-6 fatty acids in the United States during the 20th century.** Am J Clin Nutr. 2011 May;93(5):950-62.
6. Sublette ME, Hibbeln JR, Galfalvy H, Oquendo MA, Mann JJ. **Omega-3 polyunsaturated essential fatty acid status as a predictor of future suicide risk.** Am J Psychiatry. 2006 Jun;163(6):1100-2.
7. Simopoulos AP. **The importance of the ratio of omega-6/omega-3 essential fatty acids.** Biomed Pharmacother. 2002 Oct;56(8):365-79. Review.
8. Von Schacky C. **The Omega-3 Index as a risk factor for cardiovascular diseases.** Prostaglandins & other Lipid Mediators 96 (2011) 94–98
9. Ramsden CE, Hibbeln JR, Majchrzak-Hong SF. **All PUFAs Are Not Created Equal: Absence of CHD Benefit Specific to Linoleic Acid in Randomized Controlled Trials and Prospective Observational Cohorts.** World Rev Nutr Diet. 2011;102:30-43
10. Brunner E. **Oily Fish and Omega 3 fat supplements.** BMJ. 2006 Apr 1;332(7544):739-40.
11. Simopoulos AP. **The omega-6/omega-3 fatty acid ratio, genetic variation, and cardiovascular disease.** Asia Pac J Clin Nutr. 2008;17 Suppl 1:131-4. Review.
12. Burdge GC, Calder PC 2005 **Alpha-Linolenic acid metabolism in adult humans: the effects of gender and age on conversion to longer-chain polyunsaturated fatty acids.** Eur. J. Lipid Sci. Technol. 107: 426-439)
13. Ramsden CE, Zamora D, Leelarthaepin B, Majchrzak-Hong SF, Faurot KR, Suchindran CM, Ringel A, Davis JM, Hib-

beln JR. **Use of dietary linoleic acid for secondary prevention of coronary heart disease and death: evaluation of recovered data from the Sydney Diet Heart Study and updated meta-analysis.** BMJ. 2013 Feb 4;346:e8707.

14. Vedtofte MS, Jakobsen MU, Lauritzen J, Heitmann BL. Dietary {alpha}-linolenic acid, linoleic acid and n-3 long-chain PUFA and the risk of of ischemic heart disease. Am J Clin Nutr. 2011 Oct;94(4):1097-103.

15. Petrik MB, McEntee MF, Johnson BT, Obukowicz MG, Whelan J. **Highly unsaturated (n-3) fatty acids, but not alpha-linolenic, conjugated linoleic or gamma-linolenic acids, reduce tumorigenesis in Apc(Min/+) mice.** J Nutr. 2000 Oct;130(10):2434-43.

16. James MJ, Ursin VM, Cleland LG. **Metabolism of stearidonic acid in human subjects: comparison with the metabolism of other n-3 fatty acids.** Am J Clin Nutr. 2003 May;77(5):1140-5.

17. Miles EA, Banerjee T, Calder PC. **The influence of different combinations of gamma-linolenic, stearidonic and eicosapentaenoic acids on the fatty acid composition of blood lipids and mononuclear cells in human volunteers.** Prostaglandins Leukot Essent Fatty Acids. 2004 Jun;70(6):529-38.

18. Horia E, Watkins BA. **Comparison of stearidonic acid and alpha-linolenic acid on PGE2 production and COX-2 protein levels in MDA-MB-231 breast cancer cell cultures.** J Nutr Biochem. 2005 Mar;16(3):184-92.

19. Harris Harris WS, Lemke SL, Hansen SN, Goldstein DA, DiRienzo MA, Su H, Nemeth MA, Taylor ML, Ahmed G, George C. **Stearidonic acid-enriched soybean oil increased the omega-3 index, an emerging cardiovascular risk marker.** Lipids. 2008;43(9):805-11.

20. Kockmann V, Spielmann D, Traitler H, Lagarde M. **Inhibitory effect of stearidonic acid (18:4 n-3) on platelet aggregation and arachidonate oxygenation.** Lipids. 1989 Dec;24(12):1004-7.

21. Guichardant M, Traitler H, Spielmann D, Sprecher H, Finot PA. **Stearidonic acid, an inhibitor of the 5-lipoxygenase pathway. A comparison with timnodonic and dihomogammalinolenic acid.** Lipids. 1993 Apr;28(4):321-4.

22. Chilton FH, Rudel LL, Parks JS, Arm JP, Seeds MC. **Mechanisms by which botanical lipids affect inflammatory disorders** Am J Clin Nutr. 2008 Feb;87(2):498S-503S. Review.

23. Whelan J. **Dietary stearidonic acid is a long chain (n-3) polyunsaturated fatty acid with potential health benefits.** J Nutr. 2009 Jan;139(1):5-10. Review.

24. Kelavkar UP, Hutzley J, McHugh K, Allen KG, Parwani A. **Prostate tumor growth can be modulated by dietarily targeting the 15-lipoxygenase-1 and cyclooxygenase-2 enzymes.** Neoplasia. 2009 Jul;11(7):692-9.

25. Harris WS, Lemke SL, Hansen SN, Goldstein DA, DiRienzo MA, Su H, Nemeth MA, Taylor ML, Ahmed G, George C. **Stearidonic acid-enriched soybean oil increased the omega-3 index, an emerging cardiovascular risk marker.** Lipids. 2008 Sep;43(9):805-11

26. Lemke SL, Vicini JL, Su H, Goldstein DA, Nemeth MA, Krul ES, Harris WS. **Dietary intake of stearidonic acid-enriched soybean oil increases the omega-3 index: randomized, double-blind clinical study of efficacy and safety.** Am J Clin Nutr. 2010 Oct;92(4):766-75.

27. Bharadwaj AS, Hart SD, Brown BJ, Li Y, Watkins BA, Brown PB. **Dietary source of stearidonic acid promotes higher muscle DHA concentrations than linolenic acid in hybrid striped bass.** Lipids. 2010 Jan;45(1):21-7

28. Codabaccus MB, Bridle AR, Nichols PD, Carter CG. **Effect of feeding Atlantic salmon (Salmo salar L.) a diet enriched with stearidonic acid from parr to smolt on growth and n-3 long-chain PUFA biosynthesis.** Br J Nutr. 2011 Feb 8:1-12.

29. Rymer C, Hartnell GF, Givens DI. **The effect of feeding modified soyabean oil enriched with C18 : 4 n-3 to broilers on the deposition of n-3 fatty acids in chicken meat.** Br J Nutr. 2011 Mar;105(6):866-78.

30. Bernal-Santos G, O'Donnell AM, Vicini JL, Hartnell GF, Bauman DE. **Hot topic: Enhancing omega-3 fatty acids in milk fat of dairy cows by using stearidonic acid-enriched soybean oil from genetically modified soybeans.** J Dairy Sci. 2010 Jan;93(1):32-7.

Chapter 12. Oily Fish or Fish Oil? & Nutrition & Politics: The Armed Forces

1. Dyerberg J, Bang HO. **Lipid metabolism, atherogenesis, and haemostasis in Eskimos: the role of the prostaglandin-3 family.** Haemostasis. 1979;8(3-5):227-33.

2. Dyerberg J, Bang HO. **Haemostatic function and platelet polyunsaturated fatty acids in Eskimos.** Lancet. 1979 Sep 1;2(8140):433-5

3. Dyerberg J, Bang HO. **Proposed method for the prevention of thrombosis. The Eskimo model.** Ugeskr Laeger. 1980 Jun 16;142(25):1597-600

4. Bang HO. **Fish oil and ischemic heart disease.** Compr Ther. 1987 Nov;13(11):3-8

5. Danaei G, Ding EL, Mozaffarian D, Taylor B, Rehm J, Murray CJ, Ezzati M. **The preventable causes of death in the United States: comparative risk assessment of dietary, lifestyle, and metabolic risk factors.** PLoS Med. 2009 Apr 28;6(4):e1000058.

6. Wang T 2009. Industry Research Thesis, Open University, Iceland. **ISBN** 978-9979-9928-3-7 http://skemman.is/stream/get/1946/4139/11867/1/Final_fixed.pdf

7. Dutot M, Fagon R, Hemon M, Rat P. **Antioxidant, anti-inflammatory, and anti-senescence activities of a phlo-**

rotannin-rich natural extract from brown seaweed Ascophyllum nodosum. Appl Biochem Biotechnol. 2012 Aug;167(8):2234-40.

8. Kang IJ, Jang BG, In S, Choi B, Kim M, Kim MJ. **Phlorotannin-rich Ecklonia cava reduces the production of beta-amyloid by modulating alpha- and gamma-secretase expression and activity.** Neurotoxicology. 2013 Jan;34:16-24. doi: 10.1016/j.neuro.2012.09.013. Epub 2012 Oct 4. PMID: 23041113

9. Yoon JS, Kasin Yadunandam A, Kim SJ, Woo HC, Kim HR, Kim GD. **Dieckol, isolated from Ecklonia stolonifera, induces apoptosis in human hepatocellular carcinoma Hep3B cells.** J Nat Med. 2012 Oct 9.

10. Elvevoll EO, Osterud B. **Impact of processing on nutritional quality of marine food items.** Forum Nutr. 2003;56:337-40.

11. Sanders TA, Hinds A. **The influence of a fish oil high in docosahexaenoic acid on plasma lipoprotein and vitamin E concentrations and haemostatic function in healthy male volunteers.** Br J Nutr. 1992 Jul;68(1):163-73.

12. Sen CK, Atalay M, Ågren J, Laaksonen DE, Roy SHänninen O. **Fish oil and vitamin E supplementation in oxidative stress at rest and after physical exercise.** J. Appl. Physiol.83(1): 189-195, 1997.

13. Umegaki K, Hashimoto M, Yamasaki H, Fujii Y, Yoshimura M, Sugisawa A, Shinozuka K. **Docosahexaenoic acid supplementation-increased oxidative damage in bone marrow DNA in aged rats and its relation to antioxidant vitamins.** Free Radic Res. 2001 Apr;34(4):427-35.

14. Véricel E, Polette A, Bacot S, Calzada C, Lagarde M. **Pro- and antioxidant activities of docosahexaenoic acid on human blood platelets.** J Thromb Haemost. 2003 Mar;1(3):566-72.

15. Schubert R, Reichenbach J, Koch C, Kloess S, Koehl U, Mueller K, Baer P, Beermann C, Boehles H, Zielen S. **Reactive oxygen species abrogate the anticarcinogenic effect of eicosapentaenoic acid in Atm-deficient mice.** Nutr Cancer. 2010;62(5):584-92.

16. Mata P, Alonso R, Lopez-Farre A, Ordovas JM, Lahoz C, Garces C, Caramelo C, Codoceo R, Blazquez E, de Oya M. **Effect of dietary fat saturation on LDL oxidation and monocyte adhesion to human endothelial cells in vitro.** Arterioscler Thromb Vasc Biol. 1996 Nov;16(11):1347-55.

17. Berstad P, Seljeflot I, Veierød MB, Hjerkinn EM, Arnesen H, Pedersen JI. **Supplementation with fish oil affects the association between very long-chain n-3 polyunsaturated fatty acids in serum non-esterified fatty acids and soluble vascular cell adhesion molecule-1.** Clin Sci (Lond). 2003 Jul;105(1):13-20.

18. Cazzola R, Russo-Volpe S, Miles EA, Rees D, Banerjee T, Roynette CE, Wells SJ, Goua M, Wahle KW, Calder PC, Cestaro B. **Age- and dose-dependent effects of an eicosapentaenoic acid-rich oil on cardiovascular risk factors in healthy male subjects.** Atherosclerosis. 2007 Jul;193(1):159-67.

19. Seljeflot I, Johansen O, Arnesen H, Eggesbø JB, Westvik AB, Kierulf P. **Procoagulant activity and cytokine expression in whole blood cultures from patients with atherosclerosis supplemented with omega-3 fatty acids.** Thromb Haemost. 1999 Apr;81(4):566-70.

20. Johansen O, Seljeflot I, Høstmark AT, Arnesen H. **The effect of supplementation with omega-3 fatty acids on soluble markers of endothelial function in patients with coronary heart disease.** Arterioscler Thromb Vasc Biol. 1999 Jul;19(7):1681-6.

21. Arnesen H. **n-3 fatty acids and revascularization procedures.** Lipids. 2001;36 Suppl:S103-6

22. Burr ML, Ashfield-Watt PA, Dunstan FD, Fehily AM, Breay P, Ashton T, Zotos PC, Haboubi NA, Elwood PC. **Lack of benefit of dietary advice to men with angina: results of a controlled trial.** Eur J Clin Nutr. 2003 Feb;57(2):193-200.

23. Rizos EC, Ntzani EE, Bika E, Kostapanos MS, Elisaf MS. **Association between omega-3 fatty acid supplementation and risk of major cardiovascular disease events: a systematic review and meta-analysis.** JAMA. 2012 Sep 12;308(10):1024-33.

24. Mozaffarian D, Lemaitre RN, King IB, Song X, Huang H, Sacks FM, Rimm EB, Wang M, Siscovick DS. **Plasma Phospholipid Long-Chain ω-3 Fatty Acids and Total and Cause-Specific Mortality in Older Adults: A Cohort Study.** Ann Intern Med. 2 April 2013;158(7):515-525

25. Ascherio A, Rimm EB, Stampfer MJ, Giovannucci EL, Willett WC. **Dietary intake of marine n-3 fatty acids, fish intake, and the risk of coronary disease among men.** N Engl J Med. 1995 Apr 13;332(15):977-82.

26. Salonen JT, Seppänen K, Nyyssönen K, Korpela H, Kauhanen J, Kantola M, Tuomilehto J, Esterbauer H, Tatzber F, Salonen R. **Intake of mercury from fish, lipid peroxidation, and the risk of myocardial infarction and coronary, cardiovascular, and any death in eastern Finnish men.** Circulation. 1995 Feb 1;91(3):645-55.

27. Landmark K, Aursnes I. **Mercury, fish, fish oil and the risk of cardiovascular disease.** Tidsskr Nor Laegeforen. 2004 Jan 22;124(2):198-200.

28. Burr ML, Dunstan FD, George CH. **Is fish oil good or bad for heart disease? Two trials with apparently conflicting results.** J Membr Biol. 2005 Jul;206(2):155-63.

29. Cunane S. Personal communication 2013

30. Allard JP, Kurian R, Aghdassi E, Muggli R, Royall D. **Lipid peroxidation during n-3 fatty acid and vitamin E supplementation in humans.** Lipids. 1997 May;32(5):535-41.

31. Palmieri D, Aliakbarian B, Casazza AA, Ferrari N, Spinella G, Pane B, Cafueri G, Perego P, Palombo D. **Effects of polyphenol extract from olive pomace on anoxia-induced endothelial dysfunction.** Microvasc Res. 2012 May;83(3):281-9.

32. Berra B, Cortesi N, Rapelli S. 1989. **Biological significance of minor components of olive oil.** Actes du Congres

International "Chevreul" pour l"etude de corps gras 6-9 giugno 1989.

33.   Berra B, Caruso D, Cortesi N, Fedeli E, Rasetti MF, Galli G. 1995. **Antioxidant properties of minor polar compo-
       nents of olive oil on the oxidative processes of cholesterol in human LDL.** La Rivista Italiana delle Sostanze
       Grasse, Vol. LXXII, 285-288, 1995 10

34.   Carluccio MA, Siculella L, Ancora MA, Massaro M, Scoditti E, Storelli C, Visioli F, Distante A, De Caterina R. **Olive oil
       and red wine antioxidant polyphenols inhibit endothelial activation: antiatherogenic properties of Mediter-
       ranean diet phytochemicals.** Arterio. Throm. Vasc. Bio.2003;23:622–629.

35.   Covas MI, Nyyssonen K, Poulsen HE, Kaikkonen J, Zunft HJ, Kiesewetter H, Gaddi A, de la Torre R, Mursu J, Baum-
       ler H, Nascetti S, Salonen JT, Fito M, Virtanen J, Marrugat J, Group ES. **The effect of polyphenols in olive oil on
       heart disease risk factors: a randomized trial.** Ann. Int. Med.2006;145:333–341.

36.   Cicerale S, Lucas L, Keast R. **Biological Activities of Phenolic Compounds Present in Virgin Olive Oil.** Int J Mol
       Sci. 2010; 11(2): 458–479.

37.   Bayram B, Ozcelik B, Grimm S, Roeder T, Schrader C, Ernst IMA, Wagner AE, Grune T, Frank J, Rimbach G. **A Diet
       Rich in Olive Oil** Phenolics Reduces Oxidative Stress in the **Heart** of SAMP^8 Mice by Induction of Nrf-^Y Dependent
       Gene Expression. Rejuvenation Res. 2012 February; 15(1): 71–81.

38.   Ebaid GM, Seiva FR, Rocha KK, Souza GA, Novelli EL. **Effects of olive oil and minor phenolic constituents on
       obesity-induced cardiac metabolic changes.** Nutr J. 2010 Oct 19;9:46. doi: 10.1186/1475-2891-9-46.

39.   Castañer O, Covas MI, Khymenets O, Nyyssonen K, Konstantinidou V, Zunft HF, de la Torre R, Muñoz-Aguayo
       D, Vila J, Fitó M. **Protection of LDL from oxidation by olive oil polyphenols is associated with a downregu-
       lation of CD40-ligand expression and its downstream products in vivo in humans.** Am J Clin Nutr. 2012
       May;95(5):1238-44.

40.   Eilertsen K-E, Mæhre HK, Cludts K, Olsen JO, Hoylaerts MF. **Dietary enrichment of apolipoprotein E-deficient
       mice with extra virgin olive oil in combination with seal oil inhibits atherogenesis.** Lipids Health Dis. 2011; 10:
       41

41.   Dalli J, Winkler JW, Colas RA, Arnardottir H, Chian C-YC, Chiang N, Petasis NA, Serhan CN. **Resolvin D3 and
       Aspirin-Triggered Resolvin D3 Are Potent Immunoresolvents.** Chemistry and Biology 20 (2), 188-201 February
       2013

Chapter 13. Nutrition & Politics: The Armed Forces

1.   Tanskanen A, Hibbeln JR, Hintikka J, Haatainen K, Honkalampi K, Viinamäki H. **Fish consumption, depression,
      and suicidality in a general population.** Arch Gen Psychiatry. 2001 May;58(5):512-3

2.   Tanskanen A, Hibbeln JR, Tuomilehto J, Uutela A, Haukkala A, Viinamäki H, Lehtonen J, Vartiainen E. **Fish con-
      sumption and depressive symptoms in the general population in Finland.** Psychiatr Serv. 2001 Apr;52(4):529-
      31

3.   De Vriese SR, Christophe AB, Maes M. **In humans, the seasonal variation in poly-unsaturated fatty acids is re-
      lated to the seasonal variation in violent suicide and serotonergic markers of violent suicide.** Prostaglandins
      Leukot Essent Fatty Acids. 2004 Jul;71(1):13-8

4.   Huan M, Hamazaki K, Sun Y, Itomura M, Liu H, Kang W, Watanabe S, Terasawa K, Hamazaki T. **Suicide attempt
      and n-3 fatty acid levels in red blood cells: a case control study in China.** Biol Psychiatry. 2004 Oct 1;56(7):490-
      6.

5.   Sublette ME, Hibbeln JR, Galfalvy H, Oquendo MA, Mann JJ. **Omega-3 polyunsaturated essential fatty acid sta-
      tus as a predictor of future suicide risk.** Am J Psychiatry. 2006 Jun;163(6):1100-2.

6.   Hibbeln JR. **Depression, suicide and deficiencies of omega-3 essential fatty acids in modern diets.** World Rev
      Nutr Diet. 2009;99:17-30.

7.   Lewis MD, Hibbeln JR, Johnson JE, Lin YH, Hyun DY, Loewke JD. **Suicide Deaths of Active USA Military and
      Omega-3 Fatty Acid Status: A Case Control Comparison.** J Clin Psychiat 2011 10.4088/JCP.11m06879

Chapter 14. Nutrition and Politics: Sport and the 5-Ring Circus

1.   Kannel WB, Wolf PA, Benjamin EJ, Levy D. **Prevalence, incidence, prognosis, and predisposing conditions for
      atrial fibrillation: population-based estimates.** Am J Cardiol. 1998 Oct 16;82(8A):2N-9N.

2.   Burr M, Fehily AM, Gilbert JF, Rogers S, Holliday RM, Sweetnam PM, Elwood PC, Deadman NM. **Effects of chang-
      es in fat, fish, and fibre intakes on death and myocardial reinfarction: diet and reinfarction trial (DART).**
      Lancet. 1989; 334: 757–761.

3.   Leaf A, Albert CM, Josephson M, Steinhaus D, Kluger J, Kang JX, Cox B, Zhang H, Schoenfeld D; Fatty Acid An-
      tiarrhythmia Trial Investigators. **Prevention of fatal arrhythmias in high-risk subjects by fish oil n-3 fatty acid
      intake.** Circulation. 2005 Nov 1;112(18):2762-8.

4.   Jahangiri A., Leifert W. R., Kind K. L., McMurchie E. J. (2006). **Dietary fish oil alters cardiomyocyte Ca^{2+} dynamics**

and antioxidant status. Free Radic. Biol. Med. 40, 1592–1602.

5. Wu JHY, Lemaitre RN, King IB, Song X, Sacks FM, Rimm EB, Heckbert SR, Siscovick DS, Mozaffarian D. **Association of Plasma Phospholipid Long-Chain Omega-3 Fatty Acids With Incident Atrial Fibrillation in Older Adults: The Cardiovascular Health Study.** Circulation 2012, Volume 125, Pages 1084-1093

6. Kumar S., Sutherland F., Morton J. B., Lee G., Morgan J., Wong J., Eccleston D. E., Voukelatos J., Garg M. L., Sparks P. B. (2011). **Long-term omega-3 polyunsaturated fatty acid supplementation reduces the recurrence of persistent atrial fibrillation after electrical cardioversion.** Heart Rhythm. 9, 483–491.

7. Nodari S., Triggiani M., Campia U., Manerba A., Milesi G., Cesana B. M., Gheorghiade M., Dei Cas L. (2011). **n-3 Polyunsaturated fatty acids in the prevention of atrial fibrillation recurrences after electrical cardioversion: a prospective, randomized study.** Circulation 124, 1100–1106.

8. Milberg P., Frommeyer G., Kleideiter A., Fischer A., Osada N., Breithardt G., Fehr M., Eckardt L. (2011). **Antiarrhythmic effects of free polyunsaturated fatty acids in an experimental model of LQT2 and LQT3 due to suppression of early afterdepolarizations and reduction of spatial and temporal dispersion of repolarization.** Heart Rhythm 8, 1492–1500

9. Kohno H, Koyanagi T, Kasegawa H, Miyazaki M. **Three-day magnesium administration prevents atrial fibrillation after coronary artery bypass grafting.** Ann Thorac Surg. 2005 Jan;79(1):117-26.

10. Nielsen FH, Milne DB, Klevay LM, Gallagher S, Johnson L. **Dietary magnesium deficiency induces heart rhythm changes, impairs glucose tolerance, and decreases serum cholesterol in post menopausal women.** J Am Coll Nutr. 2007 Apr;26(2):121-32.

11. Toraman F, Karabulut EH, Alhan HC, Dagdelen S, Tarcan S. **Magnesium infusion dramatically decreases the incidence of atrial fibrillation after coronary artery bypass grafting.** Ann Thorac Surg. 2001 Oct;72(4):1256-61

12. Van Camp SP. **Exercice-related sudden death: cardiovascular evaluation of exercisers.** Phys Sportsmed. 1988;16:47–54

13. Maron BJ, Douglas PS, Graham TP, Nishimura RA, Thompson PD. **Task Force 1: preparticipation screening and diagnosis of cardiovascular disease in athletes.** J Am Coll Cardiol. 2005;45:1322–6.

14. Corrado D, Basso C, Rizzoli G, Schiavon M, Thiene G. **Does sports activity enhance the risk of sudden death in adolescents and young adults?** J Am Coll Cardiol. 2003;42:1959–63.

15. Sharma S, Maron BJ, Whyte G, Firoozi S, Elliott PM, McKenna WJ. **Physiologic limits of left ventricular hypertrophy in elite junior athletes: relevance to differential diagnosis of athlete's heart and hypertrophic cardiomyopathy.** J Am Coll Cardiol. 2002;40:1431–1436.

16. Bille K, Figueiras D, Schamasch P, Kappenberger L, Brenner JI, Meijboom FJ, Meijboom EJ. **Sudden cardiac death in athletes: the Lausanne Recommendations.** Eur J Cardiovasc Prev Rehabil. 2006;13:859–75.

17. Maron BJ. **Hypertrophic cardiomyopathy and other causes of sudden cardiac death in young competitive athletes, with considerations for preparticipation screening and criteria for disqualification.** Cardiol Clin. 2007;25:399–414.

18. Tester DJ, Medeiros-Domingo A, Will ML, Haglund CM, Ackerman MA. **Cardiac Channel Molecular Autopsy: Insights From 173 Consecutive Cases of Autopsy-Negative Sudden Unexplained Death Referred for Postmortem Genetic Testing.** Mayo Clin Proc. 2012 June; 87(6): 524–539.

19. Liu T., Korantzopoulos P., Shehata M., Li G., Wang X., Kaul S. (2011). **Prevention of atrial fibrillation with omega-3 fatty acids: a meta-analysis of randomised clinical trials.** Heart 97, 1034–1040.

20. Saravia SG, Knebel F, Schroeckh S, Ziebig R, Lun A, Weimann A, Haberland A, Borges AC, Schimke I. **Cardiac troponin T release and inflammation demonstrated in marathon runners.** Clin Lab. 2010;56(1-2):51-8.

21. Neuman R. B., Bloom H. L., Shukrullah I. (2007). **Oxidative stress markers are associated with persistent atrial fibrillation.** Clin. Chem. 53, 1652–1657.

22. Negi S., Sovari A. A., Dudley S. C., Jr. (2010). **Atrial fibrillation: the emerging role of inflammation and oxidative stress.** Cardiovasc. Hematol. Disord. Drug Targets 10, 262–268.

23. Jeong E-Y, Liu M, Sturdy M, Gao G, Sovari AA, Dudley SC. **Metabolic Stress, Reactive Oxygen Species, and Arrhythmia** J Mol Cell Cardiol. 2012 February; 52(2): 454–463

24. Boos C. J., Anderson R. A., Lip G. Y. (2006). **Is atrial fibrillation an inflammatory disorder?** Eur. Heart J. 27, 136–149.

25. Wacker MJ, Kosloski LM, Gilbert WJR, Touchberry CD, Moore DS, Kelly JK, Brotto M, Orr JA. **Inhibition of Thromboxane A_2-Induced Arrhythmias** and Intracellular Calcium Changes in **Cardiac** Myocytes by Blockade of the Inositol Trisphosphate Pathway. J Pharmacol Exp Ther. 2009 December; 331(3): 917–924

26. Gleeson M, Almey J, Brooks S, Cave R, Lewis A, Griffiths H. **Haematological and acute-phase responses associated with delayed-onset muscle soreness in humans.** Eur J Appl Physiol Occup Physiol. 1995;71(2-3):137-42

27. MacIntyre DL, Reid WD, McKenzie DC. **Delayed muscle soreness. The inflammatory response to muscle injury and its clinical implications.** Sports Med. 1995 Jul;20(1):24-40.

28. MacIntyre DL, Sorichter S, Mair J, Berg A, McKenzie DC. **Markers of inflammation** and myofibrillar proteins following eccentric exercise in humans. Eur J Appl Physiol. 2001 Mar;84(3):180-6.

29. Nosaka K, Clarkson PM. **Changes in indicators of inflammation after eccentric exercise of the elbow flexors.** Med Sci Sports Exerc. 1996 Aug;28(8):953-61.

178

Chapter 15. Sources of fatty acids in the diet: Your Omega-6 / -3 ratio

1. Burdge GC, Calder PC. **Conversion of alpha-linolenic acid to longer-chain polyunsaturated fatty acids in human adults.** Reprod Nutr Dev. 2005 Sep-Oct;45(5):581-97. Review.

Chapter 16. Key Anti-Inflammatory Nutrients #3: Polyphenols

1. Manach C, Scalbert A, Morand C, Rémésy C, Liliana Jiménez L. **Polyphenols: food sources and bioavailability.** Am J Clin Nutr May 2004 vol. 79 no. 5 727-747
2. Wen KC, Fan PC, Tsai SY, Shih IC, Chiang HM. **Ixora parviflora Protects against UVB-Induced Photoaging by Inhibiting the Expression of MMPs, MAP Kinases, and COX-2 and by Promoting Type I Procollagen Synthesis.** Evid Based Complement Alternat Med. 2012;2012:417346.
3. Kim SJ, Lee JH, Kim BS, So HS, Park R, Myung NY, Um JY, Hong SH. **(-)-Epigallocatechin-3-gallate protects against NO-induced ototoxicity through the regulation of caspase- 1, caspase-3, and NF-κB activation.** PLoS One. 2012;7(9):e43967.
4. Xiao J, Ho CT, Liong EC, Nanji AA, Leung TM, Lau TY, Fung ML, Tipoe GL. **Epigallocatechin gallate attenuates fibrosis, oxidative stress, and inflammation in non-alcoholic fatty liver disease rat model through TGF/SMAD, PI3 K/Akt/FoxO1, and NF-kappa B pathways.** Eur J Nutr. 2013 Mar 21.
5. Tsai PY, Ka SM, Chang JM, Chen HC, Shui HA, Li CY, Hua KF, Chang WL, Huang JJ, Yang SS, Chen A. **Epigallo-catechin-3-gallate prevents lupus nephritis development in mice via enhancing the Nrf2 antioxidant pathway and inhibiting NLRP3inflammasome** activation. Free Radic Biol Med. 2011 Aug 1;51(3):744-54.
6. Ellis LZ, Liu W, Luo Y, Okamoto M, Qu D, Dunn JH, Fujita M. **Green tea polyphenol** epigallocatechin-ᵊ-gallate suppresses melanoma growth by inhibiting **inflammasome** and ILᵎ-β secretion. Biochem Biophys Res Commun. 2011 Oct 28;414(3):551-6
7. Siriwardhana N, Kalupahana NS, Cekanova M, LeMieux M, Greer B, Moustaid-Moussa N. **Modulation of adipose tissue inflammation** by bioactive food compounds. J Nutr Biochem. 2013 Apr;24(4):613-23.
8. Bayard V, Chamorro F, Motta J, Hollenberg NK. **Does flavanol intake influence mortality from nitric oxide-dependent processes? Ischemic heart disease, stroke, diabetes mellitus, and cancer in Panama.** *Int Journal of Medical Sciences* 4:53-58, 2007
9. Mink PJ, Scrafford CG, Barraj LM, Harnack L, Hong C-P, Nettleton JA, Jacobs DR. **"Flavonoid intake and cardiovascular disease mortality: a prospective study in postmenopausal women".** *American Journal of Clinical Nutrition* 85:895-909, '07
10. Siasos G, Oikonomou E, Chrysohoou C, Tousoulis D, Panagiotakos D, Zaromitidou A, Zisimos K, Kokkou E, Marinos G, Papavassiliou AG, Pitsavos C, Stefanadis C. **Consumption of a boiled Greek type of coffee is associated with improved endothelial function: The Ikaria Study.** Vasc Med. 2013 Mar 18. http://vmj.sagepub.com/content/early/2013/03/18/1358863X13480258.full.pdf+html
11. Lorenz M, Jochmann N, von Krosigk A, Martus P, Baumann G, Stangl K, Stangl V. **Addition of milk prevents vascular protective effects of tea.** Eur Heart J. 2007 Jan;28(2):219-23.
12. Naruszewicz M, Laniewska I, Millo B, Dluzniewski M. **Combination therapy of statin with flavonoids rich extract from chokeberry fruits enhanced reduction in cardiovascular risk markers in patients after myocardial infraction (MI)** Atherosclerosis. 2007 Oct;194(2):e179-84.
13. Esmaillzadeh A, Tahbaz F, Gaieni I, Alavi-Majd H, Azadbakht L. **Cholesterol-lowering effect of concentrated pomegranate juice consumption in type II diabetic patients with hyperlipidemia.** Int J Vitam Nutr Res.2006 May;76(3):147-51
14. Tomura M, Takano H, Osakabe N, Yasuda A, Inoue K-I, Yanagisawa R, Ohwatari T, Uematsu H. **Dietary supplementation with cacao liquor proanthocyanidins prevents elevation of blood glucose levels in diabetic obese mice.** Nutrition 2007 Apr;23(4):351-5.
15. Vinson JA, Proch J, Bose P, Muchler S, Taffera P, Shuta D, Samman N, Agbor GA. **Chocolate is a powerful ex vivo and in vivo antioxidant, an antiatherosclerotic agent in an animal model, and a significant contributor to antioxidants in the European and American Diets.** J Agric Food Chem. 2006 Oct 18;54(21):8071-6.
16. Wan Y, Vinson JA, Etherton TD, Proch J, Lazarus SA, Kris-Etherton PM. **Effects of cocoa powder and dark chocolate** on LDL oxidative susceptibility and prostaglandin concentrations in humans. Am J Clin Nutr. 2001 Nov;74(5):596-602.
17. Corder R, Mullen W, Khan NQ, Marks SC, Wood EG, Carrier MJ, Crozier A. **Oenology: red wine procyanidins and vascular health.** Nature. 2006 Nov 30;444(7119):566.
18. Corder R. **Red wine, chocolate and vascular health: developing the evidence base.** Heart. 2008 Jul;94(7):821-3.
19. Caton PW, Pothecary MR, Lees DM, Khan NQ, Wood EG, Shoji T, Kanda T, Rull G, Corder R. **Regulation of vascular endothelial function by procyanidin-rich foods and beverages.** J Agric Food Chem. 2010 Apr 14;58(7):4008-

13.

20. Kohama T, Suzuki N, Ohno S, Inoue M. **Analgesic efficacy of French maritime pine bark extract in dysmenorrhea: an open clinical trial**. J Reprod Med. 2004 Oct;49(10):828-32.

21. Kohama T, Inoue M. **Pycnogenol alleviates pain associated with pregnancy**. Phytother Res. 2006 Mar;20(3):232-4.

22. Dai Q, Borenstein A. R, Wu Y, Jackson J. C., Larson E. B. **Fruit and vegetable juices and Alzheimer's disease: the *Kame* project** American Journal of Medicine 2006, *379*, 464-475

23. Mullen B, Marks SC, Crozier A. **Evaluation of Phenolic Compounds in Commercial Fruit Juices and Fruit Drinks**. J Agric Food Chem. 2007 Apr 18;55(8):3148-57

24. Scartezzini P, Speroni E. **Review on some plants of Indian traditional medicine with antioxidant activity**. J Ethnopharmacol. 2000 Jul;71(1-2):23-43.

25. Huang, M. T., Lysz, T., Ferraro, T., Abidi, T. F., Laskin, J. D, Conney, A. H., **Inhibitory effects of curcumin on *in vitro* lipoxygenase and cyclooxygenase activities in mouse epidermis**. Cancer Res., 1991, 51, 813–819

26. Jungil H, Mousumi B, Jihyeung J, Jae-Ha R, Xiaoxin C, Shengmin S, Mao-Jung L, Chung S. Y. **Modulation of arachidonic acid metabolism by curcumin and related b-diketone derivatives: effects on cytosolic phospholipase A₂, cyclooxygenases, and 5-lipoxygenase**. Carcinogenesis, Vol. 20, No. 3, 445-451, March 1999

27. Rajakrishnan V, Jayadeep A, Arun OS, Sudhakaran PR, Menon VP: **Changes in the prostaglandin levels in alcohol toxicity: effect of curcumin and N-acetylcysteine**. J Nutr Biochem. 2000 Oct;11(10):509-14.

28. Aggarwal BB, Kumar A, Bharti AC. **Anticancer potential of curcumin: preclinical and clinical studies**. Anticancer Res. 2003 Jan-Feb;23(1A):363-98.

29. Shah BH, Nawaz Z, Pertani SA **Inhibitory effect of curcumin, a food spice from turmeric, on platelet-activating factor and arachidonic acid-mediated platelet aggregation through inhibition of thromboxane formation and Ca 2+ signalling**. Biochem Pharmacol. 1999; 58:1167-72.

30. Plummer SM, Holloway KA, Manson MM, Munks RJ, Kaptein A, Farrow S, Howells L.. **Inhibition of cyclo-oxygenase 2 expression in colon cells by the chemopreventive agent curcumin involves inhibition of NF-kappaB activation via the NIK/IKK signalling complex**. Oncogene. 1999;18:6013-6020.

31. Plummer SM, Hill KA, Festing MFW, Steward WP, Gescher A, Sharma RA. **Curcumin inhibits prostaglandin biosynthesis via cyclooxygenase-2 in human blood**. Cancer Epidemiol Biomarkers Prev2001; 10:1509–9

32. Zhang F, Altorki NK, Mestre JR, Subbaramaiah K, Andrew J. **Curcumin inhibits cyclooxygenase-2 transcription in bile acid- and phorbol ester-treated human gastrointestinal epithelial cells**. Dannenberg Carcinogenesis 1999;20(3):445-51.

33. Surh YJ, Chun KS, Cha HH, Han SS, Keum YS, Park KK, Lee SS.. **Molecular mechanisms underlying chemopreventive activities of anti-inflammatory phytochemicals: down-regulation of COX-2 and iNOS through suppression of NF-kappa B activation**. Mutat Res. 2001;480-481:243-268.

34. Goel A, Boland CR, Chauhan DP. **Specific inhibition of cyclooxygenase-2 (COX-2) expression by dietary curcumin in HT-29 human colon cancer cells**. Cancer Lett. 2001;172:111-118.

35. Hong CH, Hur SK, Oh OJ, Kim SS, Nam KA, Lee SK. **Evaluation of natural products on inhibition of inducible cyclooxygenase (COX-2) and nitric oxide synthase (iNOS) in cultured mouse macrophage cells**. J Ethnopharmacol. 2002;83:153-159.

36. Hong J, Bose M, Ju J, Ryu JH, Chen X, Sang S, Lee MJ, Yang CS. **Modulation of arachidonic acid metabolism by curcumin and related beta-diketone derivatives: effects on cytosolic phospholipase A(2), cyclooxygenases and 5-lipoxygenase**. Carcinogenesis. 2004 Sep;25(9):1671-9.

37. Bengmark S. **Curcumin, an atoxic antioxidant and natural NFkappaB, cyclooxygenase-2, lipooxygenase, and inducible nitric oxide synthase inhibitor: a shield against acute and chronic diseases**. JPEN J Parenter Enteral Nutr. 2006 Jan-Feb;30(1):45-51. Review.

38. Rao CV. **Regulation of COX and LOX by curcumin**. Adv Exp Med Biol. 2007;595:213-26. Review

39. Satoskar RR, Shah SJ, Shenoy SG: **Evaluation of anti-inflammatory property of curcumin (diferuloyl methane) in patients with postoperative inflammation**: Int J Clin Pharmacol Ther Toxicol. 1986 Dec;24(12):651-4.

40. Kulkarni RR, Patki PS, Jog VP, Gandage, Patwardban B: **Efficacy of an ayurvedic formulation in rheumatoid arthritis: A double-blind, placebo-controlled, cross-over study.** Ind J Pharmacol 24:98-101, '92

41. Chainani-Wu N: **Safety and anti-inflammatory activity of curcumin: a component of tumeric (Curcuma longa).** J Altern Complement Med. 2003 Feb;9(1):161-8.

42. Sharma OP. **Antioxidant activity of curcumin and related compounds**. Biochem Pharmacol 1976; 25:1811-2.

43. Kunchandy E, Rao MNA. **Oxygen radical scavenging activity of curcumin**. Int J Pharmacol 1990; 58:237-40.

44. McCleod RF, Pabst FS. **Oral administration of a turmeric extract inhibits erythrocyte and liver microsome membrane oxidation in rabbits fed with an atherogenic diet**. Nutrition. 2003 Sep;19(9):800-4.

45. Babu KS, Srinivasan K. **Hypolipidemic action of curcumin, the active principle of turmeric (Curcuma longa) in streptozotocin induced diabetic rats**. Mol Cell Biochem 1997; 166:169-75

46. Ramirez-Tortosa MC, Mesa MD, Aguilera MC, Quiles JL, Baró L, Ramirez-Tortosa CL, Martinez-Victoria E, Gil A.. **Oral administration of a turmeric extract inhibits LDL oxidation and has hypocholesterolemic effects in rabbits with experimental atherosclerosis**. Atherosclerosis. 1999;147(2):371-378.

47. Kumar A, Dhawan S, Hardegen NJ, Aggarwal BB. **Curcumin (Diferuloylmethane) inhibition of tumor necrosis factor (TNF)-mediated adhesion of monocytes to endothelial cells by suppression of cell surface expression of adhesion molecules and of nuclear factor-kappaB activation.** Biochem Pharmacol. 1998 Mar 15;55(6):775-83.

48. Ramaswami G, Chai H, Yao Q, Lin PH, Lumsden AB, Chen C. **Effects of curcumin on homocysteine-induced endothelial dysfunction in a porcine coronary artery model.** J Vasc Surg. 2004 Dec;40(6):1216-22.

49. Chen HW, Huang HC, **Effect of curcumin on cell cycle progression and apoptosis in vascular smooth muscle cells.** Br J Pharmacol 1998 Jul;124(6):1029-40

50. Zhang W, Liu D, Wo X, Zhang Y, Jin M, Ding Z. **Effects of Curcuma Longa on proliferation of cultured bovine smooth muscle cells and on expression of low density lipoprotein receptor in cells.** Chin Med J (Engl). 1999 Apr;112(4):308-11.

51. Srivastava R, Dikshit M, Srimal RC, Dhawan BN. **Anti-thrombotic action of curcumin.** Throm Res 1985;404:413-7.

52. Srivastava KC, Bordia A, Verma SK. **Curcumin, a major component of food spice turmeric (*Curcuma longa*) inhibits aggregation and alters eicosanoid metabolism in human blood platelets.** Prost Leuk Essen Fat Acids. 1995;52:223-7

53. Mao C, Xie H, Lu T. **Studies on antiplatelet aggregation and anticoagulant action of Curcuma phaeocaulis** Zhong Yao Cai. 2000 Apr;23(4):212-3. (in Chinese)

54. Ramirez B A, Soler A, Carrion-Gutierrez MA, Pamies M D, Pardo Z J, Diaz-Alperi J, Bernd A, Quintanilla A E, Miquel J. **An hydroalcoholic extract of Curcuma longa lowers the abnormally high values of human-plasma fibrinogen.** Mech Ageing Dev. 2000 Apr 14;114(3):207-10.

55. Sajithlal GB, Chithra P, Chandrakasan G. **Effect of curcumin on the advanced glycation and cross-linking of collagen in diabetic rats.** Biochem Pharmacol 1998; 56:1607-14.

56. Arun N, Nalini N. **Efficacy of turmeric on blood sugar and polyol pathway in diabetic albino rats.** Plant Foods Hum Nutr 2002; 57:41-52.

57. Shoskes DA. **Effect of bioflavonoids quercetin and curcumin on ischemic renal injury: a new class of renoprotective agents.** Transplantation. 1998 Jul 27;66(2):147-52.

58. Mohanty I, Singh Arya D, Dinda A, Joshi S, Talwar KK, Gupta SK. **Protective effects of Curcuma longa on ischemia-reperfusion induced myocardial injuries and their mechanisms.** Life Sci. 2004 Aug 20;75(14):1701-11.

59. Ramirez-B A, Soler A, Carrion MA, Diaz-Alperi J, Bernd A, Quintanilla C, Quintanilla E, Miquel J. **An hydroalcoholic extract of curcuma longa lowers the apo B/apo A ratio. Implications for atherogenesis prevention.** Mech Ageing Dev. 2000 Oct 20;119(1-2):41-7.

60. Miquel J, Bernd A, Sempere JM, Diaz-Alperi J, Ramirez A. **The curcuma antioxidants: pharmacological effects and prospects for future clinical use.** A review. Arch Gerontol Geriatr. 2002 Feb;34(1):37-46.

61. Thamlikitkul V, Bunyapraphatsara N, Dechatiwongse T, Theerapong S, Chantrakul C, Thanaveerasuwan T, Nimitnon S, Boonroj P, Punkrut W, Gingsungneon V, **Randomized double blind study of Curcuma domestica Val. for dyspepsia.** J Med Assoc Thai. 1989 Nov;72(11):613-20.

62. Kositchaiwat C, Kositchaiwat S, Havanondha J. **Curcuma longa Linn. in the treatment of gastric ulcer comparison to liquid antacid: a controlled clinical trial.** J Med Assoc Thai. 1993 Nov;76(11):601-5.

63. Prucksunand C, Indrasukhsri B, Leethochawalit M, Hungspreugs K. **Phase II clinical trial on effect of the long turmeric (Curcuma longa Linn) on healing of peptic ulcer.** Southeast Asian J Trop Med Public Health. 2001 Mar;32(1):208-15.

64. Mohan R, Sivak J, Ashton P, Russo LA, Pham BQ, Kasahara N, Raizman MB, Fini ME. **Curcuminoids inhibit the angiogenic response stimulated by fibroblast growth factor-2, including expression of matrix metalloproteinase gelatinase B.** J Biol Chem. 2000 Apr 7;275(14):10405-12.

65. Arbiser JL, Klauber N, Rohan R, van Leeuwen R, Huang MT, Fisher C, Flynn E, Byers HR **Curcumin is an in vivo inhibitor of angiogenesis.** Mol Med. 1998; 4:376-383.

66. Huang MT, Newmark HL, Fenkel K. **Inhibitory effects of curcumin on tumorigenesis in mice.** J Cell Biochem Suppl. 1997; 27:26-34.

67. Kawamori T, Lubet R, Steele VE, Kelloff GJ, Kaskey RB, Rao CV, Reddy BS.. **Chemopreventive effect of curcumin, a naturally occurring anti-inflammatory agent, during the promotion/progression stages of colon cancer.** Cancer Res. 1999; 59:597-601.

68. Kuo ML, Huang TS, Lin JK. **Curcumin, an antioxidant and anti-tumor promoter, induces apoptosis in human leukemia cells.** Biochim Biophys Acta. 1996; 1317:95-10

69. Duvoix A, Morceau F, Delhalle S, Schmitz M, Schnekenburger M, Galteau MM, Dicato M, Diederich M. **Induction of apoptosis by curcumin: mediation by glutathione S-transferase P1-1 inhibition.** Biochem Pharmacol. 2003 Oct 15;66(8):1475-83.

70. Cheng JH, Chang G, Wu WY. **A controlled clinical study between hepatic arterial infusion with embolized curcuma aromatic oil and chemical drugs in treating primary liver cancer.** Zhongguo Zhong Xi Yi Jie He Za Zhi. 2001 Mar;21(3):165-7. (in Chinese)

71. Johnson JJ, Mukhtar H. **Curcumin for chemoprevention of colon cancer.** Cancer Lett. 2007 Oct 8;255(2):170-81.

72. Leyon PV, Kuttan G. **Studies on the role of some synthetic curcuminoid derivatives in the inhibition of tumour**

specific angiogenesis. J Exp Clin Cancer Res. 2003 Mar;22(1):77-83.

73. Ohori H, Yamakoshi H, Tomizawa M, Shibuya M, Kakudo Y, Takahashi A, Takahashi S, Kato S, Suzuki T, Ishioka C, Iwabuchi Y, Shibata H **Synthesis and biological analysis of new curcumin analogues bearing an enhanced potential for the medicinal treatment of cancer** Mol. Cancer Ther. 2006 5: 2563-2571.

74. Covas MI, Nyyssönen K, Poulsen HE, Kaikkonen J, Zunft HJ, Kiesewetter H, Gaddi A, de la Torre R, Mursu J, Bäumler H, Nascetti S, Salonen JT, Fitó M, Virtanen J, Marrugat J; EUROLIVE Study Group. **The effect of polyphenols in olive oil on heart disease risk factors: a randomized trial.** Ann Intern Med. 2006 Sep 5;145(5):333-41.

75. Serra A, Rubió L, Borràs X, Macià A, Romero MP, Motilva MJ. **Distribution of olive oil phenolic compounds in rat tissues after administration of a phenolic extract from olive cake.** Mol Nutr Food Res. 2012 Mar;56(3):486-96

76. Khalatbary AR, Zarrinjoei GR. **Anti-inflammatory effect of oleuropein in experimental rat spinal cord trauma.** Iran Red Crescent Med J. 2012 Apr;14(4):229-34.

77. Khalatbary AR, Ahmadvand H. **Neuroprotective effect of oleuropein following spinal cord injury in rats.** Neurol Res. 2012 Jan;34(1):44-51

78. Impellizzeri D, Esposito E, Mazzon E, Paterniti I, Di Paola R, Bramanti P, Morittu VM, Procopio A, Perri E, Britti D, Cuzzocrea S. **The effects of a polyphenol present in olive oil, oleuropein aglycone, in an experimental model of spinal cord injury in mice.** Biochem Pharmacol. 2012 May 15;83(10):1413-26

79. Kostomoiri M, Fragkouli A, Sagnou M, Skaltsounis LA, Pelecanou M, Tsilibary EC, Tzinia AK. **Oleuropein, an antioxidant polyphenol constituent of olive promotes α-secretase cleavage of the amyloid precursor protein (AβPP).** Cell Mol Neurobiol. 2013 Jan;33(1):147-54.

80. Visioli F, Galli C, Bornet F, Mattei A, Patelli R, Galli G, Caruso D. **Olive oil phenolics are dose-dependently absorbed in humans.** FEBS Lett. 2000;468:159–160.

81. Miro Casas E, Albadalejo MF, Covas Planells MI, Colomer FM, Lamuela Raventos RM, de la Torre Fornell R. **Tyrosol bioavailability in humans after ingestion of virgin olive oil.** Clin. Chem.2001;47:341–343.

82. Vissers MN, Zock PL, Roodenburg AJ, Leenen R, Katan MB. **Olive oil phenols are absorbed in humans.** J. Nutr. 2002;132:409–417.

83. Palmieri D, Aliakbarian B, Casazza AA, Ferrari N, Spinella G, Pane B, Cafueri G, Perego P, Palombo D. **Effects of polyphenol extract from olive pomace on anoxia-induced endothelial dysfunction.** Microvasc Res. 2012 May;83(3):281-9.

84. Campolo M, Di Paola R, Impellizzeri D, Crupi R, Morittu VM, Procopio A, Perri E, Britti D, Peli A, Esposito E, Cuzzocrea S. **Effects of a polyphenol present in olive oil, oleuropein aglycone, in a murine model of intestinal ischemia/reperfusion injury.** J Leukoc Biol. 2013 Feb;93(2):277-87.

85. Domitrović R, Jakovac H, Marchesi VV, Šain I, Romić Ž, Rahelić D. **Preventive and therapeutic effects of oleuropein against carbon tetrachloride-induced liver damage in mice.** Pharmacol Res. 2012 Apr;65(4):451-64.

86. Impellizzeri D, Esposito E, Mazzon E, Paterniti I, Di Paola R, Morittu VM, Procopio A, Britti D, Cuzzocrea S. **Oleuropein aglycone, an olive oil compound, ameliorates development of arthritis caused by injection of collagen type II in mice.** J Pharmacol Exp Ther. 2011 Dec;339(3):859-69.

87. Alirezaei M, Dezfoulian O, Neamati S, Rashidipour M, Tanideh N, Kheradmand A. **Oleuropein prevents ethanol-induced gastric ulcers via elevation of antioxidant enzyme activities in rats.** J Physiol Biochem. 2012 Dec;68(4):583-92.

88. Giner E, Andújar I, Recio MC, Ríos JL, Cerdá-Nicolás JM, Giner RM. **Oleuropein ameliorates acute colitis in mice.** J Agric Food Chem. 2011 Dec 28;59(24):12882-92

89. Acquaviva R, Di Giacomo C, Sorrenti V, Galvano F, Santangelo R, Cardile V, Gangia S, D'Orazio N, Abraham NG, Vanella L. **Antiproliferative effect of oleuropein in prostate cell lines.** Int J Oncol. 2012 Jul;41(1):31-8.

90. Cárdeno A, Sánchez-Hidalgo M, Rosillo MA, de la Lastra CA. **Oleuropein, a Secoiridoid Derived from Olive Tree, Inhibits the Proliferation of Human Colorectal Cancer Cell Through Downregulation of HIF-1α.** Nutr Cancer. 2013 Jan;65(1):147-56.

91. Elamin MH, Daghestani MH, Omer SA, Elobeid MA, Virk P, Al-Olayan EM, Hassan ZK, Mohammed OB, Aboussekhra A. **Olive oil oleuropein has anti-breast cancer properties with higher efficiency on ER-negative cells.** Food Chem Toxicol. 2012 Dec 20;53C:310-316

92. Hassan ZK, Elamin MH, Daghestani MH, Omer SA, Al-Olayan EM, Elobeid MA, Virk P, Mohammed OB. **Oleuropein induces anti-metastatic effects in breast cancer.** Asian Pac J Cancer Prev. 2012;13(9):4555-9

93. Scoditti E, Calabriso N, Massaro M, Pellegrino M, Storelli C, Martines G, De Caterina R, Carluccio MA. **Mediterranean diet polyphenols reduce inflammatory angiogenesis through MMP-9 and COX-2 inhibition in human vascular endothelial cells: a potentially protective mechanism in atherosclerotic vascular disease and cancer.** Arch Biochem Biophys. 2012 Nov 15;527(2):81-9.

94. Hur W, Kim SW, Lee YK, Choi JE, Hong SW, Song MJ, Bae SH, Park T, Um SJ, Yoon SK. **Oleuropein reduces free fatty acid-induced lipogenesis via lowered extracellular signal-regulated kinase activation in hepatocytes.** Nutr Res. 2012 Oct;32(10):778-86.

95. Drira R, Chen S, Sakamoto K. **Oleuropein and hydroxytyrosol inhibit adipocyte differentiation in 3 T3-L1 cells.** Life Sci. 2011 Nov 7;89(19-20):708-16.

96. Vazquez-Martin A, Fernández-Arroyo S, Cufí S, Oliveras-Ferraros C, Lozano-Sánchez J, Vellón L, Micol V, Joven J, Segura-Carretero A, Menendez JA. **Phenolic secoiridoids in extra virgin olive oil impede fibrogenic and**

oncogenic epithelial-to-mesenchymal transition: extra virgin olive oil as a source of novel antiaging phyto-chemicals. Rejuvenation Res. 2012 Feb;15(1):3-21
97.   Menendez JA, Joven J, Aragonès G, Barrajón-Catalán E and 30 other authors. Xenohormetic and anti-aging ac-tivity of secoiridoid polyphenols present in extra virgin olive oil: A new family of gerosuppressant agents. Cell Cycle. 2013 Jan 31;12(4).
98.   Camargo A, Ruano J, Fernandez JM, Parnell LD, Jimenez A, Santos-Gonzalez M, Marin C, Perez-Martinez P, Uceda M, Lopez-Miranda J, Perez-Jimenez F. Gene expression changes in mononuclear cells in patients with meta-bolic syndrome after acute intake of phenol-rich virgin olive oil. BMC Genomics. 2010; 11: 253.
99.   Bayram B, Ozcelik B, Grimm S, Roeder T, Schrader C, Ernst IMA, Wagner AE, Grune T, Frank J, Rimbach G. A Diet Rich in Olive Oil Phenolics Reduces Oxidative Stress in the Heart of SAMPᴬ Mice by Induction of Nrf-ᵞDependent Gene Expression. Rejuvenation Res. 2012 February; 15(1): 71–81.
100. Pizza V, Agresta A, D'Acunto CW, Festa M, Capasso A. Neuroinflammation and ageing: current theories and an overview of the data. Rev Recent Clin Trials. 2011 Sep;6(3):189-203. Review.
101. Meng Q, Cai D. Defective hypothalamic autophagy directs the central pathogenesis of obesity via the Ikap-pab kinase beta (IKKbeta)/NF-kappaB pathway. J Biol Chem. 2011 Sep 16;286(37):32324-32
102. Cai D, Liu T. Hypothalamic inflammation: a double-edged sword to nutritional diseases. Ann N Y Acad Sci. 2011 Dec;1243:E1-39. Review.
103. Cai D, Liu T. Inflammatory cause of metabolic syndrome via brain stress and NF-κB. Aging (Albany NY). 2012 Feb;4(2):98-115. Review.
104. Cai D. Neuroinflammation and neurodegeneration in overnutrition-induced diseases. Trends Endocrinol Metab. 2013 Jan;24(1):40-7.
105. Cai D. Neuroinflammation in overnutrition-induced diseases. Vitam Horm. 2013; 91:195-218
106. Fleenor BS, Sindler AL, Marvi NK, Howell KL, Zigler ML, Yoshizawa M, Seals DR. Curcumin ameliorates arterial dysfunction and oxidative stress with aging. Exp Gerontol. 2013 Feb;48(2):269-76.
107. Akazawa N, Choi Y, Miyaki A, Tanabe Y, Sugawara J, Ajisaka R, Maeda S. Curcumin ingestion and exercise training improve vascular endothelial function in postmenopausal women. Nutr Res. 2012 Oct;32(10):795-9.
108. Belviranlı M, Okudan N, Atalık KE, Oz M. Curcumin improves spatial memory and decreases oxidative damage in aged female rats. Biogerontology. 2013 Apr;14(2):187-96.
109. Latour A, Grintal B, Champeil-Potokar G, Hennebelle M, Lavialle M, Dutar P, Potier B, Billard JM, Vancassel S, Denis I. Omega-3 fatty acids deficiency aggravates glutamatergic synapse and astroglial aging in the rat hippo-campal CA1. Aging Cell. 2013 Feb;12(1):76-84
110. Denis I, Potier B, Vancassel S, Heberden C, Lavialle M. Omega-3 fatty acids and brain resistance to ageing and stress: Body of evidence and possible mechanisms. Ageing Res Rev. 2013 Mar;12(2):579-94.
111. Kiecolt-Glaser JK, Epel ES, Belury MA, Andridge R, Lin J, Glaser R, Malarkey WB, Hwang BS, Blackburn E. Omega-3 fatty acids, oxidative stress, and leukocyte telomere length: A randomized controlled trial. Brain Behav Immun. 2013 Feb;28:16-24
112. Heiss C, Jahn S, Taylor M, Real WM, Angeli FS, Wong M et al. Improvement of endothelial function with dietary flavanols is associated with mobilization of circulating angiogenic cells in patients with coronary artery dis-ease. J Am Coll Cardiol. 2010 Jul 13;56(3):218-24.
113. Nogueira Lde P, Knibel MP, Torres MR, Nogueira Neto JF, Sanjuliani AF. Consumption of high-polyphenol dark chocolate improves endothelial function in individuals with stage 1 hypertension and excess body weight. Int J Hypertens. 2012;2012:147321.
114. Ried K, Sullivan T, Fakler P, Frank OR, Stocks NP. Does chocolate reduce blood pressure? A meta-analysis. BMC Med. 2010 Jun 28;8:39.
115. Djoussé L, Hopkins PN, North KE, Pankow JS, Arnett DK, Ellison RC. Chocolate consumption is inversely as-sociated with prevalent coronary heart disease: The National Heart, Lung, and Blood Institute Family Heart Study. Clin Nutr. 2011 Apr;30(2):182-7.
116. Panneerselvam M, Tsutsumi YM, Bonds JA, Horikawa YT, Saldana M, Dalton ND, Head BP, Patel PM, Roth DM, Patel HH. Dark chocolate receptors: epicatechin-induced cardiac protection is dependent on delta-opioid receptor stimulation. Am J Physiol Heart Circ Physiol. 2010
117. Gu L, House SE, Wu X, Ou B, Prior RL. Procyanidin and catechin contents and antioxidant capacity of cocoa and chocolate products. J Agric Food Chem. 2006 May 31;54(11):4057-61.
118. Enciu AM, Popescu BO. Is there a causal link between inflammation and dementia? Biomed Res Int. 2013;2013:316495. doi: 10.1155/2013/316495. Epub 2013 Jun 6.
119. Cheng D, Noble J, Tang MX, Schupf N, Mayeux R, Luchsinger JA. Type 2 diabetes and late-onset Alzheimer's dis-ease. Dement Geriatr Cogn Disord. 2011;31(6):424-30
120. Perou R, Bitsko RH, Blumberg SJ, Pastor P, Ghandour RM, Gfroerer JC, Hedden SL, Crosby AE, Visser SN, Schieve LA, Parks SE, Hall JE, Brody D, Simile CM, Thompson WW, Baio J, Avenevoli S, Kogan MD, Huang LN; Centers for Disease Control and Prevention (CDC). Mental Health Surveillance Among Children — United States, 2005–2011. CDC Morbidity and Mortality Weekly Report (MMWR) Supplements May 17, 2013 / 62(02);1-35
121. Whittaker R. Anatomy of an Epidemic: Magic Bullets, Psychiatric Drugs, and the Astonishing Rise of Mental Illness in America. (Crown Publishers, April 2010).

122. Woodley MA, Nijenhuis J, Murphy R. **Were the Victorians cleverer than us? The decline in general intelligence estimated from a meta-analysis of the slowing of simple reaction time.** Intelligence (2013), http://dx.doi.org/10.1016/j.intell.2013.04.006

123. Rees GA, Doyle W, Srivastava A, Brooke ZM, Crawford MA, Costeloe KL. **The nutrient intakes of mothers of low birth weight babies - a comparison of ethnic groups in East London, UK.** Matern Child Nutr. 2005 Apr;1(2):91-9.

Chapter 17. Key Anti-Inflammatory Nutrients #4: selenium, Vitamins D, E and K, and the Lipophillic (Fat-Soluble) Phytonutrients

1. Huang Z, Rose AH, Hoffmann PR. **The role of selenium in inflammation and immunity: from molecular mechanisms to therapeutic opportunities.** Antioxid Redox Signal. 2012 Apr 1;16(7):705-43

2. Vunta H, Belda BJ, Arner RJ, Channa Reddy C, Vanden Heuvel JP, Sandeep Prabhu K. **Selenium attenuates proinflammatory gene expression in macrophages.** Mol Nutr Food Res. 2008 Nov;52(11):1316-23.

3. Kipp AP, Banning A, van Schothorst EM, Méplan C, Coort SL, Evelo CT, Keijer J, Hesketh J, Brigelius-Flohé R. **Marginal selenium deficiency down-regulates inflammation-related genes in splenic leukocytes of the mouse.** J Nutr Biochem. 2012 Sep;23(9):1170-7.

4. Cheng AW, Bolognesi M, Kraus VB. **DIO2 modifies inflammatory responses in chondrocytes.** Osteoarthritis Cartilage. 2012 May;20(5):440-5. Yang CY, Leung PS, Adamopoulos IE, Gershwin ME. **The Implication of Vitamin D and Autoimmunity: a Comprehensive Review.** Clin Rev Allergy Immunol. 2013 Jan 29. DOI 10.1007/s12016-013-8361-3

5. Smolders J, Thewissen M, Peelen E, Menheere P, Tervaert JW, Damoiseaux J, Hupperts R. **Vitamin D status is is positively correlated with regulatory T cell function in patients with multiple sclerosis.** PLoS One. 2009 Aug 13;4(8):e6635

6. Maalmi H, Berraïes A, Tangour E, Ammar J, Abid H, Hamzaoui K, Hamzaoui A. **The impact of vitamin D deficiency on immune T cells in asthmatic children: a case-control study.** J Asthma Allergy. 2012;5:11-9.

7. Chinellato I, Piazza M, Sandri M, Peroni DG, Cardinale F, Piacentini GL, Boner AL. **Serum vitamin D levels and exercise-induced bronchoconstriction in children with asthma.** Eur Respir J. 2011 Jun;37(6):1366-70.

8. Weisse K, Winkler S, Hirche F, Herberth G, Hinz D, Bauer M, Röder S, Rolle-Kampczyk U, von Bergen M, Olek S, Sack U, Richter T, Diez U, Borte M, Stangl GI, Lehmann I. **Maternal and newborn vitamin D status and its impact on food allergy development in the German LINA cohort study.** Allergy. 2013 Feb;68(2):220-8. doi: 10.1111/all.12081.

9. Wjst M. **Is vitamin D supplementation responsible for the allergy pandemic?** Curr Opin Allergy Clin Immunol. 2012 Jun;12(3):257-62.

10. Gregor MF, Hotamisligil GS. **Inflammatory mechanisms in obesity.** Annu Rev Immunol. 2011; 29():415-45. (Review)

11. Olefsky JM, Glass CK. **Macrophages, inflammation, and insulin resistance.** Annu Rev Physiol. 2010; 72():219-46.

12. Landrier J-F, Marcotorchino J, Tourniaire F. Lipophilic Micronutrients and Adipose Tissue Biology. Nutrients. 2012 November; 4(11): 1622–1649.

13. Ibarra A, Bai N, He K, Bily A, Cases J, Roller M, Sang S. **Fraxinus excelsior seed extract FraxiPure™ limits weight gains and hyperglycemia in high-fat diet-induced obese mice.** Phytomedicine. 2011 Apr 15;18(6):479-85.

14. Kimmons J.E., Blanck H.M., Tohill B.C., Zhang J., Khan L.K. **Associations between body mass index and the prevalence of low micronutrient levels among US adults.** MedGenMed.2006;8:59.

15. Garcia O.P., Long K.Z., Rosado J.L. **Impact of micronutrient deficiencies on obesity.** Nutr. Rev. 2009;67:559–572.

Chapter 18. Key Anti-Inflammatory Factors #5: Exercise, Carbs, Blood Sugar Control

1. BHF '10. http://www.bhf.org.uk/media/news-from-the-bhf/expanding-waistlines.asp

2. Seeman TE, Merkin SS, Crimmins EM, Karlamangla AS. **Disability trends among older Americans: National Health And Nutrition Examination Surveys, 1988-1994 and 1999-2004.** Am J Public Health. 2010 Jan;100(1):100-7

3. Sandercock G, Voss C, McConnell D, Rayner P. **Ten year secular declines in the cardiorespiratory fitness of affluent English children are largely independent of changes in body mass index.** Arch Dis Child. 2010 Jan;95(1):46-7

4. Haskell WL, Lee IM, Pate RR et al. **Physical activity and public health: updated recommendation for adults from the American College of Sports Medicine and the American Heart Association.** Med Sci Sports Exerc. 2007;39:1423–1434

5. Hamilton MT, Hamilton DG, Zderic TW. **Role of low energy expenditure and sitting in obesity, metabolic syndrome, type 2 diabetes, and cardiovascular disease.** Diabetes. 2007;56(11):2655–67.

6. Hamilton MT, Healy GN, David W. Dunstan DW, Zderic TW, Owen N. **Too Little Exercise and Too Much Sitting: Inactivity Physiology and the Need for New Recommendations on Sedentary Behavior.** Curr Cardiovasc Risk Rep. 2008 July; 2(4): 292–298.

7. Dunstan DW, Barr ELM, Healy GN, et al. **Television viewing time and mortality: The AusDiab study.** Circulation. 2010;121:384–391.

8. Warren TY, Barry V, Hooker SP, Sui X, Church T, Blair SN. **Sedentary behaviors increase risk of cardiovascular disease mortality in men.** Med Sci Sports Exerc. 2010 May;42(5):879-85.

9. Hamilton MT. **Suppression of skeletal muscle lipoprotein lipase activity during physical inactivity: a molecular reason to maintain daily low-intensity activity.** J Physiol. 2003;551(Pt 2):673–82.

10. Hamilton MT, Hamilton DG, Zderic TW. **Exercise physiology versus inactivity physiology: an essential concept for understanding lipoprotein lipase regulation.** Exerc Sport Sci Rev. 2004;32(4):161–6.

11. Healy GN, Dunstan DW, Salmon J, et al. **Television time and continuous metabolic risk in physically active adults.** Med Sci Sports Exerc. 2008;40:639–645.

12. Richman EL, Kenfield SA, Stampfer MJ, Paciorek A, Carroll PR, Chan JM. **Physical activity after diagnosis and risk of prostate cancer progression: data from the cancer of the prostate strategic urologic research endeavor.** Cancer Research 2011;71:3889–95.

13. Eliassen AH, Hankinson SE, Rosner B, Holmes MD, Willett WC. **Physical activity and risk of breast cancer among postmenopausal women.** Archives of Internal Medicine 2010;170:1758–64.

14. Holmes MD, Chen WY, Feskanich D, Kroenke CH, Colditz GA. **Physical Activity and Survival After Breast Cancer Diagnosis.** *JAMA.* 2005;293(20):2479-2486

15. Meyerhardt JA, Heseltine D, Niedzwiecki D, Hollis D, Saltz LB, Mayer RJ, Thomas J, Nelson H, Whittom R, Hantel A, Schilsky RL, Fuchs CS. **Impact of physical activity on cancer recurrence and survival in patients with stage III colon cancer: findings from CALGB 89803.** J Clin Oncol. 2006a Aug 1;24(22):3535-41.

16. Meyerhardt JA, Giovannucci EL, Holmes MD, Chan AT, Chan JA, Colditz GA, Fuchs CS. **Physical activity and survival after colorectal cancer diagnosis.** J Clin Oncol. 2006b Aug 1;24(22):3527-34

17. Meyerhardt JA, Giovannucci EL, Ogino S, Kirkner GJ, Chan AT, Willett W, Fuchs CS. **Physical activity and male colorectal cancer survival.** Arch Intern Med. 2009 Dec 14;169(22):2102-8.

18. Baker LD, Frank LL, Foster-Schubert K, Green PS, Wilkinson CW, McTiernan A, et al. **Aerobic exercise improves cognition for older adults with glucose intol-erance, a risk factor for Alzheimer's disease.** Journal of Alzheimer's Disease 2010;22:569–79.

19. Eguchi E, Iso H, Tanabe N, Wada Y, Yatsuya H, Kikuchi S, et al. **Healthy lifestyle behaviours and cardiovascular mortality among Japanese men and women: the Japan collaborative cohort study.** European Heart Journal 2012;33:467–77.

20. Zorba E, Cengiz T, Karacabey K. **Exercise training improves body composition, blood lipid profile and serum insulin levels in obese children.** Journal of Sports Medicine and Physical Fitness 2011;51:664–9.

21. Rognmo Ø, Moholdt T, Bakken H, Hole T, Mølstad P, Myhr NE, Grimsmo J, Wisløff U. **Cardiovascular risk of high- versus moderate-intensity aerobic exercise in coronary heart disease patients.** Circulation. 2012 Sep 18;126(12):1436-40.

22. Petersen AM, Pedersen BK. **The anti-inflammatory effect of exercise.** J Appl Physiol. 2005 Apr;98(4):1154-62. Review.

23. Petersen AM, Pedersen BK. **The role of IL-6 in mediating the anti-inflammatory effects of exercise.** J Physiol Pharmacol. 2006 Nov;57 Suppl 10:43-51. Review.

24. Hardie DG. **Role of AMP-activated protein kinase in the metabolic syndrome and in heart disease.** FEBS Lett. 2008 Jan 9;582(1):81-9. Epub 2007 Nov 20. Review.

25. Carling D. **The AMP-activated protein kinase cascade--a unifying system for energy control.** Trends Biochem Sci. 2004 Jan;29(1):18-24. Review.

26. Carling D. **AMPK.** Curr Biol. 2004 Mar 23;14(6);R220.

27. Bijland S, Mancini SJ, Salt IP. **Role of AMP-activated protein kinase in adipose tissue metabolism and inflammation.** Clin Sci (Lond). 2013 Apr;124(8):491-507. Review

28. Hardie DG. **AMP-activated/SNF1 protein kinases: conserved guardians of cellular energy.** Nat Rev Mol Cell Biol. 2007 Oct;8(10):774-85. Review.

29. Sanli T, Linher-Melville K, Tsakiridis T, Singh G. **Sestrin2 modulates AMPK** subunit expression and its response to ionizing radiation in breast cancer cells. PLoS One. 2012;7(2):e32035.

30. Woods JA, Vieira VJ, Keylock KT. **Exercise, inflammation,** and innate immunity. Immunol Allergy Clin North Am. 2009 May;29(2):381-93. Review.

31. Meyerhardt JA, Sato K, Niedzwiecki D, Ye C, Saltz LB, Mayer RJ, Mowat RB, Whittom R, Hantel A, Benson A, Wigler DS, Venook A, Fuchs CS. **Dietary glycemic Load And cancer Recurrence and survival in patients with stage III colon cancer: findings from CALGB 89803.** J Natl Cancer Inst. 2012 Nov 21;104(22):1702-11.

32. Orgel E, Mittelman SD. **The Links Between Insulin Resistance, Diabetes, and Cancer.** Curr Diab Rep. 2013

Apr;13(2):213-22.

33. Lee JH, Budanov AV, Talukdar S, Park EJ, Park HL, Park HW, Bandyopadhyay G, Li N, Aghajan M, Jang I, Wolfe AM, Perkins GA, Ellisman MH, Bier E, Scadeng M, Foretz M, Viollet B, Olefsky J, Karin M. **Maintenance of metabolic homeostasis by Sestrin2 and Sestrin3.** Cell Metab. 2012 Sep 5;16(3):311-21.

34. Dunstan DW, Kingwell BA, Larsen R, Healy GN, Cerin E, Hamilton MT, Shaw JE, Bertovic DA, Zimmet PZ, Salmon J, Owen N. **Breaking up prolonged sitting reduces postprandial glucose and insulin responses.** Diabetes Care. 2012 May;35(5):976-83.

35. Howard BJ, Fraser SF, Sethi P, Cerin E, Hamilton MT, Owen N, Dunstan DW, Kingwell BA. **Impact on Hemostatic Parameters of Interrupting Sitting with Intermittent Activity.** Med Sci Sports Exerc. 2013 Jul;45(7):1285-1291.

36. Peddie MC, Bone JL, Rehrer NJ, Skeaff CM, Gray AR, Perry TL. **Breaking prolonged sitting reduces postprandial glycemia in healthy, normal-weight adults: a randomized crossover trial.** Am J Clin Nutr. 2013 Jun 26. (Epub ahead of print)

37. Sitjà-Rabert M, Rigau D, Fort Vanmeerghaeghe A, Romero-Rodríguez D, Bonastre Subirana M, Bonfill X. **Efficacy of whole body vibration exercise in older people: a systematic review.** Disabil Rehabil. 2012;34(11):883-93.

38. Nguyen PH, Gauhar R, Hwang SL, Dao TT, Park DC, Kim JE, Song H, Huh TL, Oh WK. **New dammarane-type glucosides as potential activators of AMP-activated protein kinase (AMPK) from Gynostemma pentaphyllum.** Bioorg Med Chem. 2011 Nov 1;19(21):6254-60.

39. Lai CS, Tsai ML, Badmaev V, Jimenez M, Ho CT, Pan MH. **Xanthigen suppresses preadipocyte differentiation and adipogenesis through down-regulation of PPARγ and C/EBPs and modulation of SIRT-1, AMPK, and FoxO pathways.** J Agric Food Chem. 2012 Feb 1;60(4):1094-101

40. Kang SI, Shin HS, Kim HM, Yoon SA, Kang SW, Kim JH, Ko HC, Kim SJ. **Petalonia binghamiae extract and its constituent fucoxanthin ameliorate high-fat diet-induced obesity by activating AMP-activated protein kinase.** J Agric Food Chem. 2012 Apr 4;60(13):3389-95.

41. Benhaddou-Andaloussi A, Martineau L, Vuong T, Meddah B, Madiraju P, Settaf A, Haddad PS. **The In Vivo Antidiabetic Activity of Nigella sativa Is Mediated through Activation of the AMPK Pathway and Increased Muscle Glut4 Content.** Evidence-Based Complementary and Alternative Medicine 2011;2011:538671.

42. Kang SI, Shin HS, Kim HM, Hong YS, Yoon SA, Kang SW, Kim JH, Kim MH, Ko HC, Kim SJ. **Immature Citrus sunki peel extract exhibits antiobesity effects by β-oxidation and lipolysis in high-fat diet-induced obese mice.** Biol Pharm Bull. 2012;35(2):223-30.

43. Kang SI, Shin HS, Kim HM, Hong YS, Yoon SA, Kang SW, Kim JH, Ko HC, Kim SJ. **Anti-obesity properties of a Sasa quelpaertensis extract in high-fat diet-induced obese mice.** Biosci Biotechnol Biochem. 2012;76(4):755-61.

44. Shen Y, Croft KD, Hodgson JM, Kyle R, Lee IL, Wang Y, Stocker R, Ward NC. **Quercetin and its metabolites improve vessel function by inducing eNOS activity via phosphorylation of AMPK.** Biochem Pharmacol. 2012 Oct 15;84(8):1036-44.

45. Saravia SG, Knebel F, Schroeckh S, Ziebig R, Lun A, Weimann A, Haberland A, Borges AC, Schimke I. **Cardiac troponin T release and inflammation demonstrated in marathon runners.** Clin Lab. 2010;56(1-2):51-8.

46. Bassi AM, Ledda S, De Pascale MC, Penco S, Rossi S, Odetti P, Cottalasso D. **Antioxidant status in J774A.1 macrophage cell line during chronic exposure to glycated serum.** Biochem Cell Biol. 2005 Apr;83(2):176-87.

47. Bassi AM, Ledda S, Valentini S, De Pascale MC, Rossi S, Odetti P, Cottalasso D. **Damaging effects of advanced glycation end-products in the murine macrophage cell line J774A.1.** Toxicol In Vitro. 2002 Aug;16(4):339-47.

48. Olivieri F., Lorenzi M., Antonicelli R. **Leukocyte telomere shortening in elderly Type2DM patients with previous myocardial infarction.** Atherosclerosis. 2009;206:588–593.

49. Salpea K.D., Talmud P.J., Cooper J.A. **Association of telomere length with type 2 diabetes, oxidative stress and UCP2 gene variation.** Atherosclerosis. 2010 Mar;209(1):42-50

50. Taylor R. **Type 2 Diabetes Etiology and reversibility.** Diabetes Care April 2013 vol. 36 no. 4 1047-1055

51. Osler W: *The Principles and Practice of Medicine.* New York, D. Appleton and Company,1892

52. Fitz RH, Joslin EP: **Diabetes mellitus at the Massachusetts General Hospital from 1824 to 1898: a study of the medical records.** *JAMA* 31 :165 -171,1898

53. Danaei G, Finucane MM, Lu Y, Singh GM, Cowan MJ, Paciorek CJ, Lin JK, Farzadfar F, Khang YH, Stevens GA, Rao M, Ali MK, Riley LM, Robinson CA, Ezzati M; on behalf of the Global Burden of Metabolic Risk Factors of Chronic Diseases Collaborating Group (Blood Glucose). **National, regional, and global trends in fasting plasma glucose and diabetes prevalence since 1980: systematic analysis of health examination surveys and epidemiological studies with 370 country-years and 2·7 million participants.** Lancet. 2012 Dec 15;380(9859):2224-60.

54. Narayan KM, Boyle JP, Thompson TJ, Sorensen SW, Williamson DF. **Lifetime risk for diabetes mellitus in the United States.** JAMA. 2003 Oct 8;290(14):1884-90.

55. Volek JS, Feinman RD. **Carbohydrate restriction improves the features of Metabolic Syndrome. Metabolic Syndrome may be defined by the response to carbohydrate restriction.** Nutr Metab (Lond). 2005 Nov 16;2:31.

56. Accurso A, Bernstein RK, Dahlqvist A, Draznin B, Feinman RD, Fine EJ, Gleed A, Jacobs DB, Larson G, Lustig RH, Manninen AH, McFarlane SI, Morrison K, Nielsen JV, Ravnskov U, Roth KS, Silvestre R, Sowers JR, Sundberg R, Volek JS, Westman EC, Wood RJ, Wortman J, Vernon MC. **Dietary carbohydrate restriction in type 2 diabetes mellitus and metabolic syndrome: time for a critical appraisal.** Nutr Metab (Lond). 2008 Apr 8;5(1):9

57. Kaushik S, Wang JJ, Flood V, Tan JS, Barclay AW, Wong TY, Brand-Miller J, Mitchell P. **Dietary glycemic index and the risk of age-related macular degeneration.** Am J Clin Nutr. 2008 Oct;88(4):1104-10
58. Barclay AW, Petocz P, McMillan-Price J, Flood VM, Prvan T, Mitchell P, Brand-Miller JC. **Glycemic index, glycemic load, and chronic disease risk--a meta-analysis of observational studies.** Am J Clin Nutr. 2008 Mar;87(3):627-37. Review.
59. Lutsey PL, Steffen LM, Stevens J. **Dietary Intake and the Development of the Metabolic Syndrome. The Atherosclerosis Risk in Communities Study.** Circulation 2008 Feb 12;117(6):754-61
60. Knowler WC, Barrett-Connor E, Fowler SE, Hamman RF, Lachin JM, Walker EA, Nathan DM; Diabetes Prevention Program Research Group.**Reduction in the incidence of type 2 diabetes with lifestyle intervention or metformin.** N Engl J Med 346:393-403, 2002
61. Kenyon C. **A pathway that links reproductive status to lifespan in Caenorhabditis elegans.** Ann N Y Acad Sci. 2010 Aug;1204:156-62. Review
62. Kenyon C. **The first long-lived mutants: discovery of the insulin/IGF-1 pathway for ageing.** Philos Trans R Soc Lond B Biol Sci. 2011 Jan 12;366(1561):9-16
63. Magnuson BA, Burdock GA, Doull J, Kroes RM, Marsh GM, Pariza MW, Spencer PS, Waddell WJ, Walker R, Williams GM. **Aspartame: a safety evaluation based on current use levels, regulations, and toxicological and epidemiological studies.** Crit Rev Toxicol. 2007;37(8):629-727. Review.
64. Bosetti C, Gallus S, Talamini R, Montella M, Franceschi S, Negri E, La Vecchia C. **Artificial Sweeteners and the Risk of Gastric, Pancreatic, and Endometrial Cancers in Italy.** Cancer Epidemiology Biomarkers & Prevention 2009 18:8, pp 2235-2238
65. Biagi E, Nylund L, Candela M, Ostan R, Bucci L, Pini E, Nikkïla J, Monti D, Satokari R, Franceschi C, Brigidi P, De Vos W. **Through ageing, and beyond: gut microbiota and inflammatory status in seniors and centenarians.** PLoS One. 2010 May 17;5(5):e10667.
66. Biagi E, Candela M, Fairweather-Tait S, Franceschi C, Brigidi P. **Aging of the human metaorganism: the microbial counterpart.** Age (Dordr). 2012 Feb;34(1):247-67.
67. Rehman T. **Role of the gut microbiota in age-related chronic inflammation.** Endocr Metab Immune Disord Drug Targets. 2012 Dec;12(4):361-7.
68. Bengmark S. **Gut microbiota, immune development** and function. Pharmacol Res. 2013 Mar;69(1):87-113.
69. Ota T. **Chemokine systems link obesity to insulin resistance.** Diabetes Metab J. 2013 Jun;37(3):165-72.
70. Corbett EL, Watt CJ, Walker N, Maher D, Williams BG, Raviglione MC, Dye C. **The growing burden of tuberculosis: global trends and interactions with the HIV epidemic.** Arch Intern Med. 2003;163:1009–1021
71. Stevenson CR, Forouhi NG, Roglic G, Williams BG, Lauer JA, Dye C, Unwin N. **Diabetes and tuberculosis: the impact of the diabetes epidemic on tuberculosis incidence.** BMC Public Health. 2007 Sep 6;7:234.
72. Dooley KE, Chaisson RE. **Tuberculosis and diabetes mellitus: convergence of two epidemics.** Lancet Infect Dis. 2009 Dec;9(12):737-46.
73. **Workeneh B, Bajaj M.** The regulation of muscle protein turnover in diabetes. Int J Biochem Cell Biol. 2013 Jul 6. pii: S1357-2725(13)00212-4. doi: 10.1016/j.biocel.2013.06.028. [Epub ahead of print]
74. Gauhar R, Hwang SL, Jeong SS, Kim JE, Song H, Park DC, Song KS, Kim TY, Oh WK, Huh TL. **Heat-processed Gynostemma pentaphyllum extract improves obesity in ob/ob mice by activating AMP-activated protein kinase.** Biotechnol Lett. 2012 Sep;34(9):1607-16
75. Park SH, Huh TL, Kim SY, Oh MR, Pichiah PB, Chae SW, Cha YS. **Anti-obesity effect of Gynostemma pentaphyllum extract (actiponin): A randomized, double-blind, placebo-controlled trial.** Obesity (Silver Spring). 2013 Jun 26. doi: 10.1002/oby.20539. [Epub ahead of print]

Chapter 19. Foods and Cooking Techniques

1. Bengmark S. **Gut microbiota, immune development** and function. Pharmacol Res. 2013 Mar;69(1):87-113.
2. Kechagias S, Ernersson A, Dahlqvist O, Lundberg P, Lindström T, NystromFH; Fast Food Study Group. **Fast-food-based hyper-alimentation can induce rapid and profound elevation of serum alanine aminotransferase in healthy subjects.** Gut. 2008 May;57(5):649-54
3. Williams CD, Stengel J, Asike MI, Torres DM, Shaw J, Contreras M, Landt CL, Harrison SA. **Prevalence of nonalcoholic fatty liver disease and nonalcoholic steatohepatitis among a largely middle-aged population utilizing ultrasound and liver biopsy: a prospective study.** Gastroenterology. 2011 Jan;140(1):124-31.
4. Williams WM, Weinberg A, Smith MA. **Protein modification by dicarbonyl molecular species in neurodegenerative diseases.** Journal of Amino Acids 2011;46:12–6.
5. Byun K, Bayarsaikhan E, Kim D, Kim CY, Mook-Jung I, Paek SH, Kim SU, Yamamoto T, Won MH, Song BJ, Park YM, Lee B. **Induction of neuronal death by microglial AGE-albumin: implications for Alzheimer's disease.** PLoS One. 2012;7(5):e37917.
6. Luevano-Contreras C, Garay-Sevilla ME, Preciado-Puga M, Chapman-Novakofski KM. **The relationship between dietary advanced glycation end products and indicators of diabetes severity in Mexicans and non-Hispanic whites: a pilot study.** Int J Food Sci Nutr. 2012 Jul 10.

7. Guerin-Dubourg A, Catan A, Bourdon E, Rondeau P. **Structural modifications of human albumin in diabetes.** Diabetes and Metabolism 2012;38:171–8.
8. Basta G, Navarra T, De Simone P, Del Turco S, Gastaldelli A, Filipponi F. **What is the role of the receptor for advanced glycation end products-ligand axis in liver injury?** Liver Transplantation 2011;17:633–40.
9. Wu L, Ma L, Nicholson LF, Black PN. **Advanced glycation end products and its receptor (RAGE) are increased in patients with COPD. Advanced glycation end products and its receptor (RAGE) are increased in patients with COPD.** Respiratory Medicine 2011;105:329–36.
10. Fuentes MK, Nigavekar SS, Arumugam T, Logsdon CD, Schmidt AM, Park JC, et al. **RAGE activation by S100P in colon cancer stimulates growth, migration, and cell signaling pathways.** Diseases of the Colon and Rectum 2007;50:1230–40.
11. Jiao L, Chen L, Alsarraj A, Ramsey D, Duan Z, El-Serag HB. **Plasma soluble receptor for advanced glycation end-products and risk of colorectal adenoma.** Int J Mol Epidemiol Genet. 2012;3(4):294-304.
12. Kuniyasu H, Oue N, Wakikawa A, Shigeishi H, Matsutani N, Kuraoka K, et al. **Expression of receptors for advanced glycation end-products (RAGE) is closely associated with the invasive and metastatic activity of gastric cancer.** Journal of Pathology 2002;196:163–70.
13. Stott-Miller M, Neuhouser ML, Stanford JL. **Consumption of deep-fried foods and risk of prostate cancer** Prostate. 2013 Prostate. 2013 Jun;73(9):960-9.
14. Tesarová P, Kalousová M, Jáchymová M, Mestek O, Petruzelka L, Zima T. **Receptor for advanced glycation end products (RAGE)—soluble form (sRAGE) and gene polymorphisms in patients with breast cancer.** Cancer Investigation 2007;25:720–5.
15. Yu IT, Chiu YL, Au JS, Wong TW, Tang JL. **Dose-response relationship between cooking fumes exposures and lung cancer among Chinese nonsmoking women.** Cancer Res. 2006 May 1;66(9):4961-7.

Chapter 20. Internal affairs: inflammation and the microbiota

1. Sonnenberg GF, Artis D. **Innate lymphoid cell interactions with microbiota: implications for intestinal health and disease.** Immunity. 2012 Oct 19;37(4):601-10.
2. Robinson CJ, Bohannan BJM, Young VB. **From Structure to Function: the Ecology of Host-Associated Microbial Communities.** Microbiol Mol Biol Rev. 2010 September; 74(3): 453–476.
3. Bengmark S. **Gut microbiota, immune development and function.** Pharmacol Res. 2013 Mar;69(1):87-113.
4. Lew WY, Bayna E, Molle ED, Dalton ND, Lai NC, Bhargava V, Mendiola V, Clopton P, Tang T. **Recurrent exposure to subclinical lipopolysaccharide increases mortality and induces cardiac fibrosis in mice.** PLos One. 2013 Apr 9;8(4)
5. Byun EB, Choi HG, Sung NY, Byun EH. **Green tea polyphenol** epigallocatechin-ʳ-gallate inhibits TLRᶜ signaling through the -ᶦˣkDa laminin receptor on lipopolysaccharide-stimulated dendritic cells. Biochem Biophys Res Commun. 2012 Oct 5;426(4):480-5
6. Monagas M, Khan N, Andrés-Lacueva C, Urpí-Sardá M, Vázquez-Agell M, Lamuela-Raventós RM, Estruch R. **Dihydroxylated phenolic acids derived from microbial metabolism reduce lipopolysaccharide-stimulated cytokine secretion by human peripheral blood mononuclear cells.** Br J Nutr. 2009 Jul;102(2):201-6.
7. Cani PD, Amar J, Iglesias MA, Poggi M, Knauf C, Bastelica D, Neyrinck AM, Fava F, Tuohy KM, Chabo C, Waget A, Delmée E, Cousin B, Sulpice T, Chamontin B, Ferrières J, Tanti JF, Gibson GR, Casteilla L, Delzenne NM, Alessi MC, Burcelin R. **Metabolic endotoxemia initiates obesity and insulin resistance.** Diabetes. 2007 Jul;56(7):1761-72.
8. Cani PD, Bibiloni R, Knauf C, Waget A, Neyrinck AM, Delzenne NM, Burcelin R. **Changes in gut microbiota control metabolic endotoxemia-induced inflammation in high-fat diet-induced obesity and diabetes in mice.** Diabetes. 2008 Jun;57(6):1470-81.
9. Fung TT, Schulze M, Manson JE, Willett WC, Hu FB. **Dietary patterns, meat intake, and the risk of type 2 diabetes in women.** Arch Intern Med. 2004 Nov 8;164(20):2235-40.
10. Lutsey PL, Steffen LM, Stevens J. **Dietary Intake and the Development of the Metabolic Syndrome. The Atherosclerosis Risk in Communities Study.** Circulation 2008 Feb 12;117(6):754-61
11. Martínez-González MA, de la Fuente-Arrillaga C, Nunez-Cordoba JM, Basterra-Gortari FJ, Beunza JJ, Vazquez Z, Benito S, Tortosa A, Bes-Rastrollo M. **Adherence to Mediterranean diet and risk of developing diabetes: prospective cohort study.** BMJ. 2008 Jun 14;336(7657):1348-51
12. Pussinen PJ, Havulinna AS, Lehto M, Sundvall J, Salomaa V. **Endotoxemia is associated with an increased risk of incident diabetes.** Diabetes Care. 2011 Feb;34(2):392-7.
13. CDC 2008. **Principles for Appropriate Antibiotic Use for adults with upper respiratory infections**http://www.cdc.gov/media/pressrel/r010319.htm
14. Erridge C. **Stimulants of Toll-like receptor (TLR)-2 and TLR-4 are abundant in certain minimally-processed vegetables.** Food Chem Toxicol. 2011b Jun;49(6):1464-7.

15. Erridge C. **Accumulation of stimulants of Toll-like receptor (TLR)-2 and TLR4 in meat products stored at 5 °C.** J Food Sci. 2011a Mar;76(2):H72-9.
16. Huang CJ, Stewart JK, Franco RL, Evans RK, Lee ZP, Cruz TD, Webb HE, Acevedo EO. **LPS-stimulated tumor necrosis factor-alpha and interleukin-6 mRNA and cytokine responses following acute psychological stress.** Psychoneuroendocrinology. 2011 Nov;36(10):1553-61
17. Cryan JF, O'Mahony SM. **The microbiome-gut-brain axis: from bowel to behavior.** Neurogastroenterol Motil. 2011 Mar;23(3):187-92.
18. Tillisch K, Labus J, Kilpatrick L, Jiang Z, Stains J, Ebrat B, Guyonnet D, Legrain-Raspaud S, Trotin B, Naliboff B, Mayer EA. **Consumption of fermented milk product with probiotic modulates brain activity.** Gastroenterology. 2013 Jun;144(7):1394-1401.
19. Dinan TG, Cryan JF. **Regulation of the stress response by the gut microbiota: implications for psychoneuroendocrinology.** Psychoneuroendocrinology. 2012 Sep;37(9):1369-78.
20. Cryan JF, Dinan TG. **Mind-altering microorganisms: the impact of the gut microbiota on brain and behaviour.** Nat Rev Neurosci. 2012 Oct;13(10):701-12. Review.
21. Li J, Wang W, Xu SX, Magarvey NA, McCormick JK. **Lactobacillus reuteri-produced cyclic dipeptides quench agr-mediated expression of toxic shock syndrome toxin-1 in staphylococci.** Proc Natl Acad Sci U S A. 2011 Feb 22;108(8):3360-5
22. Liu Y, Fatheree NY, Mangalat N, Rhoads JM. **Lactobacillus reuteri strains reduce incidence and severity of experimental necrotizing enterocolitis via modulation of TLR4 and NF-κB signaling in the intestine.** Am J Physiol Gastrointest Liver Physiol. 2012 Mar 15;302(6):G608-17
23. Oliva S, Di Nardo G, Ferrari F, Mallardo S, Rossi P, Patrizi G, Cucchiara S, Stronati L. **Randomised clinical trial: the effectiveness of Lactobacillus reuteri ATCC 55730 rectal enema in children with active distal ulcerative colitis.** Aliment Pharmacol Ther. 2012 Feb;35(3):327-34.
24. Miraglia Del Giudice M, Maiello N, Decimo F, Fusco N, D› Agostino B, Sullo N, Capasso M, Salpietro V, Gitto E, Ciprandi G, Marseglia GL, Perrone L. **Airways allergic inflammation and L. reuterii treatment in asthmatic children.** J Biol Regul Homeost Agents. 2012 Jan-Mar;26(1 Suppl):S35-40.
25. Chiang SS, Pan TM. **Antiosteoporotic effects of Lactobacillus -fermented soy skim milk on bone mineral density and the microstructure of femoral bone in ovariectomized mice.** J Agric Food Chem. 2011 Jul 27;59(14):7734-42.
26. Jones ML, Martoni CJ, Prakash S. **Oral supplementation with probiotic L. reuteri NCIMB 30242 increases mean circulating 25-hydroxyvitamin D: a post-hoc analysis of a randomized controlled trial.** J Clin Endocrinol Metab. 2013 Apr 22. (Epub ahead of print)
27. Chenoll E, Casinos B, Bataller E, Astals P, Echevarría J, Iglesias JR, Balbarie P, Ramón D, Genovés S. **Novel probiotic Bifidobacterium bifidum CECT 7366 strain active against the pathogenic bacterium Helicobacter pylori.** Appl Environ Microbiol. 2011 Feb;77(4):1335-43.
28. Arnold IC, Hitzler I, Müller A. **The immunomodulatory properties of Helicobacter pylori confer protection against allergic and chronic inflammatory disorders.** Front Cell Infect Microbiol. 2012;2:10.
29. Perry S, de Jong BC, Solnick JV, Sanchez ML, Yang S, Lin PL, Hansen LM, Talat N, Hill PC, Hussain R, Adegbola RA, Flynn J, Canfield D, Parsonnet J. **Infection with *Helicobacter pylori* Is Associated with Protection against Tuberculosis.** PLoS One. 2010; 5(1): e8804.
30. Nakajima S, Hattori T. **Oesophageal adenocarcinoma or gastric cancer with or without eradication of Helicobacter pyloriinfection in chronic atrophic gastritis patients: a hypothetical opinion from a systematic review.** Aliment Pharmacol Ther. 2004 Jul;20 Suppl 1:54-61.
31. Lee YY, Mahendra Raj S, Graham DY. **Helicobacter pylori Infection - A Boon or a Bane: Lessons from Studies in a Low-Prevalence Population.** Helicobacter. 2013 Apr 22. doi: 10.1111/hel.12058. (Epub ahead of print)
32. Barrett JS, Gibson PR. **Fermentable oligosaccharides, disaccharides, monosaccharides and polyols (FODMAPs) and nonallergic food intolerance: FODMAPs or food chemicals?** Therap Adv Gastroenterol. 2012 Jul;5(4):261-8.
33. Shepherd SJ, Lomer MC, Gibson PR. **Short-chain carbohydrates and functional gastrointestinal disorders.** Am J Gastroenterol. 2013 May;108(5):707-17.
34. Jia R, Kurita-Ochiai T, Oguchi S, Yamamoto M. **Periodontal pathogen accelerates lipid peroxidation and atherosclerosis** J Dent Res. 2013 Mar;92(3):247-52
35. Morishita M, Ariyoshi M, Okinaga T, Usui M, Nakashima K, Nishihara T. **A. actinomycetemcomitans LPS** enhances foam cell formation induced by LDL. J Dent Res. 2013 Mar;92(3):241-6
36. Poole S, Singhrao SK, Kesavalu L, Curtis MA, Crean SJ. **Determining the Presence of Periodontopathic Virulence Factors in Short-Term Postmortem Alzheimer's Disease** Brain Tissue. J Alzheimers Dis. 2013 May 10. In press.
37. Shear MJ, Turner FC. **Chemical treatment of tumours; isolation of hemorrhagic-producing   fraction from Serratia marcescens (*Bacillus prodigious*) culture filtrate.**   Journal of the National Cancer Institute. (1943) 4:81-87
38. Yang Y, Zhang R, Xia F, Zou T, Huang A, Xiong S, Zhang J. **LPS converts Gr-1+CD115+ myeloid-derived suppressor cells from M2 to M1 via P38 MAPK.** Exp Cell Res. 2013 May 20. doi:pii: S0014-4827(13)00213-9.

Chapter 21. Genetic factors: inflammation, mutrients & telomeres

1. Masi S, Nightingale CM, Day IN, Guthrie P, Rumley A, Lowe GD, von Zglinicki T, D'Aiuto F, Taddei S, Klein N, Salpea K, Cook DG, Humphries SE,Whincup PH, Deanfield JE. **Inflammation and not cardiovascular risk factors is associated with short leukocyte telomerelength in 13- to 16-year-old adolescents.** Arterioscler Thromb Vasc Biol. 2012 Aug;32(8):2029-34.
2. Tsuji T, Aoshiba K, Nagai A. **Alveolar cell senescence exacerbates pulmonary inflammation in patients with chronic obstructive pulmonary disease.** Respiration. 2010;80(1):59-70.
3. Noureddine H, Gary-Bobo G, Alifano M, Marcos E, Saker M, Vienney N, Amsellem V, Maitre B, Chaouat A, Chouaid C, Dubois-Rande JL, Damotte D, Adnot S. **Pulmonary artery smooth muscle cell senescence is a pathogenic mechanism for pulmonary hypertension in chronic lung disease.** Circ Res. 2011 Aug 19;109(5):543-53.
4. Amsellem V, Gary-Bobo G, Marcos E, Maitre B, Chaar V, Validire P, Stern JB, Noureddine H, Sapin E, Rideau D, Hue S, Le Corvoisier P, Le Gouvello S, Dubois-Randé JL, Boczkowski J, Adnot S. **Telomere dysfunction causes sustained inflammation in chronic obstructive pulmonary disease.** Am J Respir Crit Care Med. 2011 Dec 15;184(12):1358-66.
5. Demissie S, Levy D, Benjamin EJ et al. **Insulin resistance, oxidative stress, hypertension, and leukocyte telomere length in men from the Framingham Heart Study.** Aging Cell 2006;5:325–30
6. Sun Q, Shi L, Prescott J, Chiuve SE, Hu FB, De Vivo I, Stampfer MJ, Franks PW, Manson JE, Rexrode KM. **Healthy lifestyle and leukocyte telomere length in U.S. women.** PLoS One. 2012;7(5):e38374.
7. Valdes AM, Andrew T, Gardner JP, Kimura M, Oelsner E, Cherkas LF, Aviv A, Spector TD. **Obesity, cigarette smoking, and telomere length in women.** Lancet. 2005 Aug 20-26;366(9486):662-4.
8. Tzanetakou IP, Katsilambros NL, Benetos A, Mikhailidis DP, Perrea DN. **"Is obesity linked to aging?": adipose tissue and the role of telomeres.** Ageing Res Rev. 2012 Apr;11(2):220-9.
9. Murillo-Ortiz B, Albarrán-Tamayo F, Arenas-Aranda D, Benítez-Bribiesca L, Malacara-Hernández JM, Martínez-Garza S, Hernández-González M, Solorio S, Garay-Sevilla ME, Mora-Villalpando C. **Telomere length and type 2 diabetes in males, a premature aging syndrome.** Aging Male. 2012 Mar;15(1):54-8.
10. Hou L, Wang S, Dou C, Zhang X, Yu Y, Zheng Y, Avula U, Hoxha M, Díaz A, McCracken J, Barretta F, Marinelli B, Bertazzi PA, Schwartz J, Baccarelli AA. **Air pollution exposure and telomere length in highly exposed subjects in Beijing, China: A repeated-measure study.** Environ Int. 2012 Nov 1;48:71-7.
11. Farzaneh-Far R, Lin J, Epel ES, Harris WS, Blackburn EH, Whooley MA. **Association of marine omega-3 fatty acid levels with telomeric aging in patients with coronary heart disease.** JAMA. 2010 Jan 20;303(3):250-7.
12. Kiecolt-Glaser JK, Epel ES, Belury MA, Andridge R, Lin J, Glaser R, Malarkey WB, Hwang BS, Blackburn E. **Omega-3 fatty acids, oxidative stress, and leukocyte telomere length: A randomized controlled trial.** Brain Behav Immun. 2013 Feb;28:16-24.
13. Ornish D, Lin J, Daubenmier J, et al. **Increased telomerase activity and comprehensive lifestyle changes: a pilot study.** Lancet Oncol 2008;9:1048–57.
14. Cassidy A, De Vivo I, Liu Y, Han J, Prescott J, Hunter DJ, Rimm EB. **Associations between diet, lifestyle factors, and telomere length in women.** Am J Clin Nutr. 2010 May;91(5):1273-80.
15. Kang JX. **Differential effects of omega-6 and omega-3 fatty acids on telomere length.** Am J Clin Nutr. 2010 Nov;92(5):1276-7; author reply 1277.
16. Chan R, Woo J, Suen E, Leung J, Tang N. **Chinese tea consumption is associated with longer telomere length in elderly Chinese men.** Br J Nutr. 2010 Jan;103(1):107-13.

Chapter 22. Canaries in the Coalmine: inflammation, nutrients and infertility

1. Rolland M, Le Moal J, Wagner V, Royère D, De Mouzon J. **Decline in semen concentration and morphology in a sample of 26 609 men close to general population between 1989 and 2005 in France.** Hum Reprod. 2012 Dec 4
2. Jørgensen N, Vierula M, Jacobsen R, Pukkala E, Perheentupa A, Virtanen HE, Skakkebaek NE, Toppari J. **Recent adverse trends in semen quality and testis cancer incidence among Finnish men.** Int J Androl. 2011 Aug;34(4 Pt 2):e37-48
3. Haimov-Kochman R, Har-Nir R, Ein-Mor E, Ben-Shoshan V, Greenfield C, Eldar I, Bdolah Y, Hurwitz A. **Is the quality of donated semen deteriorating? Findings from a 15 year longitudinal analysis of weekly sperm samples.** Isr Med Assoc J. 2012 Jun;14(6):372-7
4. Xie WC, Chan MH, Mak KC, Chan WT, He M. **Trends in the incidence of 15 common cancers in Hong Kong, 1983-2008.** Asian Pac J Cancer Prev. 2012;13(8):3911-6.
5. Andersson AM, Jørgensen N, Main KM, Toppari J, Rajpert-De Meyts E, Leffers H, Juul A, Jensen TK, Skakkebaek NE. **Adverse trends in male reproductive health: we may have reached a crucial 'tipping point'.** Int J Androl.

2008 Apr;31(2):74-80.
6. Mascarenhas MN, Flaxman SR, Boerma T, Vanderpoel S, Stevens GA. **National, regional, and global trends in infertility prevalence since 1990: a systematic analysis of 277 health surveys.** PLoS Med. 2012 Dec;9(12):e1001356.
7. O'Bryan MK and Hedger MP. **Inflammatory Networks in the Control of Spermatogenesis: Chronic Inflammation in an Immunologically Privileged Tissue?** In, 'Molecular Mechanisms in Spermatogenesis', Ed. Cheng CY (2008); Madame Curie Bioscience Database
8. Pérez CV, Theas MS, Jacobo PV, Jarazo-Dietrich S, Guazzone VA, Lustig L. **Dual role of immune cells in the testis: Protective or pathogenic for germ cells?** Spermatogenesis. 2013 Jan 1;3(1):e23870.
9. Russell LD, Chiarini-Garcia H, Korsmeyer SJ, Knudson CM. **Bax-dependent spermatogonia apoptosis is required for testicular development and spermatogenesis.** Biol Reprod. 2002;66:950–8.
10. Blanco-Rodríguez J. **A matter of death and life: the significance of germ cell death during spermatogenesis.** Int J Androl. 1998;21:236–48.
11. Adamopoulos DA, Lawrence DM, Vassilopoulos P, Contoyiannis PA, Swyer GIM. **Pituitary-testicular interrelationships in mumps orchitis and other viral infections.** Br Med J 1978, 1:1177–1180
12. Cutolo M, Balleari E, Giusti M, Monachesi M, Accardo S. **Sex hormone status of patients with rheumatoid arthritis: evidence of low serum concentrations at baseline and after human chorionic gonadotrophin stimulation.** Arthritis Rheum 1988, 31:1314–1317
13. Buch JP, Havlovec SK. **Variation in sperm penetration assay related to viral illness.** Fertil Steril 1991, 55:844–846
14. O'Bryan MK, Schlatt S, Phillips DJ, Kretser DMD, Hedger MP. **Bacterial Lipopolysaccharide-Induced Inflammation Compromises Testicular Function at Multiple Levels in Vivo.** Endocrinology 2000, 141:238–246
15. Collodel G, Castellini C, del Vecchio MT, Cardinali R, Geminiani M, Rossi B, Spreafico A, Moretti E. **Effect of a bacterial lipopolysaccharide treatment on rabbit testis and ejaculated sperm.** Reprod Domest Anim. 2012 Jun;47(3):372-8.
16. Sarkar O, Bahrainwala J, Chandrasekaran S, Kothari S, Mathur PP, Agarwal A. **Impact of inflammation** on male fertility. Front Biosci (Elite Ed). 2011 Jan 1;3:89-95.
17. Khaki A, Fathiazad F, Nouri M, Khaki A, Maleki NA, Khamnei HJ, Ahmadi P. **Beneficial effects of quercetin on sperm parameters in streptozotocin-induced diabetic male rats.** Phytother Res. 2010 Sep;24(9):1285-91.
18. Al-Maghrebi M, Renno WM, Al-Ajmi N. **Epigallocatechin-3-gallate inhibits apoptosis and protects testicular seminiferous tubules from ischemia/reperfusion-induced inflammation.** Biochem Biophys Res Commun. 2012 Apr 6;420(2):434-9.
19. Khorsandi L, Mirhoseini M, Mohamadpour M, Orazizadeh M, Khaghani S. **Effect of curcumin on dexamethasone-induced testicular toxicity in mice.** Pharm Biol. 2013 Feb;51(2):206-12
20. Safarinejad MR, Hosseini SY, Dadkhah F, Asgari MA. **Relationship of omega-3 and omega-6 fatty acids with semen characteristics, and anti-oxidant status of seminal plasma: a comparison between fertile and infertile men.** Clin Nutr 2010; **29**: 100–5.
21. Aksoy Y, Aksoy H, Altinkaynak K, Aydin HR, Ozkan A. **Sperm fatty acid composition in subfertile men.** Prostaglandins Leukot Essent Fatty Acids 2006; **75**: 75–9
22. Conquer JA, Martin JB, Tummon I, Watson L, Tekpetey F. **Fatty acid analysis of blood serum, seminal plasma, and spermatozoa of normozoospermic vs. asthenozoospermic males.** Lipids 1999; **34**: 793–9.
23. Safarinejad MR. **Effect of omega-3 polyunsaturated fatty acid supplementation on semen profile and enzymatic anti-oxidant capacity of seminal plasma in infertile men with idiopathic oligoasthenoteratospermia: a double-blind, placebo-controlled, randomised study.** Andrologia 2011; **43**: 38–47.

Chapter 23. RDA's and RNI's: How much Nutrition Do We Really Need?

1. Clayton P, Rowbotham J. **How the mid-Victorians worked, ate and died.** Int J Environ Res Public Health. 2009 Mar;6(3):1235-53
2. Ames BN. **Low micronutrient intake may accelerate the degenerative diseases of aging through allocation of scarce micronutrients by triage.** Proc Natl Acad Sci U S A. 2006 Nov 21;103(47):17589-94
3. Ames BN. **Optimal micronutrients delay mitochondrial decay and age-associated diseases.** Mech Ageing Dev. 2010 Jul-Aug;131(7-8):473-9
4. Schick B. **A tea prepared from needles of pine trees against scurvy.** Science. 1943 Sep 10;98(2541):241-2
5. Bolland MJ, Avenell A, Baron JA, Grey A, Maclennan GS, Gamble GD, Reid IR. **Effect of calcium supplements on risk of myocardial infarction and cardiovascular events: meta-analysis.** BMJ. 2010 Jul 29;341:c3691. Review.
6. IoM Worksop Summary. **The Development of DRIs 1994–2004: Lessons Learned and New Challenges.** November 30, 2007
7. Jiang Q, Moreland M, Ames BN, Yin X. **A combination of aspirin and gamma-tocopherol is superior to that of aspirin and alpha-tocopherol in anti-inflammatory action and attenuation of aspirin-induced adverse effects.** J Nutr Biochem. 2009 Nov;20(11):894-900

8. Royer MC, Lemaire-Ewing S, Desrumaux C, Monier S, Pais de Barros JP, Athias A, Néel D, Lagrost L. **7-ketocholesterol incorporation into sphingolipid/cholesterol-enriched (lipid raft) domains is impaired by vitamin E: a specific role for alpha-tocopherol with consequences on cell death.** J Biol Chem. 2009 Jun 5;284(23):15826-34

9. Sacha B, Zierler S, Lehnardt S, Weber JR, Kerschbaum HH. **Heterogeneous effects of distinct tocopherol analogues on NO release, cell volume, and cell death in microglial cells.** J Neurosci Res. 2008 Dec;86(16):3526-35

10. Ren Z, Pae M, Dao MC, Smith D, Meydani SN, Wu D. **Dietary supplementation with tocotrienols enhances immune function in C57BL/6 mice.** J Nutr. 2010 Jul;140(7):1335-41

11. Sen CK, Khanna S, Roy S. **Tocotrienols in health and disease: the other half of the natural vitamin E family.** Mol Aspects Med. 2007 Oct-Dec;28(5-6):692-728. Review.

12. Comitato R, Leoni G, Canali R, Ambra R, Nesaretnam K, Virgili F. **Tocotrienols activity in MCF-7 breast cancer cells: involvement of ERbeta signal transduction.** Mol Nutr Food Res. 2010 May;54(5):669-7

13. Pierpaoli E, Viola V, Pilolli F, Piroddi M, Galli F, Provinciali M. **Gamma- and delta-tocotrienols exert a more potent anticancer effect than alpha-tocopheryl succinate on breast cancer cell lines irrespective of HER-2/neu expression.** Life Sci. 2010 Apr 24;86(17-18):668-75

14. Grant WB, Schwalfenberg GK, Genuis SJ, Whiting SJ. **An estimate of the economic burden and premature deaths due to vitamin D deficiency in Canada.** Molecular Nutrition & Food Research 2010 Aug;54(8):1172-81.

15. Hanley DA, Cranney A, Jones G, Whiting SJ, Leslie WD, Cole DE, Atkinson SA, Josse RG, Feldman S, Kline GA, Rosen C. **Vitamin D in adult health and disease: a review and guideline statement from Osteoporosis Canada.** CMAJ. 2010 Jul 19

16. "Dietary Supplement Fact Sheet: Vitamin D" Ods.od.nih.gov. Retrieved 2010-03-25

17. Vieth R. **Vitamin D supplementation, 25-hydroxyvitamin D concentrations, and safety.** Am J Clin Nutr. 1999; 69(5):842-56.

18. Vieth R, Chan P-C, MacFarlane GD: **Efficacy and safety of vitamin D3 intake exceeding the lowest observed adverse effect level.** Am J Clin Nutr 2001;73:288–94.

19. Adams JS, Clemens TL, Parrish JA, Holick MF. **Vitamin-D synthesis and metabolism after ultraviolet irradiation of normal and vitamin-D-deficient subjects.** N Engl J Med.1982 Mar 25;306(12):722-5

20. Munro I. **Derivation of tolerable upper intake levels of nutrients.** Letter, Am J Clin Nutr 2001; 74:865

21. Woodhead JS, Ghose RR, Gupta SK. **Severe hypophosphataemic osteomalacia with primary hyperparathyroidism.** Br Med J 1980; 281:647-648.

22. Eguchi M, Kaibara N. **Treatment of hypophosphataemic vitamin D-resistant rickets and adult presenting hypophosphataemic vitamin D-resistant osteomalacia.** Int Orthop 1980; 3:257-264.

23. Mattila PH, Piironen VI, Uusi-Rauva EJ, Koivistoinen PE. **Vitamin D Contents in Edible Mushrooms.** J.Agric. Food Chem., 1994, 42 (11), pp 2449–2453

24. Kalaras MD, Beelman RB, Elias RJ. **Effects of Postharvest Pulsed UV Light Treatment of White Button Mushrooms (Agaricus bisporus) on Vitamin D2 Content and Quality Attributes.** Journal of Agricultural and Food Chemistry2012 60 (1), 220-225

25. Schurgers LJ, Vermeer C. **Differential lipoprotein transport pathways of K-vitamins in healthy subjects.** Biochim Biophys Acta. Feb 15 2002;1570(1):27-32.

26. Schurgers LJ, Cranenburg EC, Vermeer C. **Matrix Gla-protein: the calcification inhibitor in need of vitamin K.** Thromb Haemost. 2008 Oct;100(4):593-603. Review.

27. Knapen MH, Schurgers LJ, Vermeer C. **Vitamin K2 supplementation improves hip bone geometry and bone strength indices in postmenopausal women.** Osteoporos Int. 2007 Jul;18(7):963-72

28. Kim KH, Choi WS, Lee JH, Lee H, Yang DH, Chae SC. **Relationship between dietary vitamin K intake and the stability of anticoagulation effect in patients taking long-term warfarin.** Thromb Haemost. 2010 Jul 20;104(4)

29. Kaneki M, Hodges SJ, Hosoi T, Fujiwara S, Lyons A, Crean SJ, Ishida N, Nakagawa M, Takechi M, Sano Y, Mizuno Y, Hoshino S, Miyao M, Inoue S, Horiki K, Shiraki M, Ouchi Y, Orimo H. **Japanese fermented soybean food as the major determinant of the large geographic difference in circulating levels of vitamin K2: possible implications for hip-fracture risk.** Nutrition. 2001 Apr;17(4):315-21

30. Bolland MJ, Avenell A, Baron JA, Grey A, MacLennan GS, Gamble GD, Reid IR. **Effect of calcium supplements on risk of myocardial infarction and cardiovascular events: meta-analysis.** BMJ. 2010 Jul 29;341:c3691. doi: 10.1136/bmj.c3691. Review.

31. Bolland MJ, Grey A, Avenell A, Gamble GD, Reid IR. **Calcium supplements with or without vitamin D and risk of cardiovascular events: reanalysis of the Women's Health Initiative limited access dataset and meta-analysis.** BMJ. 2011 Apr 19;342:d2040. Review.

32. Reid IR, Ames R, Mason B, Bolland MJ, Bacon CJ, Reid HE, Kyle C, Gamble GD, Grey A, Horne A. **Effects of calcium supplementation on lipids, blood pressure, and body composition in healthy older men: a randomized controlled trial.** Am J Clin Nutr. 2010 Jan;91(1):131-9.

Chapter 24. Sunshine, shadows and showers: the dangers of living in glasshouses

1. Clayton P, Rowbotham J. **How the mid-Victorians worked, ate and died.** Int J Environ Res Public Health. 2009 Mar;6(3):1235-53.
2. Purdue MP, Freeman LE, Anderson WF, Tucker MA. **Recent trends in incidence of cutaneous melanoma among US Caucasian young adults.** J Invest Dermatol. 2008 Dec;128(12):2905-8.
3. Montella A, Gavin A, Middleton R, Autier P, Boniol M. **Cutaneous melanoma mortality starting to change: A study of trends in Northern Ireland.** Eur J Cancer. 2009 Sep;45(13):2360-6.
4. Melanoma Foundation 2013. http://www.melanomafoundation.org.uk/
5. Stahl W, Sies H. **Carotenoids and flavonoids contribute to nutritional protection against skin damage from sunlight.** Mol Biotechnol. 2007 Sep;37(1):26-30. Review
6. Dinkova-Kostova AT. **Phytochemicals as protectors against ultraviolet radiation: versatility of effects and mechanisms.** Planta Med. 2008 Oct;74(13):1548-59. Review
7. Kowalczyk MC, Walaszek Z, Kowalczyk P, Kinjo T, Hanausek M, Slaga TJ. **Differential effects of several phyto-chemicals and their derivatives on murine keratinocytes in vitro and in vivo: implications for skin cancer prevention.** Carcinogenesis. 2009 Jun;30(6):1008-15
8. Garland CF. **Symposium in Print on the Epidemiology of Vitamin D and Cancer.** Ann Epidemiol. 2009 Jul;19(7):439-40
9. Grant WB, Cross HS, Garland CF, Gorham ED, Moan J, Peterlik M, Porojnicu AC, Reichrath J, Zittermann A. **Estimated benefit of increased vitamin D status in reducing the economic burden of disease in western Europe.** Prog Biophys Mol Biol. 2009 Feb-Apr;99(2-3):104-13.
10. Yin L, Grandi N, Raum E, Haug U, Arndt V, Brenner H. **Meta-analysis: longitudinal studies of serum vitamin D and colorectal cancer risk.** Aliment Pharmacol Ther. 2009 Jul 1;30(2):113-25.
11. Yin L, Grandi N, Raum E, Haug U, Arndt V, Brenner H. **Meta-analysis: Serum vitamin D and colorectal adenoma risk.** Prev Med. 2011 Jul-Aug;53(1-2)
12. Godar DE, Landry RJ, Lucas AD. **Increased UVA exposures and decreased cutaneous Vitamin D(3) levels may be responsible for the increasing incidence of melanoma.** Med Hypotheses. 2009 Apr;72(4):434-43.
13. Adams JS, Clemens TL, Parrish JA, Holick MF. **Vitamin-D synthesis and metabolism after ultraviolet irradiation of normal and vitamin-D-deficient subjects.** N Engl J Med. 1982 Mar 25;306(12):722-5
14. Mitra D, Luo X, Morgan A, Wang J, Hoang MP, Lo J, Guerrero CR, Lennerz JK, Mihm MC, Wargo JA, Robinson KC, Devi SP, Vanover JC, D'Orazio JA, McMahon M, Bosenberg MW, Haigis KM, Haber DA, Wang Y, Fisher DE. **An ultraviolet-radiation-independent pathway to melanoma** carcinogenesis in the red hair/fair skin background. Nature. 2012 Nov 15;491(7424):449-53.
15. Umemura K, Ikeda Y, Kondo K, Hirata K, Amagishi H, Ishihama Y, Tokura Y. **Cutaneous pharmacokinetics of topically applied maxacalcitol ointment and lotion.** Int J Clin Pharmacol Ther. 2008 Jun;46(6):289-94.
16. Yamaguchi K, Mitsui T, Aso Y, Sugibayashi K. **Analysis of in vitro skin permeation of 22-oxacalcitriol from ointments based on a two- or three-layer diffusion model considering diffusivity in a vehicle.** Int J Pharm. 2007 May 24;336(2):310-8.

Chapter 25. Nutrition and Politics: The Cruelty of Business and the Persistence of Hope

1. Clayton P, Rowbotham J. **How the mid-Victorians worked, ate and died.** Int J Environ Res Public Health. 2009 Mar;6(3):1235-53.
2. Rautiainen S, Levitan EB, Orsini N, Åkesson A, Morgenstern R, Mittleman MA, Wolk A. **Total antioxidant capacity from diet and risk of myocardial infarction: a prospective cohort of women.** Am J Med. 2012 Oct;125(10):974-80.
3. http://www.ukpublicspending.co.uk/total_spending_2012UKbn

Chapter 26. Food fights, drug wars and the way ahead

1. Kelley AE, Bakshi VP, Haber SN, Steininger TL, Will MJ, Zhang M. **Opioid modulation of taste hedonics within the ventral striatum.** Physiol Behav. 2002 Jul;76(3):365-77. Review.
2. Corsica JA, Pelchat ML. **Food addiction: true or false?** Curr Opin Gastroenterol. 2010 Mar;26(2):165-9. Review
3. Corwin RL. **The face of uncertainty eats.** Curr Drug Abuse Rev. 2011 Sep;4(3):174-81.
4. Figlewicz DP, Jay JL, Acheson MA, Magrisso IJ, West CH, Zavosh A, Benoit SC, Davis JF. **Moderate high fat diet increases sucrose self-administration in young rats.** Appetite. 2013 Feb;61(1):19-29.
5. Garber AK, Lustig RH. **Is fast food addictive?** Curr Drug Abuse Rev. 2011 Sep;4(3):146-62. Review.
6. Ifland JR, Preuss HG, Marcus MT, Rourke KM, Taylor WC, Burau K, Jacobs WS, Kadish W, Manso G. **Refined food addiction: a classic substance use disorder.** Med Hypotheses. 2009 May;72(5):518-26.
7. James P 2007, International Obesity TaskForce, Geneva. Personal communication

8. Smed S & Denver S. Food & Resource Economics Ints. KVL Univ., Denmark, April 2005
9. Nader R. Unsafe at Any Speed: Designed-In Dangers of the American Automobile. 1965. Knightsbridge Pub Co Mass
10. Karppanen H, Karppanen P, Mervaala E. **Why and how to implement sodium, potassium, calcium, and magnesium changes in food items and diets?** Journal of Human Hypertension 2005; 19:S10-S19.
11. Puska P **The North Karelia Project: from community intervention to national activity in lowering cholesterol levels and CHD risk.** European Heart Journal 1999.
12. Karppanen H, Mervaala E. **Sodium Intake and Hypertension.** Progress in Cardiovascular Diseases, Vol. 49, No. 2 (September/October), 2006: pp 59-75
13. **Coxson** PG, Cook NR, Joffres M, Hong Y, Orenstein D, Schmidt SM, Bibbins-Domingo K. **Mortality benefits from US population-wide reduction in sodiumconsumption: projections from 3 modeling approaches.** Hypertension. 2013 Mar;61(3):564-70.
14. **van Baal PH, Polder JJ, de Wit GA, Hoogenveen RT, Feenstra TL, Boshuizen HC, Engelfriet PM, Brouwer WB. Lifetime Medical Costs of Obesity: Prevention No Cure for Increasing Health Expenditure.** PLoS Med. 2008 Feb 5;5(2):e29
15. Kindig DA, Cheng ER. **Even As Mortality Fell In Most US Counties, Female Mortality Nonetheless Rose In 42.8 Percent Of Counties From 1992 To 2006.** Health Aff (Millwood). 2013 Mar;32(3):451-8
16. Komlos J, Breitfelder A. **Height of US-born non-Hispanic children and adolescents ages 2-19, born 1942-2002 in the NHANES samples.** Am J Hum Biol. 2008 Jan-Feb;20(1):66-71.
17. Komlos J, Breitfelder A. **Are Americans shorter (partly) because they are fatter? A comparison of US and Dutch children's height and BMI values.** Ann Hum Biol. 2007 Nov-Dec;34(6):593-606.
18. Komlos J, Breitfelder A. **Differences in the physical growth of US-born black and white children and adolescents ages 2-19, born 1942-2002.** Ann Hum Biol. 2008 Jan-Feb;35(1):11-21.
19. CDC '09. **Chronic Diseases. The Power to Prevent, The Call to Control: At A Glance 2009**http://www.cdc.gov/chronicdisease/resources/publications/AAG/chronic.htm
20. Wu SY, Green A. **Projection of chronic illness prevalence and cost inflation.** Santa Monica, CA: RAND Health; 2000.
21. Harstall C, Ospina M (June 2003). **How Prevalent Is Chronic Pain?** Pain Clinical Updates, International Association for the Study of Pain **XI** (2): 1–4
22. Mayday 2009. **A Call to Revolutionize Chronic Pain Care in America: An Opportunity in Health Care Reform.** The Mayday Fund. 2009.
23. Johannes CB, Le TK, Zhou X, Johnston JA, Dworkin RH. **The prevalence of chronic pain in United States adults: results of an Internet-based survey.** J Pain. 2010 Nov;11(11):1230-9
24. IoM 2011. Institute of Medicine of the National Academies Report (2011). **Relieving Pain in America: A Blueprint for Transforming Prevention, Care, Education, and Research.** Washington DC: The National Academies Press.
25. World Drug Report 2005, vol. 1, Analysis (United Nations publication, Sales No. E.05.XI.10)
26. Phillips DP, Christenfeld N, Glynn LM (February 1998). **Increase in US medication-error deaths between 1983 and 1993.** Lancet **351** (9103): 643–4.
27. Lazarou J, Pomeranz BH, Corey PN (April 1998). **Incidence of adverse drug reactions in hospitalized patients: a meta-analysis of prospective studies.** JAMA**279** (15): 1200-1205
28. Leape L (May 1992). **Unnecessary Surgery.** Annual Review of Public Health**13**: 363–383.
29. Starfield B (July 2000). **Is US health really the best in the world?** JAMA **284** (4): 483–5.
30. http://www.zerohedge.com/news/2013-07-21/new-abnormal-when-200-people-have-more-wealth-3500000000

Chapter 27. Finally, an apology ...

1. Puca AA, Carrizzo A, Ferrario A, Villa F, Vecchione C. **Endothelial nitric oxide synthase, vascular integrity and human exceptional longevity.** Immun Ageing. 2012; 9: 26.
2. Ristow M, Zarse K. **How increased oxidative stress promotes longevity and metabolic health: The concept of mitochondrial hormesis (mitohormesis).** Exp Gerontol. 2010 Jun;45(6):410-8.
3. Ristow M, Schmeisser S. **Extending life span by increasing oxidative stress.** Free Radic Biol Med. 2011 Jul 15;51(2):327-36.
4. Qi C, Cai Y, Gunn L, Ding C, Li B, Kloecker G, Qian K, Vasilakos J, Saijo S, Iwakura Y, Yannelli JR, Yan J. **Differential pathways regulating innate** and **adaptive** antitumor immune responses by particulate and soluble yeast-derived β-glucans. Blood. 2011 Jun 23;117(25):6825-36.
5. Goodridge HS, Reyes CN, Becker CA, Katsumoto TR, Ma J, Wolf AJ, Bose N, Chan AS, Magee AS, Danielson ME, Weiss A, Vasilakos JP, Underhill DM. **Activation of the innate immune receptor Dectin-1 upon formation of a 'phagocytic synapse'.** Nature. 2011 Apr 28;472(7344):471-5.
6. Salvador C, Li B, Hansen R, Cramer DE, Kong M, Yan J. **Yeast-derived beta-glucan augments the therapeutic efficacy mediated by anti-vascular endothelial growth factor monoclonal antibody in human carcinoma xenograft models.** Clin Cancer Res. 2008 Feb 15;14(4):1239-47.